THE MAN WITH A COLANDER IN HIS HEAD

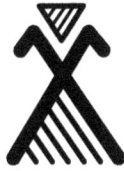

THE MAN WITH A COLANDER IN HIS HEAD

Navigating the uncharted lands of Parkinson's and Dementia

V B LANGFORD

Flying Fox Publications
2021

First published in 2021 by Flying Fox Publications

Copyright © Flying Fox Publications 2021
Text © VB Langford 2021

ISBN 978-1-5272-8938-3

Flying Fox Publications
flyingfoxpublications@gmail.com

Contents

Memento Mori

Looking back from the Age of Covid-19, the mountains we climbed seem mere foothills in comparison to navigating them now.

A pyrrhic victory you might think. To dodge the second bullet but not the first.

But side-stepping Covid-19 is not the only thing I am thankful for.

Even small battles have their place in human history. They are worth recording. And I do not want to forget.

All names and locations have been changed to protect the privacy of those who were involved in our lives during this time.

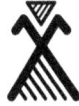

August 2020

It was his bearded face in profile on the pillow beside me that I saw in the waking/sleep borderline half-life this morning. It didn't make me sad this time. I just registered it with mild surprise. His moustache needed trimming.

The last time I saw him in a dream, we were also in bed, he is crying because he was unable to stop himself peeing. I wasn't sure, in my dream, whether it was pee, or whether he had spilled hot coffee on himself, and I desperately mopped at his thigh, trying to comfort him.

Let me tell you what I know about Prof R. Because I am his third wife. The tip of the marital iceberg.

This meant I arrived late. His two marriages, one divorce, four children and one widowhood late to be exact. We met almost by chance, but not quite. I was about to turn 50, a significant age, which deserved celebration in a significant place. For me, a New Zealander, that was almost always London. And this time Terence Conran's *Bibendum* restaurant was my first choice.

Bibendum is not somewhere you dine alone. I hadn't yet met Prof R, the brother-in-law of a friend of mine, but hoped he would be available to come as my guest, and might even be pleased to do so. Fortunately he was.

When we finally met, in the spartan reception room of the equally spartan Pen Club in Bloomsbury, neither of us felt this meeting was significant. I relaxed and began to enjoy myself. We were already late for the booking. This was normal for Prof R, which I was yet to discover. So we rode like the Valkyries through Hyde Park in his utilitarian Toyota to meet our destiny.

But even after a very good meal at *Bibendum,* beneath a glassy-eyed Michelin Man, destiny was not calling me. The restaurant, however, was significant and well worth the expense. Prof R had enjoyed his meal even more than I did. He had chosen the quail. And he had talked. And talked. And invited me for dinner at his house the next day to say thank you. I had plans, but politeness made me shelve them. I took the tube to Brixton.

———————— ∩ ————————

So, dear reader, to cut a long story short, I married him. A good man, whose list of crimes were few, and often the things he hadn't done. But procrastination and lack of motivation are not necessarily criminal. For an academic, as he was, it is almost a given. To others, it seemed simply laziness. Although he would have reacted with surprise and denial if I had asked him whether he considered himself lazy.

So I didn't meet his silent companion then, whom we later christened 'Mr Parky'. I did catch glimpses of him, in the shadows, without knowing who he was; a frozen stare, a silence where there should have been words. But there was also unconditional love. I kept waiting for him to be disappointed.

He never seemed to be. And he was caring and supportive of our shared children; if not often moved to reach out to his own. Mohammed had to come to the mountain. But he was always there. They only had to ask. A sore point with them as it turned out.

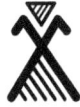

Mr Parky and Prof R

APRIL 2018 — Now Mr Parky and I are closely acquainted. And just the other day, a Saturday, there was a new unwelcome symptom; a fallen head at the lunch table, drooling, eyes rolling, so I was running for the ambulance before I realized it was momentary, not a stroke. Just a petit mal then, or a brainstorm, a fit, or whatever. I considered calling the GP, but when I worked through the possible outcomes, phone triage or a trip to hospital, neither of them seemed worthwhile or desirable. We monitor his blood pressure regularly at home. And he will see the neurologist this month.

Prof R can never remember the name of his nemesis, so it was he who irritably called it Parky — "What's this darn thing I've got? Parky something?" But we think we might be wrong. Largely because the new neurologist thinks it could be wrong.

The real Mr Parky should have arrived first with a tremor, not a catastrophic loss of memory. In November 2012, just when we were planning a return trip to New Zealand, and a Southern Lakes town we both loved and had lived in, and he said, "Why would we want to go there?"

———————o———————

Prof R had been a university lecturer. He talked like a book and his daughters rang him instead of consulting the encyclopaedia (this was pre-Google). He had the answer to everything, and even if he was wrong, he seldom admitted it until he had seen the evidence. And even then sometimes, if he didn't trust the evidence. He never let it disturb his confidence. Which was a good thing. It had got him to the top of his own tree, which was a long way from the family tree.

The remembered achievements kept him going when all else was lost; the second wife, Jan, lost to cancer, his academic life lost to caring, a child of 10 who needed him, and whom he didn't understand.

The three daughters, who were too young, even in their 20s, to understand him either, wondered why, after only two years, he needed another wife. One said to me, by way of explanation, "Dad loved Jan very much you know". But by the time she said it, we were already married.

Fertile ground for the third wife to potentially be buried in you would think. Being a third wife is an unnatural state in any case. So I was still a Ms, not a Mrs.

And the man, who had not yet met Mr Parky, carried on being himself for a very long time.

He had thought he was being himself, presumably, when he decided he was in love, just five days after we met. I boarded my flight back home in shock, telling him, "It's too soon". But we are never ourselves when we think we are in love. Both parties are insane and remain so until domestic reality sets in. We were no different to anyone else, just in more of a hurry. We had no time for taking our time. We lived 12,000 miles apart, had seven children between us on different continents, and decisions had to be made.

Learning of our intention to marry, another of his daughters said in disgust, "It's like an arranged marriage." This was technically true. We were arranging it. Eloping in fact, in self-defence, although she didn't know about that yet. My children were more relaxed, or perhaps simply more polite, the youngest positively looking forward to living in London.

So I rented out my house. Prof R came to get me with his son, and he and I alone took a ferry to another island and got married on a water taxi. The celebrant and the ferryman were our witnesses. Their wives made us a cake and decorated the water taxi with miniature white roses. We were overwhelmed. Back on land, they took us to a supermarket to buy our groceries, and then back to take the water taxi to a favourite haunt of mine in a private bay. With just the wekas and possums to keep us company and steal our shoes.

History was repeating itself. The daughter of an immigrant; I was returning to live in the city my mother had left in 1946. She had married her RNZAF Flying Officer and sailed off to New Zealand to live happily ever after.

April 4 — Today, Prof R went back upstairs straight after breakfast and his pill, to rest. Every day is slightly different but also the same. It begins with early morning medications – although to be pedantic, it actually begins at around midnight and is repeated at about 4 am before we begin the real day. Prof R then sleeps till breakfast. Breakfast might be 9.30 am or 10.30 am. Or sometimes after 11 am.

At about 1 pm or later he will reappear for his lunch. And more pills. His mobility is slow but sure. Thanks to the overnight pill-popping, there is no falling, seldom 'freezing', and not too often being lost to himself.

This routine is against the advice of the neurologist, who instructed me to reduce his overnight medications. After two falls, we ignored him. We are used to managing the medications to suit Prof R, not the textbooks. It is tempting to invite the neurologist to stay for a few nights.

After lunch, if the weather is fine, we might go to the nearby park for a short walk if he feels able. If not, we talk or look at photos to explore memory lane. We both enjoy that. But only if I edit the memories. Prof R seldom wants to watch a film or TV and no longer reads, although he can. His interests and inspirations are buried where he can no longer find them. Most of the time anyway. I tell him not to worry. The memories have temporarily slipped through his 'colander'.

Although he can still make a cup of tea and could probably empty the dishwasher, he doesn't, and as a result he cannot find the dishwasher. He still watches the news, and we discuss the issues of the day. Yesterday he asked me to remind him about his first wife. How she fits in.

By 3 or 4 pm, or earlier, he is ready for another lie-down. Lately, that has been an up-and-down lie down. And when he comes down, he is not sure quite why he bothered, as he really needs to be upstairs again. So, after a cup of tea, he goes. Which is a relief if I am in the middle of something or need to go out.

The next time I catch him awake usually is for our evening meal. A very nice time for both of us. But if his tremor is bad, I cut his food smaller or help him steady his limbs. We discuss why no one has invented a way for the offending nerves in his wrists to be isolated in some way with a mechanical wristband or pressure point. If acupressure works for seasickness, why not tremor? We have an electro-acupuncture machine, but I suspect that would simply irritate the nerve rather than isolating it. At night, if I lay my hand on his worst arm, the right one, the tremor will sometimes stop. When he sleeps, it sleeps too.

That is, until around midnight, when I need to wake myself to put a pill by his bed. I no longer wake him because the neurologist told me off. Said why would he need a pill if he's asleep? But Mr Parky never sleeps in our house and if the toilet is calling, the head needs to be on the body. Or Prof R falls. Usually, the toilet does call at about the right time and the pill is swallowed. The next one is placed by his side of the bed at about 4 am and his low light put on. Then I sleep.

Our first two years together we were busy with our two at-home sons and my efforts to freelance or find a permanent job. Both boys were studying, but with five years between them, neither were really connecting with the other. The daughters came for meals occasionally, but mostly rang to ask for help – a London bar to be fitted to a door, or a floor sanded. Understandably they didn't connect meaningfully with their little brother. And he, plagued by dyslexia, didn't connect much with school, despite the army of helpers.

So, in our third year, after two terrorist acts – 9/11 and 7/7 – that changed everything, we looked for a new beginning. It turned out not to be Wales, or Surrey or even Dorset. Prof R's son Michael, then 15, vetoed them all. He was in love with New Zealand, his mother's birthplace. And had spent his happiest times there with both parents when he was younger, before she died.

With my son Douglas about to go to university, we changed tack and flew to New Zealand on a short location hunt, leaving the boys at home. We returned with a decision – not our first choice but a good choice, with an aptly-named school – Mt Aspiring.

April 6 — This morning I found another stash of tissues in the middle drawer of Prof R's chest of drawers, in the far left corner. Used tissues. If I have no need to look in the drawer for a while, it becomes a mountain. I don't ask him why he does it. I just throw them out.

Yesterday he said to me, with wonder in his voice, "How do you know so much about my past?" "Because you told me all about it darling" I said.

And now it is my job to retell it to him. We tried to work out if anyone else had the full story of his life. Not his first wife, or even his sister, and definitely not his children. Only he knew the full story, and he had almost forgotten it. I am the repository of at least some kind of continuity.

The New Zealand solution lasted until education was abandoned and we could no longer afford to pay taxes in two countries. That took about five years, during which time we sold the London house and bought our UK bolthole on the Welsh Borders. Chosen so we could have the best of both worlds, which we did. Michael chose to stay in New Zealand.

Back home in our Welsh village, in 2009, we made the decision to remain there, and develop our cottage into a home where all the children could visit and stay and spend Christmas. All was well.

But there were signs that perhaps all was not well. Prof R was an excellent driver, but he began to make me nervous. At intersections, or anywhere quick decisions had to be made, he was milliseconds slower. He looked right, then left, and did not look right again before moving forward. I became his gatekeeper.

Some years before, on holiday in Spain with the two boys, he had turned left and remained on the left in the path of an oncoming truck. Cries of "go right, go right" from his passengers averted disaster. And after another holiday, this time in France, on the way back to England, landing at Poole in the middle of the night, he went round a roundabout the Continental way, arrows pointing towards him. This time cries of warning made no impression. He was sure he was right for what seemed like too much time, but was probably only seconds. Fortunately, there was no oncoming traffic to ram home the necessary facts of the matter. We blamed fatigue. No more midnight arrivals.

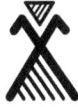

The Diagnosis

Before Diagnosis — In November 2012, we planned a trip back to New Zealand to attend Michael's wedding. Poring over the map, we talked about where we would visit after the wedding was over. Our Southern Lake home and Mt Aspiring, and the vast grasslands and mountains of Central Otago, a landscape we both loved, was my first suggestion.

And that was when, uninvited, undiagnosed, Mr Parky had popped up and said, "Why would we want to go there?" It was me who froze. Sick to my stomach. And after some gentle prompting, Mr Parky left, and Prof R returned.

On our arrival in New Zealand in February 2013, we collected our rental car. Prof R, the natural controller and ill-equipped navigator, said, "You drive." This was a red flag of a very different kind. Navigation would not be an issue. I knew the roads. But Prof R's decision that he could not drive in New Zealand was a sign I couldn't ignore. For the first time I allowed myself to think the word 'dementia'.

The trip was wonderful, and I thought no more about it. But he had also developed a minor tremor. A GP noticed it in September but had said nothing and merely tested his heart. He had always had a genetic but harmless murmur.

Back home, I now began to feel distinctly unsafe when he was driving.

I knew something was wrong, although he did not. But it would be the following year before he was diagnosed.

March 2014 (The diagnosis) — The neurologist was positive about outcomes. "At your age, you won't die of Parkinson's".

We took her word for it, and avoided the end-of-life booklet at the back of the information pack. The only sinecure was levodopa, still the best after 30 years. The neurologist prescribed 100mg, gradually increased to three times a day. A miracle, as it turned out, although only after making him so ill for the first few weeks we both wondered if it was worth it. (Now I suspect a different neurologist might have begun with 50mg).

Given there is no cure for Parkinson's, there is plenty of scope for research of the non-scientific and apocryphal kind. We tried them all – Coenzyme Q10, protein powder, kefir (I made from culture), exercise (the only universally useful remedy) and motivational thinking; none of which were instigated by Prof R, for whom lack of motivation was a major symptom. This made him reluctant to volunteer for even non-invasive Parkinson's research projects. It was also the one possible symptom of Mr Parky that I had tolerated since we met, but had understandably not recognized. Lack of motivation is quite common among the well.

Levodopa, the magic bullet, sped Prof R up. He was again safe behind the wheel. We relaxed. Towards the end of that year we planned another trip to New Zealand – house-sitting this time to enable us to stay longer. Both the neurologist and Parkinson's nurse gave us their blessing and wished us a wonderful trip.

December 2014 (eight months after diagnosis) — Not long after we took off from Abu Dhabi on the 8-hour second leg to Sydney, Prof R became anxious, then began violently shaking. And then completely lost his mind.

He did it quietly, totally unaware of where he was or what was happening; questioning my explanation that we were in an aircraft. Because there was no turbulence, we seemed stationary. It was terrifying, but only for me. We coped, by my constantly explaining, and him remaining calm, so no one else knew what had happened.

Landing in Sydney, I steered him through procedures and gates and hushed him when his remarks were clearly unrelated to our situation. We smiled our way onto a transit bus and up steps into the aircraft to Wellington. Being medically grounded in Sydney and forbidden to fly would have been a fate far worse than temporary insanity.

Halfway across the Tasman, Prof R said loudly and with wonder, "There's a bird sitting on the end of the wing." More hushing from me and a boiled sweet from the cabin crew kept his mouth busy until we crossed the New Zealand coast.

As we descended over Wellington he stared and recognized nothing. When we landed, I steered him through customs by insisting we liked to keep together. The ground staff were kind and waved us through.

Prof R still had no idea where he was. So I took him to the departure lounge, familiar territory, full of cafes and shops, and bought him a latte and we sat, and I waited. After an hour I said, "Do you know where we are now?" and he said "Yes, Wellington."

He was back.

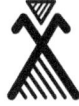

A Prof's Progress

APRIL 10 2018 — It is 7 am and we have just spent a quiet half hour waiting for Prof R's muscles to wake up so he can manoeuvre himself up onto his hands and knees holding the side of the bed. Then I can help him get up off the floor, where he has fallen. Possibly, because he has fallen asleep sitting on the side of his bed before going to the bathroom. Or he has slipped getting up. Either is possible. It is his first fall in four months. So that's quite good, but also not good, as it is so hard to prevent falls altogether, unless I never sleep.

April 12 — Sex is now a four-letter word. Too hard to attempt, even if we both still think about it. And never discussed.

We were still blissfully unaware of that as we toured New Zealand that second time, spending as much time as possible with his son Michael. But Michael was still difficult to connect with and we didn't know why. It would be a long time before I did. Prof R was lost before he was able to.

So I drove and the sun shone, and we ate gelato on the Wellington waterfront and ice cream everywhere else. I began to treat this trip as my last, without realising it. Seeking out the people I loved and the places I wanted to say goodbye to.

Christchurch was where I had been born and where two earthquakes, in 2010 and 2011, had flattened almost all of the centre and several of the historic buildings of early settlement. We had seen it on our 2013 trip in its war-zone state and now I wanted to immerse myself in the new mood of the city and its reconstruction. We had a house-sit for a month to do it.

Prof R stayed well enough to enjoy the trip and see old friends and family, although he was contributing less and listening more. And perhaps not even really listening.

This was a man who would have taken centre stage happily in any forum and pronounce his views, sometimes to a point where my cringe-factor kicked in. If anyone asked him about his career, it was the full CV rather than the executive summary. Prof R self-diagnosed as not being a team man; he preferred to lead. But now even that particular Prof R was beginning to slip away.

He loved New Zealand and would happily have returned to live there again, if not for our London families, whom we loved more, and who also had the strength of numbers. We did not talk about this as our 'sunset' trip. He didn't see it that way, confident we would return. But I was beginning already to dread the flight home.

April 24 — There is a park just a block away from our house. The latest house; in Market Town, in Kent. On nice days I either walk Prof R or the dog, but not both of them the same time. When we tried it, the dog ran around in circles and threatened to cut Prof R off at the knees.

Spring is finally moving into summer, and it is good for Prof R. In winter, he hibernated, and so did I. But his hibernation could mean not coming down until lunchtime. So he missed one meal of the day.

Keeping up his weight is one of the critical challenges. Not because he doesn't like his food. He loves his food. But even though he eats healthily, and I give him tempting biscuits with his cups of tea in between meals, he barely keeps beyond too thin. The weight has redistributed itself away from his buttocks and lower abdomen, so that naked he can look concave. And frail. Even though he is not yet. His upper body is still reasonably robust.

The tremor in his hands is a lot worse, and there is a theory that the constant movement is why Parkinson's people lose weight. No one yet really knows. But I tell him I need the 'tremor diet' and he does not. His right hand is worse than his left, because he is naturally right-handed, so I remind him to try eating or drinking with his left. It does help.

———— Ω ————

February 2015 (10 months after diagnosis) — When it came time to fly home from New Zealand – in late February 2015 – I was optimistic to his face and privately dreading a repeat of the nightmare of the outward journey.

The 3 am start from our Wellington bedsit didn't help, but all the way to Sydney he was fine. The day in Sydney was spent with two of my children – Douglas who now lived there and his older brother Alex, on a visit from London. We walked and talked in blinding heat, but I was sure the hours on the ground and the exercise were going to help his brain cope with 35,000 ft for the next 20 hours.

When we reached Abu Dhabi, he was still okay. But there came a moment in the transit lounge when he looked at me and said, "where are we"? And it all began again.

As we entered the departure lounge, there was a second cabin baggage search and the customs staff decided to give me the forensic one. I ushered Prof R forward while I grappled with the barked request to find all my electronic devices and turn them on. I had no idea where my UK devices were. The entire contents of my backpack were spread across the counter before I found them. No bomb, but the extra phone, fortunately still charged, and enough sweat from me to suggest a guilt complex. There were no smiles from any of us. Except from Prof R, who had not moved and was watching with interest.

The following 12 hours were endured by encouraging him to sleep. We were both exhausted. There was an incident with a cup of water that required me to put a blanket on his wet seat to hide the apparent loss of bladder control. Every trip to the toilet was an anxious wait from my seat for him to emerge, followed by frantic waving until he found me again.

My neighbour in the window seat, a young businesswoman, was discreet, but eventually I felt she should have an explanation. Her warm concern was strangely comforting. Here was an ally of sorts. And I could stop worrying about what she might think. Or whether she would say something to the cabin crew.

Prof R was asking where the bags were, constantly searching for his cabin bag every few minutes and unable to confirm for himself that we would be reunited with our suitcases when we landed. I was still trying to avoid an emergency landing to an alternate airport and removal from the plane.

Finally, we crossed the coast of England. Always a welcome sight, but this time doubly so. As if to reward our endurance, we were put into a holding pattern over London. This would normally be a joy to both of us. As we banked sharply at what felt like 45 degrees, I pointed out the Thames and enthused about the view. Prof R later told me he thought I had arranged a sightseeing flight, just for him.

This time Customs was a breeze. Midday on a Sunday is the perfect time to land at Heathrow. The terminal was almost empty, long evacuated from the previous arrival. And being Heathrow, there was no checking for illegal fruit or drugs, or tests for mental competency. We were allowed to proceed through together and waited patiently in the baggage hall for our bags.

Prof R was still flying high, but now on a flight path back to sanity. He knew he needed his bag. We waited and we waited. My bag came through; his did not. He stood wistfully by the revolving dregs of unclaimed bags, until a gentle ground-staffer came up to ask him if he was alright. It took a few more rides on the carrousel before we spotted it, naked and unrecognizable without its distinctive belt.

We were almost home free. Except I had made an error with the arrival date and time zone calculation. The cheap minicab which had brought us to Heathrow three months ago had been booked to return for us, in error, on the following day. I had to ring him to cancel.

After which, we paid a fortune for a black cab to get to Walton-on-the-Hill and a bed with his sister Doris and her husband Brian. It was their daughter's house, and Prof R could not navigate it for the entire three days we were there. He was ill, but not in the sense that anyone could do anything about it.

I rang the Parkinson's nurse and she suggested reducing the levodopa for a day or so. She had no idea why flying had caused his reaction. He had a nightmare during the first night and woke me in fright, showing me the wreckage of our room. "I dreamt I had killed you!" He had been looking for the bathroom. But as it turned out, I discovered he had peed on the snow-white shag pile carpet in the corner of the room. I lied and told him it was water; and lied about it to his sister too.

Before he was really well enough to travel, we had to. Our welcome had been timed to fit in before another guest. That meant first driving down to Kent to pick up our car from his sister's house, where they had left it. The battery was flat. And while his brother-in-law was charging it, Prof R became shocked and chilled, shaking uncontrollably. A hot water bottle and blankets and my arms around him failed to make much impact.

When we finally got into the car, he assured me he remembered the way back to his niece's house, and then discovered, as I drove up a slip-road onto the motorway, that he didn't. Fortunately, I then discovered that I almost did, so we carried on. It was necessary to stop in an emergency zone on the motorway when he became desperate to pee. Abusive horns from passing traffic as he climbed the bank. And then we had to stop again at a motorway service station for him to pee again. Even if the car battery was not fully charged, we both decided a cup of tea was the least we deserved and the most we needed. And then we continued our journey until my nose led me to our destination.

When we finally walked in the door, my sister-in-law said, "Where on earth have you been?" And when I explained, she said, "You took a risk with that battery," to which I replied, "It was a lesser risk than a ruptured bladder; and nothing compared to mental incapacity for 12 hours at 35,000 ft." [1]

May 8 — His stepdaughter is coming for lunch next week. We haven't seen her for eight years, so I'm very pleased she has got in touch. She is the daughter of Prof R's second wife, Jan, and today I was thrilled to find a box of her mother's things. A Chinese marble chess set, a silver dressing table set and a silver tea set.

We have carried these things with us for 18 years. At every house move, I have found other treasures that I know Jan's children should have. While I am racked with concern, Prof R feels no such emotion. Although I know he loved his wife very much. So, was this Mr Parky? An empathy by-pass that is much more evident now.

---

1.   *Postscript: No one but Google solved the problem of Prof R's little misadventure with levodopa. Apparently a very small number of people react the way he did, and no one warns you that it is possible, probably because the medical people we consulted did not know. I'm glad they didn't, or we might never have gone.*

When I had first arrived to live at his house, after our wedding, I discovered he still had not moved Jan's clothing from my side of the wardrobe. Now it seems even more odd than it did then. As a third wife, I was prepared to be adaptable; to blend seamlessly into someone else's home; respecting a lost mother who had been adored.

But I had been with him more than two years before a headstone was finally bought and engraved – the wording chosen by her children – and installed at the head of an ever-sinking strip of grass on an unmarked grave. His stepdaughter had been asking him to do this for several years.

May 10 — Once a year, since we arrived in Market Town, Prof R has an appointment with a gerontologist. It has to be one of the most pointless things we ever have to do. Once a year seems too often and comes around too quickly. it entails a 45 minute drive to the hospital where he, the gerontologist, is located. Then we spend 45 minutes answering his questions and telling him what he doesn't know, and then we leave. He contributes nothing. We should charge him for the consultation.

We chose Market Town because we believed it to be well-connected. And in so many ways it is. The railway station is two blocks away, the shops and town centre just three blocks. There is a cinema, high on our list. We have been twice, but now Prof R is no longer able to sit through an entire film.

Our medical practice is four blocks away. There is one even closer – two blocks – but their list was full because they are the best practice in town. There is a drop-in out-of-hours nurse-led clinic until 8 pm. But when we arrived in 2017, Market Town did not have a Parkinson's nurse. Why? It depended who you asked. But probably two things – lack of funding and lack of available Parkinson's nurses. *(Finally, in 2018, they were given a base at the polyclinic. See below)*.

So, whenever Prof R has an appointment for anything relating to

Parkinson's, we have to drive – 15, 20 miles or more. The nearest A&E is also 45 minutes away. But there is a polyclinic 6 miles away that is in growth mode to meet demand, and may become a lifeline.

When Prof R's memory loss began to make itself felt, long before we moved here, he was started on a cognitive drug called Rivastigmine; another miracle for a while, and another one we self-managed when time between medical appointments was too long or were not available.

It took months for me to figure out how to pronounce Rivastigmine properly. Rather embarrassed, the Welsh neurologist said, "don't tell anyone I said this, but the easiest way to remember, is to think of Reva Steincamp". Reva Steincamp was famous for having been tragically killed by her lover, a well-known paraplegic Olympic athlete.

Prof R is now on the maximum dose. In fact, just a milligram over, because we split his dose through the day to three, rather than the recommended two doses. We're afraid to increase it, and won't risk it, even though now he now has huge chunks of his past hidden from him. Except occasionally when a 'file' opens.

The levodopa we also largely self-manage. Most Parkinson's people and their carers do. Because there are so many different types of Parkinson's – as many as 90 plus – we become the only experts on the symptoms and management of our own unique disease and its progression.

Prof R takes seven standard-dose 100mg pills a day. We've no desire to increase the dose because once, when we tried, he experienced hallucinations. So his tremor and mobility we have to manage in other ways. We self-diagnose him as 'stable'; although perhaps 'manageable' might be more accurate. Whatever step of the ladder we are on, we refuse to look either up or down. Some days, like today, he is just tired and only shows up for meals and a chat.

Sometimes I try to remember what he was like 'before'. I have become so used to my current husband, it can be difficult. Conversation is the biggest loss. Now I talk to him and for him mostly, tired of my own opinions but needing to connect with him intellectually. And often hoping he will find the issues of the day as interesting as I do. He is still present in the present, aware of the news and with a lingering short-term memory that sometimes impresses me. He says he loves talking with me. Which is just as well.

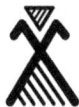

Love, War and New Zealand

2000 (Before the wedding) — What stays with me now is his unconditional love. If we argued or disagreed over an issue it was not because he was disappointed in his choice of a wife. With him, I could be myself and myself was good enough. It took time to relax into this new security, even if our occasional power struggles seemed risky.

This did not mean he was prepared to relinquish any power, just that he felt I was worth persevering with. Prof R had a wealth of experience and knowledge that he was eager to share. New arrivals from the Antipodes who were no longer young or inexperienced nevertheless had a hard job reminding him of the fact.

It could be both mundane and amusing. Dishwashers in the UK need salt but those in New Zealand do not. I had never heard of putting salt in a dishwasher, a fact he refused to believe. How could this be? And how could I possibly do a cold-water clothes wash? And in a top-loading washing machine called Gentle Annie, that was not designed for a laundromat and made very little sound? If it didn't exist in Prof R's world – the mother country – it simply didn't exist. Proving him wrong in the small things was a sport I never tired of, because there was so much I did need to learn. It was fun to be sometimes right.

Before we decided to get married, while we were each on separate continents, Prof R asked me to come and live with him. To risk all. To give up my lucrative consultancy, my home, my daughter Hope (who was at university and could not come) and move to the UK. I said, "It's not enough." To create a secure new family, we needed to show them we were serious. Committed. He agreed, and asked me to marry him. It was the first time a man had proposed to me, so naturally, I said yes.

Prof R invited me over to London for that first Christmas in 1999, and secretly planned our elopement – not in New Zealand, but in January 2020 in Poole. We would stay at Corfe, which he loved. I went for Christmas, but did not marry him then. Although I didn't know that when we went to Corfe.

In the hotel, the night before our wedding, we talked. But mainly he talked – about his past loves; things he needed to say, but as he talked, I felt less and less ready to become his next love.

The next morning, the day we were due to be married, after confessing my unreadiness to Prof R, I rang the Registry Office at Poole to cancel. The registrar was a man of empathy and wisdom. No doubt he had conversations like this from time to time, though hopefully not very often. We were very welcome, he said, to rebook at any time.

Prof R was very unhappy with my decision, but still confident of our eventual union. I wasn't, but could not bear to say so. He wanted to join us up as a family with the National Trust. I managed to talk him out of it, feeling sure that this was pointless. I just wanted to maintain my secret, not hurt him, and fly home as planned.

We were in possession of two wedding rings. And Prof R suggested we try them on. As he slipped mine onto my finger I was suddenly overwhelmed by unexpected emotion. A feeling of both premonition and fate. A surrender to whatever lay ahead. As I in turn put his ring on his finger, it was as though the ceremony had already taken place. The die was cast. And it had been all along. But I had lost sight of it. I miss that man more now than I might have done then.

———◠———

August 2020 — This whole business of ageing is very odd – the need to still have purpose not easily understood or explained. Especially where retirement is imposed more than chosen. It is mostly about a sudden sense of loss – of a future, of any relevance perhaps, other than to be available free labour for mundane purposes in communities, or charities. Not usually offers of a seat on the board. And if it is, it will be because no one else is prepared to be seconded.

We're told this is the time for us to "give back", as if we hadn't spent our lives giving, one way or another. More appropriate to tell us not to "give in" to lethargy and daytime TV. Write a book, paint a picture, plant a border or take in a boarder.

Age and retirement had never bothered Prof R the way it did me. He had taken early retirement from the university at 58 to care for his wife and Michael in her last year. When I met him, two years after her death, he impressed me by saying he was never bored. I was guilty of being easily bored. To such an extent that my first husband once accused me of always expecting to be entertained.

Prof R was happy either working with his photographs or cameras, or reading about history or archaeology. He was far better with technology than I was, even though I had earned my living with a computer for several years. He also appeared to be a whiz with his impressive filing system and the management of the household finances. There were few things he could not mend, even if he didn't feel like bothering. And he loved gardening, even if he didn't feel like doing it. "There's not a big enough garden here to bother."

The lack of motivation only showed on the surface – the broken whiteware at the back of the house blocking the French doors, the front room set up as an office with an old blanket covering a ceiling-high pile of files. And upstairs, after his stepdaughter had found a new home, her front bedroom stacked to the roof with furniture or anything else that didn't have an obvious home.

I had married a rock, not a rocket. But I knew he must have been a rocket once. He had the certificates to prove it.

⸰

Prof R's War — Prof R spent the first seven years of his life, or the five he could remember, at war, living in a London where bombs were normal. Broken windows from blast damage frequent. And even, he recalled, once being strafed in the street by a presumably lone German fighter pilot looking for targets on his way back to the coast and home.

His father was working in a reserved industry, at the gas works, and was a St Johns first aid volunteer at work and out-of-hours.

He is extremely proud of his father. When the bombs fell, and the family scrambled into the Anderson shelter, his dad would climb to the top of the house to spot where the bombs were landing, before jumping on his bike with his first aid kit and racing to where he thought he could be of most use.

When peace was declared, the future professor said to his parents, "Will there still be newspapers?" Thinking "what will there be to put in them?"

Young Prof R knew all about vegetables, because he had helped his father with their two allotments during the war. His parents had a tandem bicycle, and he would ride off on the back seat with his father in the early evening to tend them.

He grew up enjoying eating as well as growing vegetables and would drink the cabbage water in which his mother had boiled the victim to its death. But he wanted more than just a small plot. He dreamed of acreage. Not excessive, but enough to be able to boast about; or to be able to emulate his father's achievements.

When we decided to move to New Zealand, in autumn 2003, I made it my mission to find Prof R a garden big enough to realise his dream. Our first house, in the Southern Lakes – close to the water but not close enough to see it, that being too expensive – did have a garden that was big enough for him to make himself a vegetable plot. And he did.

_____Ω_____

May 15 2018 — We learn our defensive behaviours in infancy. Instead of getting angry, Prof R withdraws and occasionally cries. His daughters tell me he has always done this. It works for him. But I always wanted him to project his feelings outwards. Turning inwards is a pathway to depression. I wanted him to get angry and argue his case. My initial sympathy at his tears gave way to tough love. "Stop crying. I'm not interested in tears. I want to hear what it is you need to say."

He cries much less now, when he actually has more to cry about. But he still retreats into 'sad face' and silence if he is challenged. And then I feel distressed and guilty, because it is not good for him. It makes his tremor much worse.

His mother was an oasis of calm. Or as far as I can tell. Her photos show a woman who is clear-eyed and intelligent. Sure about her purpose, but content not to lead. At some point when he was in his early teens, she came to Prof R and said she felt she might have to leave his father, who was having an affair with a neighbour. Prof R tells me he replied, "If you do, I'll throw myself out of the window." She stayed. I sometimes wonder what decision I would have made if one of my children had said that to me. Fortunately, none of them did.

2006 — Our second property in New Zealand had three acres, a lovely little colonial-styled two-storey house and a summerhouse. The day we viewed it, Prof R was smitten. But he would not or could not make a decision. We drove to a nearby spa town for the weekend and I walked him to the top of Conical Hill. It is pine-covered and steep and the perfect way to prepare the 'little grey cells' to do some thinking. At the top, we sat admiring the valley, with its small picturesque alpine town and nearby mountain-fed river. And eventually I said to him, "so what do you want to do? You must decide now in case we lose it to another buyer." Uncharacteristically, he made the decision "I want to buy it."

May 20 — Now that the weight is failing to cling to him, no matter how much food I put in front of him, I find it hard to remember 'big Prof R'. I was 'Shallow Hal' in those early days. Very slim myself and not impressed with the rotund, although I never said so. We probably looked a little incongruous together then. Now I fear he is catching up to me. Soon we will weigh the same, and eventually no doubt he will streak towards frail. I would stop it if I could. But his body is a walking chemical cocktail, burning fuel like a shooting star.

Yesterday was the wedding of Prince Harry and Meghan Markle; 19 May 2018. It was also my eldest son Alex's 41st birthday. When I called him, he returned to the question which concerned him very much. How could I live a life while still caring for Prof R? He wants me to find respite care. I assured him I had compartmentalized it. I don't think about what we could be doing – travelling, going up to London for the day, even visiting the cinema. It's parked. I'll make a judgement about respite care if and when I really need it.

While we were talking, Prof R appeared from the toilet, struggling to do up his trousers. I helped him with one hand, determined not to relinquish my son in the process.

Last night, Prof R was rising every few minutes in the small hours of the morning. It happens sometimes and he doesn't know he is doing it. He goes to the bathroom usually, although occasionally will veer off and head down the stairs. I have to be alert for falls. It makes no difference if I ask him to try to stay in bed. He is driven to rise. It's possible his muscles are tense, although fortunately he has no pain. He will not remember if I ask him about it this morning. I had to wake him for his early pills and at 11 am he is still not down for breakfast. He is exhausted and so am I.

———————— ∩ ————————

Prof R was always a night owl, never retiring before about midnight. In our first few years together, we subsisted on about 6 hours sleep a night, which suited him, but slowly drove me to exhaustion. I began falling asleep on the sofa after meals. He would be upset if I didn't greet him at bedtime like the new bride I was. But this Cinderella was turning into a pumpkin. Literally.

I began to gain weight. Prof R made the best curries in the world and I was not accustomed to them. In the beginning, he had left me to do all the cooking, until I asked him to share. And now I was being hoist by my own petard. What fed the gander was now feeding the goose.

———————— ∩ ————————

May 23 (The 'new' neurologist – Kent) — Finally, I think Dr V understands what it is like to be Prof R, if that's possible. It took only 15 minutes today for him to realise there is no more medication that can be prescribed and only perhaps occupational therapy for the tremor. Dr V is puzzled by Prof R's sleep patterns, suggesting, again, that I should not wake him for his medications. I invite him to come and stay with us for a week and he laughs. But he understands.

We discuss new research developments with pressure gloves designed to still the nerve impulses to Prof R's hands, although these are far from production. Too late for Prof R.

I also tell Dr V about the *petit mal*, after deciding this morning that I would not, in case he blamed me for doing something wrong. He reassured me, saying neither the brain supplements nor stress would have caused it, and probably there was an interruption in his heart or blood pressure.

***

2006 — When we bought that three-acre property in the heart of the wheat fields of Canterbury, we were thoroughly pleased with ourselves. Full of motivation, we signed on for a course in tree cultivation and planned what we would grow and which animals we might graze for local farmers. We began with three sheep and very quickly learned to hate them. They ate a small corner of one paddock to a dustbowl and ignored the rest. They were stupid and too heavy to move without a bribe.

Friends suggested we rent out the grounds for weddings. There was a white gazebo beyond a small bridge over a stream, in a lush green dell and with rose bushes in abundance. The front lawn was capable of housing two tennis courts. The string quartet could play on the veranda. The friends who suggested it would supply the string quartet.

There were two paddocks and outbuildings on one acre that we eyed for subdivision. But the land was zoned rural so that was out. Instead, I cut the tinder-dry grass with the ride-on mower, until someone mentioned one spark would set a grass fire fit to devour the neighbouring farm. And on the way take the huge macrocarpa windbreak trees with it. In the end, we did none of it. Not even the vegetable patch. Prof R was motivated to dig one, briefly, but disturbed a wasp nest and retreated, like the Pied Piper, bringing them with him. Thoughtfully, he raced towards me, calling a warning. I was clearing the rose beds in front of the house of thistles taller than I was. We managed to keep ahead of the escort and escaped indoors.

Prof R did clear the undergrowth of the small woodland behind the house, which was a job in itself. And never went near the fledgling veggie patch again. We had bitten off more than we could chew. Especially as we were now spending the Antipodean winters in our bolthole in Wales.

But we loved the property. And Prof R loved nothing better than to watch me scuttling out of sight on the lawn mower leaving a trail of dust behind me. The more I worked, the happier he became. And I became progressively more irritated. He was the boy who held the lantern while his mother chopped the wood; happy in his work, whistling probably, and sure of his value. I didn't have the heart to tell him the truth.

There were trees – quite a few – large enough and close enough to crush the house, so the tree doctors came and swung around them at 100 feet, removing any branches that seemed hazardous. Then they tackled the boundary trees that could crush cars. It cost a fortune.

When it was time to go back to the UK for the southern winter, we found a man who wanted to graze horses on the land and promised he would, in return, mow and do groundwork. When we returned after five months, the neighbours complained that the horses were ill-treated, and we discovered that the grounds were too. It could be embarrassing to be part-time members of a close-knit small community.

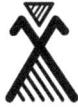

Spring–Summer 2018

MAY 25 2018 — Prof R's stepdaughter, when she came to lunch yesterday, reminisced about a man who, once on task, was always slow and methodical. When he cooked, he took his time and every ingredient he could muster. It was how he unwound after a day with his students. Her mother, his second wife, didn't really enjoy cooking and was also seeing physiotherapy clients in the evenings, so she was grateful. Until it came time to clean up after the meal, when the whispered wail would go up, "Does he really have to use every pot in the house?"

The complicated combined family I walked into, with my youngest son, had a history it was impossible to fathom.

On the surface, all was well. There were three apparently well-adjusted daughters from his first marriage, a newly-graduated stepdaughter, still at home, but about to fly. Only the young son was obviously struggling; too young to be close to any of his grown-up siblings. Lonely, bored and sad.

As time progressed, things became no clearer. But the actors became more obviously just like any other family. There were undercurrents from the past. I knew all about undercurrents, having just escaped a rip tide of my own. But these were affecting the senior siblings' relationships with their father. He had left their mother when they were still pre-schoolers, and time had not cured their pain – simply made space for the enormity of things unsaid to grow.

I had left my own children, to ultimately make a second home for them elsewhere, so I could share them with their father. I understood what may have driven him. But I struggled with the enormity of this loss for his children; so young, with a father desperate to escape. To them, there had been no clear cause, no crime committed, except his own. He had begun another relationship when the youngest, Julie was a new-born.

When we first met, he had not told me the truth of this, because he was afraid, he said later, that I would be unable to accept it. My husband's affair and the subsequent fallout that led to my own departure from the family home had shattered my foundations, and I was far from recovered from the experience.

At the time, it was necessary for me to interpret Prof R's flight as a crisis of the head; even while the realisation of what his wife had suffered was unbearable. It was a lesson in forgiveness that I struggled with for years. And when the lie surfaced, eventually, I felt he had been right not to tell me.

Now, Prof R needs me to remind him of all these things he told me about his life. I used to tell him honestly, but now I leave out all the bits that could cause distress. Remorse for past deeds that cannot be undone uses up emotional energy that is needed to face each day.

May 27 — Prof R has just weighed himself at my suggestion. As he says, "I am getting more bones". He weighs 65 kg, my own weight. And that is not enough. We joked that 18 years ago he would have given almost anything to be so slim. But he would not have given away his life to Parkinson's for the privilege.

Our already healthy and substantial diet will have to include some Prof R-only additions. More cake, more cream, more pasta. He has a sweet tooth so it should be easy. After years of austerity, Prof R now has permission to break out of jail.

———o———

Between the ages of 11 and 18 Prof R discarded his Peckham vowels, embraced RP and developed a love of languages and the theatre. He was the 'poster boy' Grammar Schools were established to help, and he did not disappoint. At Haberdasher Askes, he went beyond his parent's wildest dreams and discovered his own. Motivation then was not an issue.

He always knew he was lucky, then. Class mattered and education was the way up. That, and Received Pronunciation. This was before Estuary English and Northern Soul. There was nothing fashionable about a Peckham lexicon. He needed elocution and in drama classes he got it.

His eye was firmly fixed on university, which was a foreign country to his parents but which they wholeheartedly supported. He became fluent in German and French. There were student exchanges to the continent and Prof R went to a newly post-war Germany. He stayed with a family whose English mother had somehow managed to out-live her wartime there. And he found the Germans welcoming to him as well.

When he was 19 or so, Prof R side-stepped compulsory military service by getting himself a job as an assistant teacher at a French école for one year. The école was at Compiegne where, in a railway carriage in the forest, the First World War armistice was signed.

From there he was only one step away from reading English at Nottingham.

———o———

Prof R has just called quietly to me from the downstairs bathroom. He says "help"! This is the first time he has been unable to lever himself up from the toilet seat. There is the basin for him to grip with one hand, or two, but today he needs more. And he is not happy to report that he still needs to wipe himself. But with a helping hand onto his feet and my departure he is able to complete his task with his dignity intact.

He has been stuck in bathrooms many times for different reasons, but this was something new, and while the handbasin is easy to grasp for leverage, he may need a handrail as well. There will come a time when he will need me to clean him too, but neither of us needs to think about that just yet. It is important to remain positive and find a joke inside the black holes that sometimes appear.

I'm a bit tired today because I got up at 5 am. This is because he was quite confused at 4 am and I needed to stay alert while he went to the bathroom. He was there a long time and I had to try not to fall asleep. When he finally came back to the bedroom, and levered himself back into bed, I was wide-awake.

When this happens, or if I wake earlier, I go downstairs and make myself a cup of tea, without disturbing our new puppy. She sleeps the way a baby should, without sound all night, and only gets up when I tell her she can.

I usually choose not to read, but to watch the BBC overnight news. Reading makes me tired and I don't want to sleep on the couch. If it's 2 or 3 am I go back to bed after an hour or so. But at 5 am there's no point. So, after an hour I go and have a bath with Dead Sea salts to sooth my skin as well as my soul.

After the bath, I check Prof R and then dress and do my 'face'; the face that meets the day and anything else that might be encountered. Without my 'face' I am ironically not myself. The same with my clothes, which must be comfortable but still reflect a woman who is living for today, not yesterday.

When Prof R is reminiscing, he remembers this: Taking a school theatre troop on tour in Europe with Shakespeare's *Coriolanus*. This choice would be a challenge for any thespian, but they were undaunted. He was in charge, and this was the triumph of his life at that point. They received rave reviews in the local papers. He has never truly topped the sheer joy of this achievement, it seems. It dominates the early memories that remain. It is the path he did not follow and sometimes regrets; working in theatre management. There was less kudos and less income than an academic career.

He was also interested in journalism, and accepted his first job with an industrial journal selling their advertising. (*By the time I met him, this had been edited to, "I worked in industrial journalism".*)

The job required a lot of travel, and he didn't have a driver's licence, so his boss took him on a sales trip in his mini and after a while, tired, told Prof R to drive. So well did the pupil take to the wheel, the instructor went to sleep.

When I first knew him, Prof R could drive eight hours in a day without even thinking about it. It had been a normal day's work for him, as a visiting lecturer, to give a talk at a university campus in Wales at 11 am and drive back to his London campus in the afternoon.

By the time he was first married, in 1962, he had returned to teaching. But after a while, still not satisfied, he began a second degree in Educational Psychology part-time. He wanted to do more than teach younger students in a classroom.

—

Now, Prof R cannot drive at all, and hasn't done for three years, but he seems not to miss it. He doesn't get engaged, even as a passenger. Always terrible at navigating, he is content to just sit and allow me to work out routes or listen to me rant when I get fouled up by the Satnav.

This is a welcome change. Before his illness, he would begin to give me directions for the exit from a roundabout 500 yards beforehand, and describe every other detail of the intervening 500 yards in doing so. When we reached the roundabout, I would have to say, "Quickly, just tell me which exit. I need to know NOW". Succinct instructions were outside his natural teacher's remit to "explain in full".

Mysteriously, being terrible at navigation never seemed an issue for him when he drove alone, all those years ago, to universities far and wide. Did Mr Parky intervene there too, before I met him?

As therapy, I have been asking him to remind me about his career; the four London campuses, his colleagues and his milestones. It's a pleasant way to help him jog his grey cells. Sometimes he will just say what meant the most to him in the end. "I was Dean of the department." That was his last post. He was Dean when, only 58, he took early retirement to care for Jan.

It helps him when I say, "Which university did you meet Jan at?" or Pam, or Maggie for that matter. Pam and Maggie came after his first wife, Susan, and before his second wife Jan. There were only two years between Jan and me, so there were no other names in between.

—

Currently, I am obsessed with the malfunctioning of our pill regime. It seems impossible to be sure either of us will always be alert when the next one is due. It means we cannot get mentally absorbed in an activity or become lost in a book.

Being lost in a book is mostly my problem. Prof R only occasionally glances at a magazine. Also, in the night, my sleep is hounded by the fear of not waking at the correct times. So far, I have managed quite well, but only by sleeping on the edge of a proverbial cliff.

So, I am on the hunt for an alarm watch, preferably not something that makes me look like a person with a problem, even though I am. There is no point in Prof R wearing it, although we could both wear one.

He still needs help to access his pills, as the box does not clearly tell him what he needs to know.

The box we have settled on has 'morn', 'noon', 'eve' and 'bed'. There is no slot for early morn or overnight. I used a permanent pen to write times next to those words, but they rub off, or there is a day he is later having his early morning pill, so the whole day has to be altered to remain in step. In which case, an alarm would be only an irritation.

I have bought a child's blackboard for the bedroom to chalk up his ideal regime of meds. If I should drop dead, or be absent for any other reason, the paramedics will have something to refer to. We're also registered on an emergency hotline. And have a small cylinder with a green cross on it that takes his prescription and which we must keep in the fridge where they can find it.

It's interesting when you are adapting to a new reality of life to discover the things that someone really needs to invent. Usually someone, somewhere, has, but it is not always easy to find it. But you can almost guarantee that when you do find it, it will be 'not quite right'.

This has happened with his personal alarm, which hangs from the rail by his bed. It took some finding, because we did not want one that is connected to a call centre or other relative. We have one now that rings three numbers in our house in succession if he has fallen and needs help. But first he has to be able to reach the button on the alarm. You might think it sensible for him to wear it, but believe me, it isn't. How easy it would be to press it in error when it is around your neck or on your wrist; you wouldn't even need to have dementia. A good scenario for comedy, but not for the nervous system.

I might not have been aware of that tripwire if I had not watched an American comedy series called *Grace and Frankie*. It stars Jane Fonda and Lily Tomlin. Grace and Frankie have an incident when both are prostrate on the floor with bad backs. It's temporary, but their children insist on buying them alarms to wear around their necks. However, Grace and Frankie run a business. Selling 'personal items'. And the next time they have an online meeting with a client, Frankie (Lily) leans against her computer keyboard and presses her alarm button by accident. The disembodied voice from the call centre asks her if she is okay. Does she need an ambulance? She cannot turn it off of course, and so it becomes farce, and an ambulance is dispatched. It was a salutary lesson to me.

When it comes to the alarm watch, I can report that all of them are ugly. I will keep looking.

—

As I face my own mortality, I have Prof R to thank. Without him, I would still be pretending I am young. As it is, in the spirit of surrender, I have grown out my blond tresses and now sport a rather unfetching grey. Next year I will be 70. The worst nightmare of our youth really does come true. Amazing.

A friend of mine, much older, told me to suck it and get used to it. She claims no one gets grey hair that doesn't suit them. Our natural colour is always going to match our complexion. Her reference for this is a course she once did on colour matching. I also did a course on colour matching years ago and remember nothing being mentioned about hair colour. It was all about what material suited my face. Whether I was a winter, summer, autumn or spring. No one mentioned the hair. I keep trying to surprise myself in the mirror to see if it will tell me a different truth, but no luck so far.

—

May 28 — I have bought a smart watch. Not the expensive kind, but a nice one that will vibrate when twinned with the alarms on my phone. Smart watches – the very smart kind –are something I have previously sneered at. The first time I saw someone flip his wrist to use it to pay for an item, I quietly smirked. "Pretentious jerk".

I also thought them insecure. Because Prof R and I once had a 'Trojan' in our online account. There is nothing more unnerving than watching your money moving between your accounts, as if by magic. The ghost in the machine. And unless you have been cut off from civilisation or had your head in a bucket, you will know that if your phone suddenly goes dead your SIM ID has been hijacked, and with it all your personal data.

None of this has anything to do with Mr Parky, and therein lies its fascination. It is one of the things that engage my brain during days filled with equally pointless administrative activities.

—

Prof R is being fed cake, at least once a day. Fortunately, he likes it and seldom says no, even if he is not hungry. It is ironic we are on opposite trajectories with our weight. Basically, Mr Parky and I are incompatible. Even though I am not tempted by cake or biscuits, or even rice crackers. I seem to be staying fat on meat and veg and dairy products – even the zero fat ones.

Our breakfasts are identical – muesli and grapes for breakfast with goats' milk and yoghurt. Our lunch is often one slice of artisan sourdough wheat and rye bread with eggs and salad. (Prof R cannot eat leaves so the salad is every colour but green).

I do snack on a handful of dates dipped in humus, while Prof R snacks on anything I can tempt him with. Plus one latte, and several cups of tea, and a small glass of wine after dinner. And the dog loves it when I make popcorn. No butter. But salt, yes.

"So, exercise" you would think. I have bought a cheap Fitbit, and if I make it to 6000 steps it tingles on my wrist in a not altogether pleasant way. This target is surprisingly hard to achieve for the home-based, even with dog walking, stair running and a trip to the shops.

The house is not Buckingham Palace, or even semi-detached. It is a 'town house', otherwise known as a terrace; one room and a hallway wide and three floors high, including the attic, so I would need to continuously walk around both it and the 'low-maintenance' garden to get to the desired 10,000.

I have any number of exercise DVDs and YouTube guidance on the Five Tibetan poses. They are less appealing in summer weather. This is England. Summer weather is precious and to be savoured outdoors.

———————————

Exercise has never bothered Prof R. But when he was young, he could cycle from London to Brighton. He may only have done that once, but he did do it. With his best friend Dennis. They stayed the night with his aunt and uncle in Telscombe, hidden in a fold behind the cliffs above Peacehaven, "the village that time forgot"; so old it is recorded in the Doomsday Book. Prof R has taken me there. His uncle worked on a farm and his aunt did cream teas in summer for passing walkers.

Prof R spent a lot of time there, with their sons, his two cousins, during the war. He has a memory that should not be his own, of his aunt and uncle returning from church one day to say that it had been announced on the radio that war had been declared with Germany. Prof R would have been less than 2 years old.

———

People are dying ahead of me in ways I don't want to think about. No one seems to be dying quickly. You have to ask yourself why dying is so much less efficient than being born. And a lot more painful, or at least painful for longer. My elder sister Stella has plans to circumvent the last chapter. But what if the chapter you thought was the last was actually the penultimate chapter? I would be afraid to beat the gun. So by the time I recognised the last chapter, it would be too late to do anything about it.

We, the Baby Boomers, are blocking up the natural order of things by living longer without necessarily being healthier. The young are impatient. When are we going to die and relinquish all that wealth they are sure we are sitting on? We're just soaking up resources and contributing nothing. I agree with them. Because the only thing we can contribute is money, babysitting and wisdom, and they only need the money and the babysitting; and if you don't live close enough for that, it's only the money.

Prof R thinks less about all this than I do; probably one of the advantages of the creeping fog of dementia and a younger wife. We don't talk about the end game, because I want him to be content with the now. And he, thankfully, stopped looking for the last pamphlet in the Parkinson's information pack some time ago.

The woman from Carers Support has just made her bi-monthly phone call to me. So kind, so welcome but so unable to be any use whatsoever. Except perhaps in an emergency. The monthly meetings they hold for carers are more like confession time at AA than friendly chats with like-minded souls. Beware the well-meaning facilitator with the sympathetic expression.

―――――――⌒―――――――

June 2 — Saturday. Our dog managed to upend me on the grass in the park today. She is less than two, medium-sized, and very strong, but I like to think I am also strong. Another dog raced across the grass to make friends and my dog took fright. I must have been hanging on to her lead tightly or I would not have fallen. As she disappeared from the park in the direction of home, I assured the owner of the other dog that it was not his fault. I lied. My true opinion is that a dog that does not respond to its owner's call should be on a lead.

I don't chase after my dog on these occasions, and they have been multiple. A fatalist, I know she will only return if a) I am cunning and b) if a car doesn't get her first. I followed calmly on foot until I came upon a good Samaritan who had her in his grip. My hero. Her loose lead had become tangled in the tyre of a parked car.

Let that be a lesson to her.

My sister is horrified and says I must give the dog some serious training. "What if you had broken your hip?!" She is sending her advice from 12,000 miles away, in New Zealand. She knows a thing or two about dogs. But I'm not so sure that a frightened dog would stand still while another bears down on it, no matter how good the training. However, I will take the advice. Although training my dog to lose her initiative is something I am ambivalent about.

The most satisfying part of this incident is that I fell, rolled and got up like a whippet. Or more accurately, the Wobbly Man. Just try doing that on a normal day. Beats me.

—

Prof R's son is not communicating. I spend far too much time thinking about this and wondering what would enable him to do so. His wife, quite rightly, refuses to do it for him, although usually she will communicate to thank us for gifts.

If I had a chance to speak to him, the beloved son, I would only say, "I know you have things you wanted to say to dad, and now he is too ill. But it would be sad if you were left with regrets in the future." As a stepparent, I can only say so much, and it is a fine line to tread. When I asked Prof R whether he was upset or worried by not hearing from his son he said that generally, he was not, but that he would be very pleased to.

He feels more and more out of the loop with his children; unable to keep up with their lives on so little information. I tell him you don't need to have Parkinson's disease to feel that way. When they are no longer under our roof, we can feel left out, on the side-lines, cast adrift in the outer stratosphere of their orbits. There seems to be no cure for this.

Quite often, we have had them under our roof, for several days or occasionally several months. I get pleasantly accustomed to it, especially when they become part of the household and share in the daily feeding routines. But if they don't, the burden of work is such that I count the days till they depart.

I choose to remember the ones I wish would stay. The ones who make me cry when they leave, but hopefully not in front of them. In other words, my own. My three beloveds. When the house is full of the new generation, my grandchildren or Prof R's, their intelligence and energy excites and exhausts me equally. There would be tears before bedtime if visits were too prolonged, and they might be mine.

June 4 — Prof R is 'off air' this morning. It's not always easy to know when this is happening. I only discover it when I begin to try to tell him something about the dog or the Funfair setting up in the park. And when I look for a response, he is busy gazing intently at the little pile of supplements in the pot by his breakfast bowl, deciding which one to pick up next. Sometimes I feel unreasonably upset about this. It feels more lonely and isolating to be living with him than usual.

So, to cope, I have left the room to get the dirty washing basket. Doing household chores might be boring but they are also reassuringly normal. And better than getting cross or sad.

June 5 — After avoiding the issue for four years I have finally been persuaded by an accusing display in my library to take out a book on dementia. Prof R's is unusual, or so it has appeared, so I never expect to get information that is relevant to his situation.

This book, with the fetching title *When Someone You Love Has DEMENTIA*, claims it covers the lot – Alzheimer's, Lewy Body (possibly

Prof R) and vascular dementia (also possible). So I have hidden it in my office for sneaky reading when Prof R is resting.

Yesterday he missed his dinner altogether. He was too tired to tackle the rattling cutlery and shaky spoon. I would gladly help him eat but he, for once, had no real appetite for it. Sometimes when that happens, I will say "just go over and sit on the couch for a while and see how you feel in a few minutes", and he can recover. But last night he went off to bed at 6.45 pm. I went up to him twice to find him feeling okay and not hungry. Just sleepy.

—

It is now after 10 am and he has not come down for breakfast yet. I would trade his ability to fast with him, but that's all. This is not an appealing way to lose weight. He can have his neglected dinner for lunch today, and I will be funnelling more cake into him to make up for the precious lost calories.

When I sleep, I dream that I need to be awake, and when I am awake, I dream of sleep. Last night I dreamed we were in New Zealand and had to catch a plane to the UK. The plane was due to leave at 7 am and we were still at the motel at 6 am. Checkout time for international flights is three hours before take-off. I woke to find I was keeping tabs on time because I wanted to give Prof R his morning meds. He had been awake-asleep and rising and reclining again for the previous hour or so. I lose track but try to sleep in the intervals. It seems to work, mostly.

The theory about weight and stress is interesting. Because if the stress hormone Cortisol remains switched on, it causes havoc with your digestive and other systems. Ghrelin, the appetite hormone, is switched on too. Hence the midnight munchies, always seen in American sitcoms but never experienced by me. My cravings are restricted to daylight usually. Although in winter, daylight hours are not long enough to cover all my 'munch time'. And I have all sorts of tricks to outwit them.

I have a store cupboard full of 'healthy' snacks. Dates, popcorn (which

I make myself), humous (fattening apparently but good), sugar free baked beans, fat free yoghurt, kefir quark, sparkling water (*full of sodium I later discover*), lean cold meats, eggs.

Now, writing this, I have made myself hungry again. It might be time to walk the dog. The myth about dog walking is that it forces you to exercise. Anyone with a dog will tell you that they stop and sniff at regular intervals, preventing you from getting a decent stride going long enough to get short of breath. Aerobic it is not.

Of course, a very well trained dog is not allowed to stop and sniff or run or pull, or talk to other dogs in a loud voice, or chase cats or children or birds. But that is a dog with the stuffing knocked out of it. I realise I probably should be the owner of a dog with the stuffing knocked out of it for reasons of safety.

We both thought we had bought a small dog, but she has turned out to be taller and more than 11 kg and very strong. And impulsive. And a dog that licks both me and the upholstery. She's adorable.

My library book tells me that Lewy Body dementia can mimic Parkinson's disease, but also that Parkinson's sufferers can have Lewy Body dementia. I see a chicken and egg situation here, but the neurologist said that, given Prof R responds to levodopa medication, he probably does have Parkinson's as well as probably Lewy Body.

Certainly, one piece of information in this book seems to match Prof R's experience. It says, "dramatic fluctuations in mental function". Prof R takes rivastigmine to delay his loss of cognition and it has seemed miraculous at times. When he is 'on board' I usually give credit to the medication. Another chicken and egg. The book goes on to say, "This can be a bewildering situation for relatives".

They can say that again, and again, and again. I can be mid-sentence with my 'on-board' Prof R and suddenly be confronted by 'man-overboard'. It must be the most infuriating part of this illness of his.

Although only to me. As the woman who wrote the book, *Susan Elliot-Wright*, says so eloquently, they "may have periods of being alert and coherent, alternating with periods of confusion and unresponsiveness". She doesn't say yet what to do about my own responses.

As if to illustrate Susan's point, Prof R has come down from our attic bedroom holding the medic alarm that hangs by his bed in his hand. I said, "Why have you brought that down?" and he said, "I want to know what it is." There are moments of despair that turn to laughter, they are so absurd, and this is one of them. The lesson is, if your beloved has random dementia buying an alarm button is probably wishful thinking.

The hybrid smart watch arrived, and I have almost programmed it. The only part I have had trouble with is the function I bought it for – the alarm. So I have written to the help desk and asked for more instructions. Meantime, the watch, which is about the size of a small dinner plate, has to be worn on the inside of my wrist as it is so heavy it slithers in that direction if I try to wear it on the outside.

However, being so large it is easier to read in the dark, when I can so easily make a mistake with the time. A few nights ago, I put his midnight pill by his bed at what I thought was 12.20 am, but by the light of the toilet I discovered was only 11.20 pm. So I took it away again. And then worried I would not wake when it was in fact 12.20 am or thereabouts. I may have to relent on not having the mobile phone by the bed, and let it wake me up directly rather than via the watch.

By the time I have become good at this stuff things will have moved on and I will then be no good at a whole lot of new stuff.

Yesterday he said "I'm sorry you are being pulled into living your life in a way you don't want". In these rare moments when he expresses concern about me I feel so touched, I say something like, "Thank you darling but really, apart from going on holiday, what else would I be missing?" If I have to lie a little to be kind, I will lie.

Another delicate delve, dear reader, into the subject of sex. Sex has not been in our vocabulary or our bed for over a year now. It's not that we don't still both desire it, but that Prof R does not remember that his physical functioning is now impaired and that he hurts me if we try. If it is ever discussed, he assumes that the solution to the mystery must reside with me. Perhaps I have 'gone off' sex. Where his self-esteem resides is clear, and because I love him, I am always sensitive to that in my responses.

—

For the last three days I have been sneaking in an extra half-dose of levodopa in mid-afternoon. Not keeping this information from Prof R, but agreeing that the neurologist does not need to know. We will try it for a week or so and see if it helps the tremor and the fatigue. It is always hard to tell because Mr Parky changes Prof R's routines and headspace so frequently, it would be an unscientific experiment unless longer than just a few days. And I haven't the time or energy to muster a control group.

I watched Prof R eat a piece of carrot cake this afternoon using a spoon. This is part of my fat-building offensive. Tomorrow will be the first weigh-in. He refuses to use his fingers to eat cake, as I unashamedly will. Given I am not eating cake at all at the moment, it is doubly frustrating watching him trying to get each portion to his mouth, as it teeters dangerously *en route*. Then he unthinkingly proved the exception to his own rule, when he picked up a portion in his fingers. But the next mouthful travelled by spoon. My motto is to let him do things his own way unless it is going to harm him. The fact that watching him harms me is not relevant.

So far today I have reached 5,813 steps on my Fitbit. To achieve even that I have gone out either for business or pleasure three times. The dog has been walked and that is both business and pleasure, depending on how she behaves. Today she was on the brink.

—

It's time Prof R had another shower. We are very secretive about how seldom he has them, as most people would be horrified. I'm not anymore, since Matthew Parris has given me permission not to. Matthew Parris is a political writer and broadcaster with strong views and a habit of seeing which way the tide is heading in order to swim in the opposite direction. I have always been a fan of his.

Matthew says that we all bathe far too often, and it is totally unnecessary. He apparently stopped washing his hair 10 years ago when he was on location somewhere where no shampoo was available. Deep in the jungle I believe. This is not to say that Matthew does not like water. On the contrary, he likes wild swimming and was once told off for getting the tides wrong and putting himself in danger while swimming the Thames. I imagine he may well have taken a shower after he'd been rescued.

Prof R and I cannot claim to clean ourselves by wild swimming. If we don't shower or bathe, we are not immersing at all. I have caught on to this with great enthusiasm and use bathing wet wipes to remain clean where it matters. There's no need to spell that out. I may have to find another way to keep clean if wet wipes are banned for environmental reasons, and there is every chance they will be. Although I will happily bin them. Like the Greeks.

My deodorant is made of crystal, which is non-chemical. My hair and body get washed twice a week, although I love a bath and would bathe a lot more often if I could. It unwinds me in ways nothing else does. Not even a glass of red wine.

Prof R is more experimental than I am and is going for the full Robinson Crusoe programme, but without any access to salt water. He refuses the shower every time I suggest it. But I am keeping an eye on him – personal washing and putting out clean underwear every day. So far, there appear to be no obvious reasons to interfere, which astounds me. I am offering to 'check' his skin where it is hidden from view, but he declines politely.

The other reason I offer to check his skin is because it finally became obvious he wasn't washing his face. I interfered, washed it thoroughly, though just with water, and advised him he might see better if his eyelashes were not matted in dried mucous. Mr Parky is definitely taking a turn for the worse, even if Prof R isn't. It's possible to take any new fad too far.

June 7 — Fatty and Skinny are going downstairs. It is 10.30 am. Skinny is told to stop off in the main bathroom to be weighed. He overshoots and is headed down the next flight before being recalled. There is no increase beyond 65 kg. Fatty also weighs herself. No decrease. In fact, a 1 kg increase to 67 kg. Wednesday is apparently the best day to check your weight, as we are reportedly at our lightest. There is no scientific reason for that as far as I can see, but I was 66 kg on Thursday. Today, Skinny is winning by 2 kg. But Skinny still needs more cake.

By lunch, he had eaten his breakfast, plus a large scone, followed quickly by a lunch of last night's leftovers – two venison sausages and veggies with butternut mash. I had two eggs on a piece of toast. Then we both had a cup of tea out on the deck and he had another biscuit.

After all that, he fell over while heading for the back door to go and lie down. He fell on paving bricks, on his side. Miraculously nothing was broken. But I had to devise a military-style manoeuvre to get him to his feet. That involved going indoors for a long carpet runner, which I placed alongside him so he could roll onto it and up onto his hands and knees. I put a garden chair by his head and held it steady so he could grab the seat to pull himself up. His only wound is a graze on one elbow and perhaps, later, a black and blue hip. I, on the other hand, feel this has been another lucky escape, and wonder how many more falls he will have before our luck runs out.

June 9 — Another fall in the bathroom at 6 am. This time I cry with frustration. It takes so long for him to get up and if I try to lift him it hurts him. Not that I can lift him, but I try to act as leverage he can push against. So, the usual routine, asking him to focus on getting onto his front first, then onto his knees.

In a small space this requires slow and careful thought. After more than half an hour we finally achieve it, and he is able to grab the basin and get to his feet. We discuss the possibility of his waking me every time he goes to the toilet in the night, until we realise that unless I actually go into the bathroom with him, that won't prevent a fall. Only he can do that by making sure he has a handhold at all times. And he doesn't do that when he is tired, or his head is not yet on.

After the fall he took a pee and then stood in the bathroom without a handhold and added another used tissue to the bulk that is already in his pyjama pocket.

The three radios I ordered on Amazon have arrived. This is not what it seems. We actually do need three new radios. We have been going 'without' except in the kitchen and bathroom. Now we have two little Roberts — one for my office and one for Prof R's bedside table — and an August, whoever they are, for the living room. These are our first digital radios that actually work. We bought one several years ago before we realised that where we were living, in the countryside, there was no digital signal. We remained without a signal until we moved here, to Kent, over a year ago. The radios cheered me up enormously, once I worked out how to programme them.

It's sad to see Prof R unable to use these electronic wonders now. But fortunately he doesn't care about that. When I showed him the new radio for his bedside I said, "Of course, you may not want to use the radio, but the clock should be nice and clear to see in the dark." He said, "The old one is just a clock." It isn't, it's a clock radio and it is the size of a tank, probably a collector's item by now. At one time, he would have been showing me how to programme the new one.

Prof R knew how to use everything to do with the computer, or appeared to. He had been an 'early adopter'. As time passed, he remained apparently able to do all these things, while quietly losing the thread. His bank account, I eventually discovered, was operated in overdraft. So he tallied his balance to include it. Fortunately, he paid off his credit card every month. But he continued to believe he had a great deal more available funds than he actually did.

What he *did* have was a portfolio of investments, under the watchful gaze of his 'personal banking adviser'. None of these Blue Chips increased in value over the 20-odd years he had them. But several decreased. And when he finally sold the majority of the shares, at a loss, the very attentive personal banking adviser, who would visit him at home, suddenly lost interest; or so we liked to joke.

Another little surprise for me came about when I took over doing Prof R's tax returns. He had always done them online, but paid for a TaxCalc programme rather than using HMRC's free one. I understood why, when the free one defeated me. But when I was checking his work pension, I discovered that he had neglected to name the person who would receive a portion of it in the event of his death. Did this mean his second wife had not been named either? Nor his first presumably, although under the terms of the pension he could name anyone. It didn't have to be a spouse.

When I told Prof R about the oversight he was amazed and rather shocked. When exactly had Mr Parky first shown his colours? Although it's probably not fair to blame Mr Parky for everything. More accurate perhaps to blame Mr Lewy Body or his dementia doppelganger. Now there's a name that trips nicely off the tongue.

With Mr Lewy Body on board, last year we needed a Power of Attorney and a financial adviser to help me offload the remaining investments. For this purpose, having them all online was worse than not, with proof of identity a nightmare of lost passwords and misfiled tiny dividends that it is apparently a crime to mislay.

It took six months to unravel it and during that time, I almost unravelled myself. We also had to pay the adviser, but it can be a small price to pay. I have always been a great believer in the value of a 'third party' to keep the hounds from baying too loudly at the door.

<hr>

June 11 — A bad day for Prof R. He said to me "I feel as though I am dying". But later, when his medications had kicked in, he felt a little better. But still not well enough to go for a walk.

This man wrote love emails to me in volumes that would have defied the post. Twice a day, every day, while we were apart and hardly knew each other. And I wrote back. Twice a day. We also spoke by phone twice a day. Prof R printed out our emails and put them in a file. He felt they might be worth keeping.

I came across them, several years ago, while we were still living on the Welsh border, and began to read. It was a shock to see how self-absorbed and 'Mills and Boon' we were. This was not literature, or even very interesting. It would be toe-curling if any of our children had ever set eyes on them. So, with his permission, I burnt them in the garden incinerator.

While I was feeding each sheet into the flames, Prof R suddenly said, "I hope you are not burning anything valuable." I assured him I wasn't. But later he said he thought I had burnt a very important document – a letter his second wife Jan had written, to be given to their son. I was horrified he would think I had done such a thing, but he was adamant it might have been in the file of our emails. This seemed, if not insane, at the very least odd. I was very shaken by his accusation, because accusation it was. And later, when he eventually found it, in a hard-backed manila envelope that could not possibly have been unseen or misidentified, we were both very relieved.

Much later, when we moved house, again I could not find it where he told me he would put it, in his file drawer in his desk. I still have not found it. One day I hope to.

(That day came in January 2020. And the place turned out to be a side pocket of one of his old laptops, which I was preparing for disposal.)

I wonder if any love letters are worth preserving, in hindsight. They are a means to an end, building bonds between souls who hope to become kindred but are principally obsessed with unrequited sex.

There are other letters I have read that bear this out. Letters Prof R was happy for me to read and had totally forgotten existed. We were sorting the files in the shed in Wales when I found them, and he had no memory of them or why he had kept them. Letters from his lover. the lover who gave him an excuse to leave his first wife. She wrote just as excruciatingly as we had, about her longing for him (and with some sexual detail which, being only human, I did find interesting). Her letters, like ours, did not reflect well on her state of mind, but I recognised the complete selfishness that accompanies obsession. I suggested they might not be nice for his daughters to read, and he agreed. We burnt them.

June 13 — The weather is warm, calm and sunny. After breakfast at 11 am and a sleep and lunch at 3 pm plus carrot cake and another sleep until 6 pm, Prof R was suddenly able to go for a walk after dinner. An impressive distance at a respectable speed without holding onto me;

right around the perimeter of the park, which some claim is almost a mile. I doubt it, but I was impressed and very relieved to finally get him outside again.

When I said to him that perhaps it was the extra half-strength levodopa he is taking mid-afternoon; that it had given him 'legs'; and perhaps when his medicine wears off, he can "fall off the cliff", he said "I hope not", and I had to explain it was figurative not literal. Then we talked about what early signs of his illness there may have been in the past, until we were both exhausted. Pointless but somehow necessary.

June 15 — I awoke at almost 7 am to see Prof R sitting on the side of the bed, having taken his top off, as is his wont, and for the first time saw the full extent of the bruising on his back and side from the two falls he has had. I wondered if I should photograph them and decided against it. They are best forgotten.

—

Why do I feel guilty if I return home to find Prof R sitting in the living room, expectantly? Not occupied, just sitting. It is always a gamble to hope to be back from a routine trip to the shops before sleeping beauty descends.

Today, I had gone out a bit later – around 3 pm – after working on some proof reading of the family 'tome'. I expected to be back within half an hour. But I tarried a while in the market, because it's pleasurable, and then, when I returned, I had an encounter on my doorstep with the previous owner of our house, which took another 10 minutes. And I was lucky to escape with that. So of course, when I finally came in, there he was. Expectant. So I felt guilty.

There is also an issue for me of feeling less than lively physically. I cannot understand why this is. A short walk around the town and I am glad to sit down. My legs ache. Everything aches. It is as though I am out of kilter and my muscles are being used in new ways. Perhaps I *am* out of kilter and walking badly. Is this what they call 'bone tired'? If so, it is a good description.

Correspondence with friends and acquaintances by email are my main contact with the outside world and it is what suits me best. There is no timetable to follow, no obligation to rush. I'm reading a book about letters – real letters – but to me the email is under-valued. It can be just as deep and philosophical and intimate as anything handwritten on paper. My latest correspondence of note has been with my cousin, whose husband has just died. That sort of writing has to be thought through with great care; a sensitive blend of sympathy and lightness. And her replies show she also needs the lightness.

June 16 — Our house gives us an urban view akin to Hitchcock's *Rear Window*, except it is our front window. It is not our intention to be nosey or intrusive. But when we are at our table eating our three meals a day, that is where our eyes are directed. Whether we like it or not, we are witness to snapshots of the lives of the family who live opposite – or what we imagine to be their lives. It's an idle pastime, making up stories about their day. They are waiting for guests, or taking rubbish to recycling. Or the baby is going to nursery and they are going to work. The husband likes to cycle seriously. We know that.

Of course, if we had a life ourselves, we would be too busy to look at theirs. But I like to think it is a game of give and take. That they can see me up in my office, drying my hair or sitting at my computer, or catch me taking the dog out for a walk, or heading off for the shops. I don't mind if they do notice because I have nothing to hide.

Today began well. Prof R was early to breakfast and ready for a walk before lunch. It was downhill from there. When he feels as bad as he does this afternoon, he says, "I think I feel worse than I've ever felt", and

I gently remind him that when he is feeling really ill, he forgets he has probably felt as bad before. And it will soon pass.

Again he said, "I feel like I am dying". That is the second time he has said that this week. I never know what to say in reply to that. Other than soothing platitudes. I could have said that the same goes for me, even if I am dying more slowly than he is. Although some days I wonder if I am going to beat him to it.

June 17 — A red letter day. A perfect summer day. This afternoon Prof R felt like going to Whitstable, by the sea, famous for its oysters; although we weren't going there for them. It's only a 20 minute drive from home but we haven't been for about eight months. I wasn't sure I wanted to go at all. Months of conditioning was having an effect.

But we went. And we over-did it. Prof R got tired beyond the point of exhaustion, but we both declared it was worth it. And we watched the lifeboat go to sea. I sat Prof R on top of an upturned dingy right by the slipway so he could enjoy it.

The launch of a lifeboat can be, for me, better than all the Christmases and birthdays put together. Although it is better if they go down a ramp, fast, rather than get pushed to sea by a tractor. However, I was not in a mood to be critical. It was magic. Even when Prof R needed me to hold his lemonade so he could drink from it through a straw.

We agree we will do it again.

The other two reasons it is a red-letter day are 1) My eldest son Alex had his citizenship ceremony and now has a British passport; and 2) my daughter Hope and her partner have decided to get married. I am both over the moon and on notice. That is my signal to begin to think about respite care.

June 18 — The drought has broken. I wanted to run down to my computer to write about it even while it was still happening. Prof R has had a shower. The first in several weeks. It happened by accident. He came down from a short nap rather earlier than expected and after I got over feeling mildly cross, because I was drying my hair, I said "if you are feeling awake why don't you have a shower"? and he said, "Okay". Good idea."

I carried on drying my hair for another 10 minutes, listening for the water. So I could supervise. Nothing. But when I went up, there he was, only just divesting himself of his last piece of clothing, his singlet, in preparation. I could see where his bruises were healing, now a less livid shade of yellow. I didn't mention them. Then it was necessary for us to remind ourselves how his shower operated, and in he got. I stayed nearby, on call, to help if necessary, but he managed to wash himself, including his hair.

Prof R, when he is on task, is meticulous and methodical, and that hasn't changed. Anyone living with him knows this and must be patient. It is one of the reasons he was seldom asked to vacuum the living room. He has taught me to enjoy the delay; to see waiting as time out to be with my own thoughts.

And when he was ready to get out, I helped him to dry himself, although he did most of his front. And his meticulous methodology meant he took his time and did it properly. He always begins with his flannel. Removing the excess water while standing in the shower box. I have always found this fascinating. Considering he was never in the armed services.

This is the first time it has been necessary for me to help him and it is a return to old skills – drying the children. Of course, it is a sign of the slipperiness of the slope, but it is also a sign of love. I felt satisfaction in the task.

Now he is resting, as it is exhausting to do all that undressing and washing and drying and dressing, again, even when we are well.

—

We now have a drought of the usual kind with baking hot, humid days and no rain, even at night, although the black clouds gather and form and then change their minds and go. I have watered the pots. Everything we have is in pots – trees, shrubs, climbers and not many of any of them. Next week the men come to rip everything out and start again with the decking and railing and our little picket gate onto the grass. It will be wonderful.

June 20 — Prof R's sense of humour can pop out like an unexpected ray of sunshine. This morning, when he can be at his most unresponsive and not quite with it, I was giving him his pills when he brought the water cup up towards his mouth and landed it on his nose. I said, "no, no, your nose is not your mouth" and he said, "speak for yourself".

My eyes are red and sore from the effort of not crying. I am proofing the copy of my book about the family and have just read the part about my mother's death. Prof R came down at the point when my eyes had filled, so I was at great pains to suppress the threat of tears.

Because we are so isolated physically from our friends and even our families, I rely a great deal on communication by email and text. If a day passes when I've not had a 'chat' with someone there is a danger of feeling deprived and even lonely. Prof R is both unperturbed and undisturbed by any of this. He was always isolated and prefers it that way. As long as he has a loving companion, he is happy enough.

June 21 (the summer solstice) — I am thinking about respite care. And how difficult it is to even think about, let alone organise. I cannot imagine anyone caring for Prof R overnight in the watchful way I can. Unless they spend the night in a chair in the room, in which case he would perhaps be horrified and unable to sleep himself.

So I am hoping my darling daughter decides on a midday wedding in

London so I can jump into my train carriage for home before it gets dark and the carriage turns into a pumpkin. In fact, I am secretly hoping she will get married on the longest day of the year, which would have to be next year, so I can go home in the evening, in daylight. I have managed to organise a huge worry for myself a year in advance. That must be a record of some kind.

In reality, I have a neighbour who works in the care sector who should be able to point me at a reliable care provider. Then I can begin to introduce Prof R to the idea over time. Because there will be time enough. And we can select a carer whom we can book well in advance and get to know. This will all work beautifully if Hope and Simon get married in London. If they choose anywhere else, I am cooked.

There have been no more falls this week. Prof R is being very careful and so am I. But it is only a matter of time before Mr Parky trips him up again. And each time, I discover a new method for retrieving him from the floor. His alarm button is still sitting on my desk, where I put it when he brought it to me to ask what it was. I'm trying to decide if it's worthwhile returning it to the railing by his bed.

June 23 — Yesterday I felt desperate. I've no idea why. I felt behind bars and busting to get out. It was such a bad day for Prof R. One of those days when you cannot see the point of this disease. If it wants to kill him, why doesn't it just get on with it? Why torture him? And me? Why the tease of a good day?

I tried to improve the tension in the violin strings in my body by running up and down the stairs four times. It is supposed to be as good as going to the gym. Certainly, it wastes less time. I believe it helped. But what helped more was Prof R suddenly springing to life in the evening and saying he would like a walk.

These summer evenings are a blessing. We will have forgotten how they feel when winter comes around again. The soft soothing balm of the air on our skin and the smells – is it Jasmine, or Daphne? Or the carefully tended rose bed in the park?

Today is a good day. Yesterday is forgotten. Tomorrow the men come to replace our rotten decking and install a new rail around it. I am as excited as if I had been sent tickets to fly to Sardinia or Santorini, or Crete or Sicily. Or a hundred other Mediterranean islands I haven't been to and would love to visit. Getting new decking is big in a world that narrows by the day.

—

Surprise! Just when I thought Mr Parky was sleeping, he came down to my office all confused mid-afternoon thinking it might be the middle of the night. The reason for his confusion was the fact that he had taken two doses of levodopa, it appears almost together, plus for good measure, his evening dose of Rivastigmine. Thinking it was night-time you understand. He is now banned from managing his own medication pot.

Later, contrary to expectations, he has recovered in ways that make me think he should overdose more often. I took him outside in the garden and began feeding him in an effort to soak up the drugs. Ice cream followed by an apple and some cheese. Then a cup of tea and two biscuits. He would normally be tired again by 5 pm but he isn't, and I want to wash my hair, so I have taken the risky step of letting him remain on his own in the garden enjoying the heat, which is considerable, from within a shady corner. When I returned, clean and dried, he was fortunately still there.

Where it can come unstuck is if I don't feel well. Then my patience thins to a wafer and I have to be very careful. Today is such a day. Just headachy and generally not feeling positive, no matter how hard I try. Hay fever makes me feel this way.

It's actually a good week because the nice new timber for the decking is the colour of light honey and smells of the forest, even though it is laden with preservative.

Today the builder is bringing his 13-year-old daughter. It is "go to work with your dad" day. Or presumably also "go to work with your mum". I don't think dad really knows how he is going to keep his daughter busy and I just hope she is not bored.

I suspect my headache and malaise is because I am bored. And boredom can be either creative or a colossal waste of time, depending on your circumstances. Currently, I cannot escape into my own brain very often.

June 25 — The thought of my daughter's wedding finally propelled me next door to talk to my neighbour. I asked if she could recommend someone, as I need to begin to introduce Prof R to a companion he will be happy to be with when I am away. She said yes, she knew the perfect person.

Today V rang. I am also a V. The same V. At least he won't have to learn a new name. She sounded lovely and will come and meet us over coffee. She asked if I would like to meet at a café at 2 pm, and was nonplussed when I said that could be difficult as Prof R's schedule was rather unreliable. He had just arrived down for lunch and it was almost 2 pm. She tells me she has never cared for anyone with Parkinson's before, so I'm not sure about her skills with falls or dementia. If she cares for older people it should not be a problem, but I will need to ask all those questions. It's possible she just takes people to the shops. She won't need to worry about that with Prof R.

The builder is finishing off the new decking. Tomorrow the dog can be released from her prison on the first floor. At least one of us gets out of prison occasionally.

June 26 — I have noticed a marked deterioration in my attitude. Perhaps I would be happier if the weather was not so glorious. When it is like this, bright blue, people bustling everywhere, children laughing and playing, barbeque smells wafting over our fence – maybe that is when I feel my solitude the most. Because now solitude is the right word, whereas before, up until just a few weeks ago, I had still been able to feel the companionship of Prof R.

June 30 — Saturday. The hoped for carer, V, is coming for coffee on Thursday. I had so many questions when she rang, but she said, "We can talk about that on Thursday". But I wanted to know things that might determine whether she even needed to come on Thursday. For instance, she did say that she does not do weekends at all. I can see this is going to be a problem because the only special occasions with the family will more than likely be on a weekend.

Yesterday I noticed sap running down the back wall of the fairly-newly painted house. I contacted the contractor and asked if she knew why this might be happening. She said, "When the wall was first painted, they can't have sealed the knotholes properly", and I'm thinking the obvious "Why did the knotholes wait for 14 years and a new paint job to weep"? But I didn't say that because it was obvious she would take no responsibility for the problem. But when I said I would need to get someone in to fix it she replied, "Can we help with that"?

A beautiful hot day today. Someone may be getting married, because the church bells are ringing in that uplifting way that cannot signal a funeral. Prof R arrived down for breakfast at 10.30 am and went back to bed at 11.30 am.

After repairing the white paintwork on the windowsill where the builder man passed each length of the decking through from the front of our house to the back, I went down to the market. An Italian man, incredibly beautiful, just like the day, was singing opera, presumably to pay for his supper. A student perhaps. The market is bustling and it lifts my spirits. How lucky we are to live so close to everything.

Next weekend Hope and Simon are coming down, so I can take them out for a celebration lunch. Prof R says he doesn't mind staying here. I will feed him first and we won't go until after he is settled and medicated. It is still relatively safe during the day for him to be left for up to two hours. (The judgment of that is made almost minute by minute, by 'reading the runes'. There is no opportunity to be scientific about this.)

But last night was one of his 'early hours wandering' nights. Just to the bathroom and back, and fortunately I was not sleeping and had that pleasant sort of wakefulness that is just relaxing, not stressful. On his last meander he didn't come back after half an hour, so in the end I had to go and get him. He was standing in front of the handbasin and had taken off his pyjama top. He doesn't remember doing that today.

All this reinforces my feeling that anyone who cares for him overnight needs to do so from a chair in the room. That is costly and not nice for him, but it may not be necessary ever, hopefully. I don't want to think about the future wedding.

I'm hoping to get Prof R out for a walk today. He hasn't felt like it for several days. He seems to be getting thinner, so I have bought a lot of cake and biscuits from the delicatessen.

Wimbledon begins next week. I have been known to down tools and ignore all requests for help during Wimbledon fortnight in the past. Now I seem to have lost that passion, although it can be aroused if I watch a really good match. Somehow all these things are now too slow for my attention span, which is always thinking about the next thing I could be doing. I have decided it is healthy to choose to believe that none of it matters – the paintwork, the weeks of electrical work, the next thing to break, the continual gathering of the dust in every corner.

July 1 — Sunday Last night Prof R was in his element talking about his father and the Anderson Shelter in their garden. So many things

Prof R doesn't remember. He no longer pines for New Zealand or even his children. But we are both fascinated by history, and bemoan the likelihood that the lessons it can teach us are forgotten by succeeding generations.

We had been talking about it – the loss of a legacy of wisdom that death brings – and that conversation led to our parents; and suddenly his face lit up. There followed a detailed description of how his father constructed the Anderson Shelter. The escape route through the back, held shut by screws, the deep earth cover over the curved iron roof, planted in flowers. How it was furnished. Every detail. This is what is lost when memory goes, and nothing is written down. Of course, he is telling me, and I am writing it down, but that is a poor record.

———————

A saviour of sorts arrived in Britain just before the Second World War. The Mass Observation programme was set up to track information and attitudes of populations facing war. It's still going. Nella Last, a housewife living in Barrow-in Furness, was persuaded to take part. Her wartime daily record came alive to me when Victoria Wood dramatized her life on TV in 'Housewife 49'. The title was how Nella described herself for the Mass Observation team. It is an unintentional consequence that the outcome was a memoir for the masses, and it's a wonderful thing.

———————

We got the giggles before bed when his hand shook too much for him to hold a glass to his lips to take his bedtime pills. I always say, "use the other hand!" and occasionally he does. But last night he said, "Where are those straws?" and I said, "You don't need a bloody straw, you can do this", and eventually he did. It also made me giggle when I heard him in the downstairs loo trying to do up his belt. Jingle, jingle, jingle means he is playing the castanets again. And I go to help.

But I don't laugh when I help him to take his pills in the morning, when he is not himself or anyone else either. Just zombie-like and needing total care to take them and lie down again, after an age in the bathroom staring at nothing. Then I feel afraid that I will not be able to leave him with anyone else, no matter how good they are. Because they must expect the unexpected, or even that nothing unexpected may happen at all.

July 2 — Lately, just occasionally, Prof R has begun to get attacks of the 'frights'. As an expert in these things, I am well placed to soothe and reassure that it will pass; to tell him to relax and slow his breathing. Last night he got them at 2 am. I noticed he was awake and asked what the problem was and he said, "I am dying". When he is in this mode his tremor is violent. I try to hold his hands and sometimes suggest he puts them underneath his body. Eventually it passes and he can sleep, but not usually before another sequence of trips to the loo. I don't allow myself to doze when he is like this. I'm fearful of a fall.

What is particularly disconcerting in the night is his unresponsiveness to my questions, unless I press him. He must try to tell me what he needs and how he feels, otherwise I am in danger of helping him back into bed when actually he needs a pee. In which case he will attempt to get up again almost immediately.

This morning, at 8.20 am, I went to check if he was sleeping before having my breakfast and taking the dog for a walk. He was half dressed. And was down before 9 am to eat his breakfast. I cannot remember the last time we were at the breakfast table almost together, even if in tandem. He was quite happy for me to take the dog for a walk while he ate, with a promise of coffee on my return.

It wasn't until 11 am that he needed to go up to rest again. We had sat outside on our newly milled decking with our backs to the sun and my hat on his head. Although he had no idea it was mine, as it is equally suitable for a man. I pottered with the rubbish bins and watered the shaded plants while he sat, and we talked when I sat too. Although mostly I talked.

As soon as he went to lie down again, I was off like a whippet. That seems to be my favourite description for any higher level of motivation that drives me into action. This time I wanted different food to go with this different weather, which turned out to be fresh corn on the cob, fennel and wild boar sausages. I had a sore hip, which miraculously recovered after a pleasant conversation with a man who needed directions to the Physic Garden. Perhaps the garden works its magic within a radius yet to be determined. I was very gratified and decided my pains are mostly determined by my head. That doesn't stop them being unpleasant.

———————————

We have a very flimsy gate full of gaps between us and our neighbours. This might not matter, but they have a lovely but challenged 18-year-old son who has both Downs and Autism and who keeps trying to open our gate or peer through. And he calls out to Prof R. Again, this might not be a problem if he did not have the potential to become very violent when he is stressed.

Once, when we were returning to our front door, he and his father emerged from their door in a rush and his dad said to us "stand back, he's being violent". Whereupon, on seeing Prof R, the boy became immediately placid and happy because he loves Prof R, even though he hardly knows him. I have a theory about white hair and beards. They are very comforting. Shades of Father Christmas perhaps.

We have the 'backside' of the gate so presumably any repair is down to them, but I am happy to decorate it with a series of tin signs placed strategically. This is quite challenging but a lot of fun. So far, I have four signs in place, a round one for Castrol, an everlasting calendar, an advertisement for chicken feed and a lovely vintage ad for the Messerschmidt car, Prof R's favourite. He took some time to make the effort to look at it, but was gratifyingly pleased when he did so. I need some long thin signs now to finish the job.

———o———

July 3 — We've just been to the GP. The appointment was made for us by the practice because the neurologist has handed (offloaded) Prof R over to them for his ongoing care.

—

We go in and Dr T says, "So how can I help you today?" So I said, "You asked Prof R to come in" at which point he decides to read the notes. I say, "The tremor is the major problem" and ask about recent studies with Botox, to which he says "It's not in the public domain", whatever that means, and offers support groups and clinics that put railings in your loo etc.

Then he asks, "Is memory an issue?" And I say, "He's on the maximum dose of Rivastigmine so, yes". I have managed all this with smiles. The strain is killing me. But I just chose to enjoy teasing him. He means well. He is made happy by my jokes and less of a failure presumably, although he has no reason to feel pleased with the consultation.

July 4 — I have had the meeting today, not tomorrow as planned, with the woman, also called V, who is a trained carer/personal assistant. She magically makes two hours disappear for me in delightful conversation. Whether it was delightful for her I don't know, but I was impressed.

Instead of coming down at some point from his loft to meet her, Prof R hid. I totally understand why. He is lying prone on the bed quietly distressed when I go upstairs to tell him all is clear. He needs to understand that we cannot operate without a back-up person and the sooner we get to know and like V the better it will be. I didn't tell him that at one point in the conversation, something that was said made me cry.

—

Prof R's youngest daughter Julie will finally come down on Thursday for lunch. She last came in February. She said, "Do let me know if I can bring anything?". Don't you hate that? What you want to hear is "I'll bring something for lunch. Is quiche/salad/antipasti ok?". So I just said, "Don't bring flowers!" I should have added "or chocolates".

But I'm looking forward to seeing her nevertheless.

My sister rang me for a rare chat from Dunedin. Only when her phone went dead did she admit she had not used WhatsApp. Neither of us can afford not to use WhatsApp. But we talked for an hour and I know she is worried about me and I am worried about her. She is at the loose end of life and wondering what she is meant to do next. I at least have a purpose, even if I am fenced in by it. V may release me for yoga once a week for £13 an hour. She is worthy of that and probably more.

July 5 — Julie brought chocolates. She asks me what I like to do for myself. And it is a kind question, but one which also upsets me. There is no suggestion from her that she or her sisters could come down to visit one day and sit with Prof R, instead of just eating lunch.

During lunch, her father runs out of steam and needs to withdraw to lie down. Realizing, suddenly, the difficulties of planned activities, she suggests that I could form a book group and host it from home. The temptation to say," That's a novel way of getting a break", is resisted. Then she says, perhaps I would like to share my experiences on an online chat room? I change the subject.

After lunch she left with promises to return with the children very soon. Prof R came down to say goodbye and has now gone back to bed. It's hard to see why they would want to visit at all. Only I seem to see the real Prof R still lurking within. We are an exclusive club and likely to remain so.

July 8 — The heatwave continues, and a shower becomes more urgent. Because Prof R is feeling tired, I suggested he have his breakfast in his pyjamas and shower afterwards. Showering with my supervision is still relatively new, and he manages most of it himself. I simply stand by and hand him the soap or adjust the water temperature.

Watching him naked becomes more shocking. The concave abdomen and loose skin on his stooped frame makes me think of him as he was before. And even before that, when I first met him, and he was overweight. Now he is truly frail, but still has pride in a thorough hair wash and a flannel dry afterwards before he will take the towel from me. But first he has to be persuaded to shower at all.

I am bonded to him by this conspiracy of the new reality of our intimacy in very different ways. It's a love that contains much more now; tenderness, protectiveness, fear, loss. Sometimes still a little 'tough love' when I feel he could push himself a bit more and me less. I have to be careful, because he might almost be afraid of upsetting me, now that he is so vulnerable. It's unbearable to think of that.

There is still the intellectual intimacy that continues to grow over time. He truly is my best friend, when he is himself. Only we can know how it is for us. It feels more lonely when he is not himself.

At one time I could have separated my love for him clearly from my other great loves, my children; but now the lines are blurred, and I'm conflicted by the desire to see them and the desire to protect him. The care situation is not going to be straightforward.

The prospective carer V, when asked, said she would not attempt to lift him if he fell. (I agree). She would wait for him to recover and then help him get up. Or she would call an ambulance. That part seems less useful than what we are able to achieve ourselves, with strategic thinking. Ambulances are a last resort.

In between all this, I watch the players at Wimbledon and the PM Theresa May in their separate battles for a win. There is plenty to occupy the 'little grey cells'.

July 9 — Last night he raised a fist to me again because I entered the shower room unannounced. This happened because I saw him through a gap in the door, frozen at the hand basin. I wanted to help him return to bed but I gave him a fright. I must signal my approach in future. He was horrified when I cried out "Oh" in my own fright, and was abject in his apologies. I know he hasn't the strength to hurt me physically. But I still felt a little afraid and hurt, even though I know it is simply a reflex action.

There is an email from his son, and I am so relieved he has begun to be in touch. There are things he would like to have said to his father – issues he once needed to raise – but now it is too late.

Another surprise late afternoon to find all his medications have disappeared from the pill pot. He can't remember taking them. We laugh and don't try to resolve the issue. He can't remember, he is still standing, and in no danger apparently of hallucinating or frothing at the mouth. He eats a hearty meal and now has ice cream twice a day after meals.

July 10 — I have found the brochure for the stairlift company that I sent for last autumn. Now seems a good time to retrieve it. Prof R agrees. Things are becoming rather less reliable in the 'wobbly leg' department. The increasing effort to pull himself up the stairs using the rail. And I am not far behind him in finding the climb exhausting when I am tired.

9.15 am and I can hear Prof R coming downstairs. But all is not well. He is confused about the time of day and whether I am real, although a good long hug and reassurance helps him with that. He is back up in his bed now and I will check him in half an hour. I tell him it is just the levodopa. It has messed with his head and it will pass.

It is 12.30 pm before he reappears, although I have been up several times to check him and give him his mid-morning levodopa. So today he has breakfast followed in quick succession by lunch, and I forgot to offer him ice cream as he has gone back to bed.

In his little supplement pot each morning Prof R now has a full strength St John's Wort, a multi-vitamin, D3, Omega 3, two slippery elm tablets (for his bowel), one magnesium, and one high strength probiotic. *(Research has since identified one particular probiotic called Bacillus subtilis has protective effects against the toxic proteins that build up in the gut of Parkinson's patients.)*

I have all the same pills except for the St John's Wort, plus thyroxine and an antihistamine. We have no idea if any of it is doing us any good. I also put nutritional yeast on our breakfast cereal. A friend says it gives her energy and I tend to agree.

I've done nothing about the stairlift as I want to wait until he is introduced to V the carer. When I reminded him of her visit, he couldn't remember anything about her. This is going to be a big challenge for each of us. As he grows more vulnerable, I grow less courageous about leaving him.

July 11 — Quite a lot has happened. David from the stairlift company, extremely unfit, came to survey our stairs. He needed to sit down at the top of each flight. He took two hours. I had forgotten to ask how long it would take when I made the booking.

He also kept me ages pondering the problem of how to fit the lift track – which fixes to the carpet – where it reaches the top of the first landing. The handrail is on the other wall. The wrong wall. No solution coming from him. After about half an hour I asked if it would be very expensive to move the handrail to the opposite wall and he said, "No. The cost would be the same."

He hadn't mentioned it, he said, as he felt that it would add an extra layer to the complexity of the issue. Except that he used different words. He said, "It seemed like a step too far," which I took to mean that either he hadn't thought of it as a solution until I asked, or he couldn't be arsed.

So next Tuesday, two different men will come at two different times to fit two different stair-lift rails. The upper loft stair will be curved and twice as expensive as the straight stair. Prof R and I conferred for all of 30 seconds before deciding we really didn't want to move from our loft bedroom down to the first floor.

It will cost us £7,645. I'm glad we had the decking replaced two weeks ago or it would have been postponed. I'm also glad we relinquished the small investments.

And this afternoon, Michelle the speech therapist rang. I had consigned her to my 'Do Not Resuscitate' file. It is five months since she gave Prof R his assessment. She was as lovely and bright and cheerful as I remembered and not at all apologetic. Prof R has an appointment for later this month.

July 13 — More surprises. Saturday was perfect. Almost too perfect because it was so hot. After wondering, without enthusiasm, if he could manage a walk to the park, Prof R was persuaded to try to make it a lot further, to the creek. It is full of boats and bunting for the nautical festival.

He felt wobbly, and we talked about looking for a walking frame if we made it as far as the market. There's always a stall for wheelchairs and walking frames. It's a niche market that has become a bottomless pit. There's big money in it.

Because it was nearly 4 pm before we set out, the market was packing up, so we kept going. We reached the closest part of the creek, a grassed landing where the Sea Scouts vintage hut stands. It was full of people and stalls under tents and a music stage. I looked for his response, but there wasn't one. The Thames barge was moored alongside many other smaller boats. It has a sail the colour of Devon soil on a wet day. I love it.

Worried I was pushing Prof R's boat out a bit far, I asked if he wanted to go back home or try for the bridge. He said, "I don't mind." So we tried for the bridge and made it. I took a Prof R selfie – a side profile of a man apparently loving the sight of all those boats – to prove he was there. On the way home I felt a surge of something that was almost grief but was also joy. I had missed these moments; being out with him.

The tiredness has punished us today. We had a disturbed night, and by 6 am, when I had put Prof R's feet back into the bed for what seemed like the tenth time, I began to smell a rat. His 4 am pill was still on his bedside table. Worse, reaching into the pocket of his trousers I discovered his pill pot rattling ominously with his bedtime pill of the night before. We will play catch-up today.

It's the Wimbledon Gentlemen's Final (whom they call 'men', never 'Gentlemen', during the tournament, although they insist on saying 'Ladies' throughout) and they will be playing in 30 degree heat. Good luck with that.

President Trump has stirred up a hornets' nest among the good people of Britain this week. And those of us who are a little bored and without the energy to protest have been mightily entertained. The Queen, pictured between Donald and Melania, was a sight to behold. They could have chatted across her head without seeing her. Even the mighty shrink in older age. And how she managed to negotiate the grass at Windsor to inspect the troops at 'The Donald's' pace in this heat fills me with admiration.

July 15 — When I stroke Prof R's back to comfort both of us, I am reminded of how good he was at massaging painful muscles. He may have learned it from his second wife, who was a physiotherapist. He called it 'tiring the pain' and it is a technique I use often on myself. Hurts like hell but it works.

We are still very attracted to each other beneath all the things that keep us apart. But the Parkinson's excess saliva 'drool' makes kissing difficult. I find if he is on his back it is safer for me. Though I don't share that with him. I never want him to feel physically unattractive to me.

—

I am reminded of a joke I shared with my first husband when we both announced our pending second marriages – me to an older man and he to a younger woman. He said, "I am robbing the cradle and you are robbing the grave". It still makes me laugh. Even though now it looks as though we are closer to the grave.

Now I must go and clean the stairs so that the installers of the stairlifts can wreck them.

July 17 — Sometimes it feels as though I've bitten off more than I can chew. Prof R had to be moved from our room in the loft to the guest room on the first floor before 9 am to beat the stairlift installers – but also before his head and body had synchronized. There was a perilous descent from the loft, me issuing instructions Prof R could not understand. Then, a perilous trip to the guest room ensuite toilet. His vision is affected, and he cannot determine distance and space easily.

At this time of the day, until his medication kicks in, looking for fresh handholds is difficult. On the first attempt he could not pee. Nor could he speak properly to tell me what he needed. There was a discussion about did he want to sit or stand? First he wanted to sit but didn't trust his handholds. So then he stood and eventually, with me issuing useless advice, stroking his back, he peed. Then it was a marathon back to the bed, which is higher than our other bed and difficult for him to judge. I told him I was sorry for my lack of skill. That I wanted to be his mentor, not his tormentor and he smiled.

This was an unwelcome window on the future, and I have shut it again firmly. It's obvious I will not be able to look after him alone at some point. We will deal with that when we get to the impasse.

This afternoon the lower stairlift is to be fitted and the man who is doing the loft stair, Bob, thinks it can't be done to the design David the surveyor claimed it could. This could make my day a little more interesting.

July 18 — The straight stair installer, Jon, was creative and not afraid to move the handrail, but he couldn't until I had assured his boss on the phone that I would not sue for any damages from our 'deviation'. We were lucky with Jon. He did what Bob (he of the morning shift) would not have done. And while the rail is now a little high for me it is perfect for Prof R. The chairs will sit idle while Prof R remains motivated to avoid them. The grandchildren are waiting impatiently in the wings for their turn.

When Prof R acted as test dummy for his upper stairlift, we could not stop him placing his hands on the armrest controls while I was using the remote. The result was a 'two steps forward, one back' to the top, until I eventually won. He's not terribly impressed with the lifts but agrees that the extra rails make good secondary handrails when climbing the stairs.

—

The weight is still dropping off his frame. Today I made a special trip to find fattening but good muffins or cake. I daren't bake or I would eat it. When I returned he greeted me downstairs when he should still have been up. I had been out for 30 minutes and had left as soon as he ascended the stairs.

I am swamped by him the minute I walk in the door; his plaintive, "Feel my hands, they're cold," rather than, "Hello darling". For some reason, moments like this can fill me with overwhelming emotions – frustration, anger, fear at my loss of liberty; at his loss of faculties. These emotions can turn into an urge to cry.

And when we go outside – because the weather is so warm – so that he too can warm up, he soon has to move into the shade because he is too hot. I feel both the heat and the cold, so I understand it, but sometimes his need for me is hard to take. If I had remained out longer – heaven forbid, perhaps had a coffee – I would have returned to find him sitting on a chair gazing into space. And his hands would be cold. And I would feel guilty, which in turn would make me feel frustrated, angry, afraid... etc, etc.

He also did not want to eat the chocolate muffin I bought him. It was too dry. Maybe later with ice cream. Maybe.

July 20 — A text from a stepdaughter at 5.30 pm yesterday asking if we have forgotten her youngest child's birthday. (But not worded so bluntly.) *"This is absolutely not meant to be a prompt, more concern that something has gone missing as you are normally the queen of efficiency!"* We would not always hear from her if he *did* receive a present.

I feel nothing – I'm flat-lining on emotions over this. But I did ask what we could send, did *not* apologise and before it is time for me to put dinner on the table, I have told Amazon to dispatch a bike bell disguised as a ladybird. I have not sent her a text to confirm this has been done. I hear the deafening sound of my royal crown hitting the floor. Nice Queen is Ice Queen.

The nice thing is, I can still share all these little events with Prof R, and he will enjoy the irony of the situation. Although if a story is too long, he may drop off to sleep.

The main event today will be the dentist for Prof R this afternoon. I am seriously looking forward to this. All good dentists will be remembered on my deathbed.

—

Every time I walk into the hall and see the stairlift I get a shock. They demand attention and I keep forgetting they are there; especially the one at the top of the stairs in our loft bedroom. It feels slightly inappropriate. Like a third person who is watching us in bed. It has a flashing light telling you that it's not asleep. I wonder if the KGB use stairlifts to spy on people?

July 24 — It's hot again. The dog is feeling lazy in the park as early as 9 am and so am I.

Cocking a snoot at the stairlifts, a 'window' opened for Prof R at 10 am and we shot through it, at his suggestion, to the market. This can make me nervous. Every few yards I'm asking if he's okay. Do we need to go back? And he says no. He's on a roll. We're always arm in arm, slow, shuffly, and we get in everyone's way, but we don't care. The mobility scooters shoot past, impatient. I would like to disable them properly.

When we got home, he said he had enjoyed the trip more than anything in ages. I would agree with that. We also have two new cordyline palms for each side of the front door. The hot weather killed the last ones. At £5 for two we can afford a few fatalities.

We reminisce together about why we chose Market Town and why it was the best decision we have made in a long time. In spite of his sister refusing to visit currently because, correctly, she feels it's "our turn"; although those quote marks are mine. She doesn't put it like that. She says, "Do come over any time". I have told her so many times that Prof R is seldom well enough to visit anyone, that I am considering putting it on a loop on the answerphone. There is a game here with rules that escape me. I have, a few times, asked if they will be home on a particular day, when Prof R seems well enough, but there is always, for them, another commitment of some kind. Remember, remember, "Never hit the ball back".

In the market we bought Doris a present for her pending birthday next month. It will be wrapped and added to the one we bought her husband for his birthday in March. They have an invitation to call in tomorrow. They are busy, but may be able to fit us in. We'll look forward to that.

The new dentist, a woman of a certain age, old enough for me to worry she may retire, was a hit with Prof R and asked us if we have been socializing since we moved to town. There's no answer to that question that will not reflect badly on us.

July 28 — Doris didn't visit, and I am more than grateful. Instead, an old friend rang. By that I mean a friend who is also old, not a friend of long-standing. So, an hour on the couch laughing with her was much more rewarding.

Phil the graphic designer assures me he is racing to the finish with the book. He asks me about a title for Part Four, which he surmises is mostly about the children. I have totally forgotten my structure for the book, so I have to check. I tell him it is actually about the family finale, and am tempted to tell him to call it, *"One affair, one escape and a divorce"*. But instead, I say, call it *"Snap, Crackle and Pop"*.

—

I almost threw a lemon pie at Prof R yesterday. We were having tea and cake outside in the shade on the new decking. The pie was a small one and he was having difficulty. It crumbled as he ate it. I didn't notice until he had handfuls of crumbs and the dog was feasting on the overflow below. Unreasonably, I became quietly furious that he hadn't said anything. "I need a plate" would have done. At which point I flounced off to get one. But not accepting his helplessness in these situations is both fruitless and a waste of energy.

So, the perfect afternoon tea continued, with an attempt to put one of the new silicone covers on his tea mug so he could drink through a straw.

We hardly ever have to use them and it's just as well. They are the size of a boastful condom and just as hard to put on any normal small mug. It is necessary to put them on after you have put the liquid in the cup or glass. This is like fitting a cover on a ship's swimming pool in a storm. And the swimming pool is hot. Prof R then attempted to hold the cup while drinking from the straw. This is not possible when the reason you have a straw in the first place is because your tremor is out of control. Laughter, as usual, saved us.

August 1 — A letter from the company who sold us the personal alarm. At first glance, I have no recollection of who they are. Their company name, *Friends and Family*, doesn't provide a clue. But the text of the letter reminds me we are supposed to sign up to pay for the sim in the alarm; £6 a month. Prof R has never used it, although he now recalls what it is for. But he is unlikely to use it if he falls upstairs because he is unlikely to be able to reach it. Wearing it is not an option for a sane life. I am going to ignore the letter and leave the alarm to become useless from 18th August.

Also today, a call from *Acorn* who put in the stairlifts. *Acorn* is also an interesting choice of name for a business that has nothing to do with seeds or squirrels. I am in the middle of making Prof R's latte, but I answer the phone because I don't know they have an entire sermon to deliver. At the point where she commiserates with me that Prof R has not used the lifts yet, I begin to lose focus. And when she says "Well hopefully he will get more use from it before too long" I decide this conversation is not fruitful, because she has lost focus as well. I already know her next piece of script will cover the four-year maintenance plan, which will cost £250 a year. For each stairlift. I have seen the advance letter warning me about that. So I tell her I am in the middle of making my husband a coffee and can she call back. I made a note of the number, so I remember not to answer the phone. But I should have blocked it.

—

On Monday the weather was cooler and Prof R, instead of saying "no" to an invitation to go out, said "yes". I said, "Shall we go and see your sister?" and he said, "That would probably be a friendly thing to do". So we went, carrying two birthday presents; one for her husband Brian, whose birthday was in March and the second for her, whose birthday is next week.

The car had not been out for six weeks. I found myself excited to be behind the wheel for something other than a medical appointment. We phoned first and left a message (me secretly relieved they were not home). When we arrived at their house, they had still not returned (me secretly relieved again) so we left the presents concealed by the front step and headed for the beach.

We hadn't been to the beach at Seasalter, which is about 10 minutes from our house, for more than six weeks; despite, or perhaps because of it being the hottest summer since 1976. Prof R can be in his element when he is in his element. We walked along the sea wall into the head wind and returned with the wind behind us. Always the best policy I find. The wind on this occasion was a rare and welcome balmy breeze from the South West. We allowed ourselves some elation, although the stony beach with its bleak breakwaters would win no prizes. For us, it was a few moments of bliss.

August 3 — I have a wonderfully kind friend, whom I knew first at school. She sends me metaphysical healing links. Sometimes she is off the scale with this stuff, but today, she has sent links to YouTube guides on how to use healing codes. I have the ability to ignore the jingoism and focus on process with these things. I learned Reiki with the same mental approach. But healing codes require the person who is ill to be engaging with the process and Prof R will not and could not do this. It is, to me, a form of self-hypnosis and he has never engaged with that.

And I too have lost all energy for alternative treatments. It is as helpful to Prof R that I talk positively to him and suggest he sit on his hands to rest them. Or fold his arms. His body visibly relaxes, and he looks almost confident. I tell him he is the person in charge here. If the hand isn't behaving, he should make it toe the line. Of course, that's only when he isn't eating or drinking, but it's enough to feel in control some of the time. We're not looking for perfection here. Good enough is good enough.

The heat is back. Today it will be 33deg. We have the dentist for Prof R at 2.45 pm.

August 4 — The dentist was cancelled. Prof R was too hot.

But my book is finally published. Uploading it onto the publisher's website was almost as difficult as giving birth. Technology needs to be tricked into doing what we need it to do. In this case, as they are based in the US, I waited till they were asleep in the hope that my job would stop freezing and "breaking", as my chat helper so usefully put it. She said yesterday, "Your job is broken, you will have to start again."

It was not our fault – hers or mine. Even though I needed guidance there was no reason for it to bail out of the process. Too many cooks perhaps. But Phil has taken over, with more success. Two proof copies are on their way to me. The proof will be the pudding and it better be good. I feel flat. Post-partum blues perhaps.

—

Prof R used the stairlift today with great reluctance. He needed it but would rather have fallen two flights of stairs than admit it. I told him that I need to practice using them, so this was a good opportunity. He was not to see himself as a lesser man, blah blah blah. No better or worse than a war hero with no legs. It probably didn't help when I added that small children who are paralyzed have to use these chairs without thinking they have failed somehow.

I forgot not to answer the phone when *Acorn* called back yesterday. But I was ready for them this time. She made a lot of small talk before asking me if I had considered the maintenance programme. I said I had, and thank you, we would not need it until the guarantee has run out in a year, so call back then. She pointed out we would get a discount if we bought the four-year contract now. So, for the straight stair, it would be about £600 and for the curved stair it would be £1200. And this was payable up front. For that they would come out on command, even on Christmas Day. My response was to laugh unkindly and tell her it was "extortion". Surely the chairs are a product they are proud of that will not need that degree of maintenance. She promised to pass on the feedback, and I said I hoped the next call she made would be more rewarding.

August 8 — Two falls, three hours apart, this morning; the first in two months. We are getting better at our spatial ability to extract him from the bathroom in various ways. He is sore, but not broken. It was a relief to discover I can hear him fall in the loft when I am in the kitchen, two floors down. So the alarm probably wasn't necessary in any case.

And strangely, he had a better day than normal. He seems to be sleeping less during the day. Which is both good news and bad news. It meant he was on deck for his eldest daughter Hannah when she came to lunch with her son, aged 11. He, the grandson, has luxurious long dark hair and is incredibly beautiful. But shy. "He is his own man" I tell my eldest son Alex, when he says someone should make the boy cut his hair. I disagree. The roles are reversed with our generations. The new conservatism shocks me. "I would have let you have long hair" I rebuked him. And he had the perfect answer, as always, "The school would not have allowed it".

—

The rains finally came. We need it but I get easily bored. My book is finished and printed and will hopefully be read by my intimate circle – or at least they will say they have read it. The advance proof copes are late arriving. A third cousin in the USA has already ordered her copy. I tell those who are not family to just look at the pictures. That will probably tell them everything they want or need to know about my family.

The most interesting responses have been the absent ones. Silence from the two siblings. No matter how much we consult, memoir is a bed of thorns tiptoed across at great risk. But I am glad I've done it.

The half of the family who belong to Prof R are not in it, so they don't need to be either consulted or told about it. We do well, Prof R's children and I, but there are many things, like the book, that I don't tell them about. I fear their power to diminish it. They are kind to me now, very kind. But this has only grown more recently, since their father became ill. The advantages of this last step-parent have become more apparent to them.

And I have had some very pleasant surprises lately from the girls. "Dad is very lucky to have you", was one of them. And just this week, a first; "Would you like me to bring some food down for lunch"? This is a huge step forward in my step-relationships.

August 11 — Today I have been planning my own 'expiry'. It's not the first time I have tackled this issue. There is already a so-called *Life Book* in the in-tray on my desk. This time it began with worrying about Prof R's death – what he would want, and the process required – and naturally, being selfish, I then began to think of myself.

The children already have my Will and their instructions. "No funeral". But they might need more help. Google, as usual, has all the answers. I have now found out how much it costs to have a 'Direct Cremation' and exactly what that involves. It's not pretty. But it only costs about £1200. When we had our previous dog put down there seemed to be more care and love involved; although it was about £1000 cheaper. But we got a very attractive wooden box thrown in for the ashes. In the direct cremation world you don't even need a coffin. You can have a shroud. The image is chilling, or at best, 'in your face'. I would need to go on a diet before I would want anyone seeing a silhouette of my body in a sheet.

It's not even necessary to pick up the ashes. In fact, you had better request it specifically if you want them back. There will be an extra charge. There is no guarantee of when the body will be cremated as they schedule it for downtime. A bit like a night-store heater.

If you would like a small ceremony it will cost extra and if you want a specific time it will cost even more. But it would be nice to think someone was present to see me off. And preferably not at midnight, or whenever. How much notice would they get? "Madam we have had a cancellation. Can you be here in 10 minutes?"

A 'less direct' cremation does have the small ceremony if you wish and perhaps a funeral director to do all the leg work, so you don't have to get an Uber to pick your loved one up from the hospital or the slab or wherever, and take it to the crematorium. I'm leaning towards that option currently. If only because it would be nice to know that I hadn't been cremated in an oven built for ten. It looks as though you could still come in under £3000. Cheaper than having the LED spotlights installed throughout our house. Much cheaper.

The link to the information site has been saved on my desktop as "What to do when someone dies". So I can find it for Prof R and someone else can find it for me. There is no point sending this information to the children now, as they will have lost it if I last another 20 years. And the link won't work then either. I'm still not confident they will find anything they need on my desktop when the time comes. Or that they will find my *Life Book* in the in-tray. Or that it won't be out of date. They might be organizing everything from another location. There is no obvious solution to this.

No doubt this topic engages me so much because I feel Prof R's mortality more than my own and I know it will be my responsibility to follow all the correct steps at the appropriate time. Strangely, I seemed to manage to do all this when my father died, but I suspect the funeral director provided a lot of guidance. My father had already been taken to a morgue in a hospital, so I only had to decide which funeral director to choose. Even that was easy. I chose the same one who had buried his mother six years earlier.

But that was 26 years ago and 12,000 miles away. I live somewhere else entirely. I will need to do some more research.

—

Our path today to the Physic Garden, past the great church, was blocked by shiny cream Daimlers and silly hats. There was a wedding, and the bride was about to enter the church. A man approached us kindly to explain everything we could already see with our own eyes. He said he and his family had done the flowers and his daughters wanted to see the bride. He wasn't really into brides, he said. I said, joking, "Do you prefer the grooms?" and his eyes widened with shock. "Just joking" I said, and he laughed, slapping me playfully on the arm to show he didn't mind really.

So we managed to see the Physic Garden and stayed long enough for me to take a photo of Prof R on a bench to prove he had walked that far, although it is only two blocks from our house.

August 12 — I have, at 7 am, woken bone tired, barely able to stir my body enough to help Prof R return from the toilet and to give him his morning pills. I can feel very grumpy and far from the perfect caring wife at these moments. After climbing back into bed, I realise I won't go back to sleep. My mind has woken up without me, so I'm up, putting out clean trousers and underwear for Prof R and collecting my own from the drawer.

Last night, for the first time since all this began, I scoffed a third of a bar of dark 85 percent chocolate. If I lose control of my body, there is the fear I might lose control of my mind.

Tidying my desk, I have come across a notebook that doesn't need to be kept. But before I throw it out, I read a list I made when making Prof R happy seemed to be a top priority for me. It's headed "Prof R likes to do…"

The first item on the list is "Play with V". Not much else has changed either. Except that now he cannot indulge his former love for photography, history, archaeology and films. He also no longer wants to go out for coffee. Or travel. So now I can throw out the notebook.

Why was/am I so obsessed by what made Prof R happy? No doubt a psychologist would say it takes the heat off me to make myself happy. But I think if the people we love are happy, we are very often happy.

In the notebook there are also pages and pages of Scrabble scores. That is another thing he can no longer do.

August 13 — A very unsuccessful conversation today about our new carer, whom Prof R has of course forgotten under duress. And he does not improve with further explanation, becoming more and more stooped and hands flapping uncontrollably even when I take him in my arms to steady him. He cannot understand why we need a carer, even when I call her a Personal Assistant. He says he is perfectly okay on his own when I go to Pilates. He is a person who used to lecture students. He has momentarily forgotten he is ill.

After some calming time on the couch his mind opens up again and he begins to recall the other V. And he eventually accepts the idea that we need her as another team member. We have no one else and we cannot operate safely without her. He says, "And how do you fit in?" knowing he loves me, but briefly not sure why. He clings to the fact that he loves me and repeats it. I say, trying to lighten things up, "I love you more". He needs to check occasionally where the anchor is.

I can see a possible issue ahead with our carer having my name. Will he, in six or eight months, know which V is which? A sickening thought.

He has been up for five hours today. It has depleted his memory chip.

Overnight I discover he didn't have his last levodopa before bed. He seldom forgets this, but it's a reminder that I need to do more than shake his pill pot to check. It was beside his bed; along with the slippery elm which most definitely helps him have no further fears of constipation. Except when he forgets he has been, and tells me that people with Parkinson's only pass a poo every three days.

August 14 — My book arrived in hard copy. I am thrilled but in a low-key sort of way. It seems so totally unimportant in the scheme of things. And then we discover a huge software error on page 16, and another one on page 26. So it's back to repair, upload and two more proof copies to wait 10 days for.

This is strangely good, because I want things to settle a bit. I want my siblings to forget about it and whatever it was that unsettled them when I announced it was finished. Their silence no longer matters. And if they never mention it again, I will be happy. And if they ask where it is, I can explain the delay. Either way is a good outcome.

August 16 — I break out in a 'boredom sweat' with the effort of talking on the phone with a fixed smile to tradespeople, medical people (much rarer), and well-meaning relatives (almost extinct). But the grocery delivery company Ocado I am always pleased to hear from; even when, like today, they are late.

Also overdue was the blood test today for my underactive thyroid (three years overdue). It will not detect my boredom. Even though boredom makes me tired.

Prof R is drifting off. I'm not sure where. Perhaps he is drifting in.

Either way, he tends not to listen anymore. He will say he is…but it is harder for him I suspect to actually connect to what I am talking about. I speak too quickly and jump from subject to subject and I need to change how I'm speaking to him, without taking on that 'nursey' patronizing tone. Because the intelligent Prof R is still in there, even if he is in a labyrinth. It seems not to frighten him anymore.

August 17 — A New Zealand friend has sent me this piece of research done in 2009.

"Results of this national longitudinal study of 3,376 elderly married individuals showed that spending at least fourteen hours per week providing care to a spouse predicted decreased mortality for the caregiver, independent of behavioral and cognitive limitations of the care-receiving spouse, and of other demographic and health variables."

On the face of it, it's full of holes. How could controls for such a high number of variables be achieved? And then be removed from the calculation?

My conclusion is equally unscientific; "bullshit". Who in their right mind would believe that caring for a loved one over the long term is anything other than extremely stressful? The rewards are there, because we love them and we dread their loss, but the cost is high; a life for a life. Caring is definitely still a life, but while we can acknowledge that the 'now' is our real life, we have to hope the life we had before is still out there, waiting in the wings. But it won't be the life we had before will it?

With that in mind, I woke at 5 am and emailed V the PA to book her for Saturday 15th September. *(It appears I had forgotten that V did not work on the weekend.)* Then I emailed my daughter to tell her I can visit on that date. I will take the train to London and I will have lunch with her and admire the new flat.

The Prof R hurdle will be overcome. He will come to like the new third member of our team. He will not get upset and go silent and shake uncontrollably when it is time for me to leave. I have to believe this. And even if he does, I have to walk out the door. Otherwise, there will come a day when we need backup, and no one is there.

August 19 — I can feel isolation creeping up slowly, like a cold fog. It is three months since I have seen my elder little family. They are so preoccupied now with other serious issues. Ophelia's mother is in danger of being deported. To New Zealand, so not a disease-ridden archipelago somewhere. Some problem with her visa and perhaps she has not met the requirements for it to be extended permanently.

So my darling daughter-in-law is clearly beside herself. She makes rash offers of visits to see me at the last moment, which I make elaborate excuses to help her get out of. They will be relieved when I can visit them. The children cannot possibly feel a relationship with this Nana. I've become the Nana who makes jaunty comments on the photo stream.

When winter comes, so soon now, visits will be off by mutual agreement. It is too cold and miserable and the days too short. There will be another pre-Christmas-Christmas here in mid-December no doubt, so they can meet their other obligations on the real day.

I love Christmas, in spite of my feelings that it is an artificial construct, and becomes a day of mourning for so many. Something you want to escape, but can't, because it comes to you. No one is spared the intrusion of other people's celebrations. *(Except, as it turns out, in a pandemic).*

Last night Prof R forgot who Boris Johnson is, so today I asked him again to see if it was a momentary glitch. He still could not remember, although he said the face was familiar.

Then I changed tack and asked him instead who the Prime Minister is. But still he could not remember, although he knew she was a woman. Warmer but not up to date. Neither loss seemed to concern him.

This marks a step change in his loss of memory. The tide has been held back for two years but is now starting to force its way through the holes in our rivastigmine defences. "The colander is holier than thou."

August 20 — This morning I noticed his soiled pyjama pants as he returned to bed, and changed them for him without saying why. He was very dopey. Self-care is becoming much more difficult for him.

A friend, trying to be supportive, suggested I dispense with the cost of the carer and take Prof R everywhere with me in his wheelchair. I almost cried at the lack of understanding. But she's a good friend so I explained that he did not always want to go out and respite was what I needed, not just mobility.

But her comment made me reassess what I am doing. Carer Support offered me a carer assessment a year ago. I said no thank you; we were fine. Now we're not fine. It's time I took them up on that offer.

August 23 — The electricians have finally finished rewiring 74 faulty spotlights in our ceilings. And a few other things, some of which I have now forgotten. They have been visiting for almost six months. The invoices add up to £5000. But we can sleep safely in our beds. Well, unless they missed something.

Prof R spent most of yesterday in his bed. But he seems happy and engaged when he is up. Except he still can't remember the name of the PM. I am missing my dose of the BBC *Daily Politics* at lunchtime. Brexit – or the politics of it – has been a godsend for me, but I don't tell anyone that. My ever-diminishing social media circle will have to see me through another winter. But no matter how desperate I become, Facebook will not be revisited.

August 24 — Planning for the carer assessment has concentrated my mind. Today I realized Prof R had no emergency plan for my absence. Whether I'm on the floor or out the door. So we have practiced what he would do. First, try next door, both sides. Failing that, he had to demonstrate to me that he could dial 999. He would not be able to find other numbers easily. Another box that we did not see has now been ticked. But only temporarily.

August 26 — Twin step-grandsons aged seven tore through the house, rode the stairlifts and brightened things considerably. They exhausted Prof R though, and he needed a lie down straight after lunch. When, hours later, he emerged again, one said, "It must be quite good to have a shaky hand for cleaning your teeth". They are old enough to begin to understand what grown-up illness can look like. But young enough not to let it worry them. Rather like the dog, they are liberating to play with.

Their father, cornering me in the kitchen, said "Rachel has mentioned that she and the girls would like to come down and sit with their father so you could have some time off." But later, Rachel asked me if I planned a trip to London to see my daughter's new flat, and when I said "yes" she only said, "that's good". So I told her we were trialing a carer and she said again "that's good" and I said, "Well, yes, otherwise I wouldn't be able to go to London". And she said, "I didn't really think about that". At which point, half under my breath, I said, "No one does". To which she made no comment at all.

To come to terms with these realities I have to place myself as close to being in their shoes as it is reasonably possible to get. And when I do, I see fear and denial and a natural desire to run for the hills. If I can just hold that thought I will lose the resentment which may turn me to stone if I'm not careful.

August 27 — After a disturbed night and waking Prof R for his early pills, it is now nearly midday and he has not arrived for breakfast. Exhaustion from yesterday.

I find I am bored, and decide this is good practice for motivation if living alone. Having said that, I'm probably getting rather more practice than is good for anyone.

On my desktop I have a rather tattered old mantra for motivation which says, "The cure for boredom is curiosity. There is no cure for curiosity." Sometimes, for the largely housebound, there is even a shortage of curiosity. Although there are people who solve that by peering out of their own windows to see what the neighbours are up to. Curtain twitchers. How I sympathise. People are at least more interesting to watch than birds.

There are other cures for boredom besides curiosity. My caregiver skills got a boost this afternoon when I found Prof R flat on his back in the bathroom. He had not appeared for lunch after promising he would be down for breakfast by lunchtime. I didn't hear him fall this time. He claimed to have been down for only a few moments. (Tempting to paraphrase the philosophical cliché; "If a man falls in a loft but no one is around to hear him, does he make a sound?" Discuss.)

We manoeuvred him to the best recovery so far, but he was not yet *compos mentis*. He was also odorous. Without protest he let me change his pyjama pants and clean him with a wet wipe. Poo has seldom repelled me. And once clean, he agreed to have some ice cream before taking more pills. By the time he had been fed his ice cream he realized he needed the toilet again. And this time, when he had finished, he gave in and let me clean him.

I now feel a fully qualified *bona fide* personal carer. Because while it has never bothered me, wiping a bottom, this was my first adult bottom, other than my own, so it was the exam I had been afraid of failing. I feared he would be humiliated by it, but frankly, I'm good at it. And dementia has its blessings. It can be kind to both the afflicted and their loved ones. This is a relief.

August 29 — At 1am I did what I always do at various times during the night – I peer through the crack in the bathroom door to see if Prof R is okay or needs a wake-up call. This time I saw him combing his hair carefully, checking himself in the mirror. I waited till he had finished and then asked, as usual, if he was okay. Before helping him back to bed.

—

A New Zealand cousin, Liz, and I have quite a correspondence going. We have shared experiences that bind us in ways that is both comforting and very useful. And we can laugh. She is three months into her widowhood, so she is beginning to defrost and feel again. This can be as painful as thawing out your fingers on an icy morning. But we can defrost each other.

She told me her husband had to be nursed in a special hospital bed in their home for the last few weeks of his life, because the regulations in New Zealand do not allow the medical staff to care for someone in a standard bed. This, if it also applies here, in the UK, is a major blow to me. Where would Prof R go? There is no room in our bedroom, and we would have to get rid of the spare bed to put him in the guest room. The living room?? My 'nightmare of nightmares' is to have a sickbed where the dining table should be. There is no separate dining room. I'm going to try not to think about that just for now. But I have another question for Susan from Carer Support who will assess my needs next Tuesday.

—

It's almost September and officially autumn. And mysteriously, the 'artificial construct' of our calendar is matching the weather. It's cooler. I am requiring a bit more discipline to take the dog out in the morning. Soon I will need a lot more.

Now I must make up a briefing sheet for V the carer, even though she hasn't asked for one. How she can care for someone without knowing their pill regime, or where the cups and plates are, and whether Prof R needs to be woken for meds or not, is beyond me. She has her first two-hour stint next Wednesday so it's all new territory. And I keep imagining worst-case scenarios for the Saturday in two weeks' time when she will care for him for most of one day.

August 31 — Ophelia's mother is definitely being deported. She would qualify for her passport with the correct paperwork but has left her run too late. Her husband already has his UK passport, but has no option but to follow. She is pragmatic and seems quite content with the thought of a summer in New Zealand. After a decent interval – the first sign of winter being ideal I imagine – she can reapply for a new visa. Why does their departure make me feel even more alone? Because they are the only friends – and family too – from my own generation who are within reach perhaps.

—

In spite of my resolve to park the issue of Health and Safety and the hospital bed, I have been scared out of my wits by my kiwi cousin. The dreaded hospital bed – and presumably a hoist and levers to elevate and recline upper and lower body. The cheerful notion of others, that he can recline happily, flanked by all this equipment, in the living room, fills me with horror. This is not for a few weeks. This is a long term and possibly slow end-of-life care situation.

In desperation I have been looking at the space at the foot of our bed with an eye to how a hospital monster on wheels might fit there. My cousin also said her husband was upset about being moved from his own bed to the high hard prelude to the morgue slab. I will not cry now, but I might later.

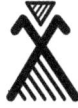

Autumn–Winter 2018

SEPTEMBER 3 — I can almost cry every time I have to deal with any of the various 'auto-persons' masquerading as medical specialist's secretaries. The presumably lesser-paid receptionists, in contrast, are caring and considerate.

The Neurology Department, which we had hoped to have banished from our lives, popped up again in the letterbox, this time for the Movement Clinic. It is at the same hospital where neurology lurks, in mid-Kent, which is a 45 minute drive from here. An unnecessary trip, when I know they have a clinic in Canterbury. Because a previous neurologist's referral letter to their Canterbury clinic told me so.

Phoning these departments calmly does not necessarily help me to stay calm. When Ms Auto-Person says 10.30 am is the only time available, in a tone I haven't heard since schooldays, a wave of childish emotional response engulfs me. But I tell her politely that 10.30 am is not possible. It is too early for Prof R, who is still asleep upstairs at 11 am. And I explain it is the dementia that causes this problem, not his movement disorder.

But apparently the new Movement Disorder doctor cannot be messed with. We must take it or leave it. With the familiar unspoken threat, 'or else'. It's in the small print of your referral letter. If you turn down an offer of treatment, the NHS cannot guarantee you will be offered care in future. So I stay calm, and tell her not to worry, I will make some enquiries and see if we can see the Movement Disorder doctor at Canterbury.

The NHS understandably believes it is only their staff who are at risk of bullying, not the patients. They have huge signs saying they are entitled to be treated with respect. And there are indeed patients the staff have good reason to fear.

But we, the non-violent, are also afraid. An urgent or distressed tone, and for the particularly sensitive, even a raised eyebrow, can be enough to trigger their defences. So I will do nothing, until I have counted higher than 10 and then I will call again, and wait for them to tell me whether I can change Prof R's appointment to Canterbury.

And when we do eventually see the Movement Disorder doctor, I will ask if anyone is interested in Prof R's memory loss. His 'elephant in the room'. The D word. His 'colander'. The unmentionable. Where is the referral to the so-called Memory Clinic, which remains a mystery to us, even though several well-meaning people have written several referral letters on Prof R's behalf over several years? Since 2014 in fact.

September 5 — What a difference a woman called Susan can make to my view of my future with Prof R. She came to do my Carer Assessment, and she made me feel safe – or at least safer. No one can know how the way forward will be, but at least she gave me signposts and people to call. I hadn't realized how isolated I had felt.

This visit was after an episode in the night when Prof R had his eyes open but did not respond to me. I called and touched and kissed and eventually he took some notice of me. And then he said, "Who are you?" But that was an episode and it passed.

Today we have V the carer beginning work with a two-hour test run. It is now 11.30am and Prof R has not woken up, other than to pee. I have just had to wake him to give him his mid-morning levodopa. My guess is he will be eating breakfast, then lunch and then ice cream as V walks in the door at 1pm. This at least means he will probably not hide in his bedroom while she is here. Because he won't be tired. But as he will have forgotten she is coming, there is no guarantee.

September 7th — At the dentist this afternoon Prof R's session stretched from my anticipated 30 minutes to a marathon hour. He had three fillings, and when the dentist, the divine Mrs L, finally emerged from her surgery to speak to me, she reported one filling was so deep he may eventually lose the tooth.

It took me several minutes to help him move from the dental chair to the waiting room, and then seat him while I paid. During this process, her next patient, a man, entered the room and watched us sympathetically. When I had finally settled Prof R into a chair, I turned to him, feeling a need to lighten the mood, and said, "When my husband arrived here an hour ago, he was an athlete. Good luck in there!"

—

We've got my great escape planned for Saturday 15th but I'm getting cold feet. It will now be his eldest daughter Hannah who comes, not V. I had forgotten, V doesn't do Saturday. Hannah agreed to my request because I used my birthday as an excuse. It won't be my actual birthday, but it will be in lieu of my birthday.

What will she do if he needs help after toileting? Should I warn her? Should I first ask Prof R if he would mind if she helped him? But in his state of mind how does the world look?

Wednesday's care session with V went well. Prof R retreated upstairs after half an hour and she twiddled her thumbs and washed up the lunch dishes in the sink. What a treat. And I had my first lunch with a friend when I could truly relax.

Food is becoming more troublesome than toileting. There are so many things now that feel strange in his mouth. Anything stringy or of a texture he finds hard to swallow. I cut up the chicken, and I feed him like a baby bird if necessary, but that is not the end of it.

September 8 — So, the good news is, I asked Prof R if he would mind Hannah wiping his bottom and he said "no". When I asked Hannah if she minded wiping her dad's bottom and she said, "no problem". Drama over.

Little meltdowns for me come right out of the blue. I'm fine, I'm cool, I'm having a laugh watching some silly comedy, and then I hear the squeak, squeak, squeak on the floor above. My heart takes the lift to the basement. He's half an hour early. I want that time. It's mine. And I'm all talked out.

And that's the thing. The talking is all I can do now to keep him company. And sometimes I'm just so tired of doing nothing, sitting and trying to find things to talk about that might entertain or engage him. So, after a two-hour stint on the couch or in the garden I'm all talked out and I long for him to go upstairs for a rest. And fortunately for me, and the reason probably why I have managed so long without a break, he mostly does.

September 10 — The cumulative effect of these never-safe nights must start to affect my brain. It can switch into neutral if I'm trying to remember something when I am in a different context. Lunch out with my friend last week, whom I hadn't seen for years, and suddenly I couldn't remember the famous name of one of my favourite shops in London. Worse, it was Conran's, who also owned *Bibendum*, where Prof R and I had our date with destiny so long ago.

September 13 — My sister in New Zealand has dropped a bombshell. She has decided to come over and help for two months. In order to do this, she is taking out a loan for the air fare, and I am not at all confident that she is doing the right thing. This is a woman on a restricted income – pension and additional benefits. And two months wintering over here, the way we live, will drive her to distraction, even if it does reduce her living costs. I am hoping she will see her way to wisdom before she forks out for the tickets.

Yesterday was my first Pilates day and it was such a revelation to rediscover all the parts of my body ultimately connected to my head. I tend to focus only on the 5 kg or whatever that is balanced on my neck. The remaining 62 kg is exercised occasionally, intermittently, and even though I always feel so much better after Pilates, my 5 kg of scrambled egg on top never learns the lesson.

The blessed 30 copies of my book are sitting in a brown box on the floor of my office waiting to be posted out. This is the easy part. I'm going to thoroughly enjoy it, even if Royal Mail will rob me for the privilege.

September 16 — Sunday. I'm being hounded by the hound. She wants a walk, and I am so knocked out I am ignoring her.

Yesterday was magical and it might be better if I didn't experience that level of enjoyment again too soon. The after-crash is a downer and last night, like an over-excited 5-year-old, I could not sleep.

My Saturday began as usual, but once I had settled Hannah with her father and a two-page briefing sheet, and got on that train, I was flying. It was a slow train and stopped at every station, but my head was in a very nice space. It was my first trip on a train in three years and my first day away from Prof R in I-don't-know-how-long. Fortunately I could still remember how to get around the platforms.

Once safely in Crofton Park, it was lunch with Hope and Simon in a café, a tour of their 'hood', cake at the new flat with all the other darlings, and a love fest for me. Cinderella for a day.

I may never get over it. I keep feeling like crying. And Hannah did not need to wipe her father's bottom.

September 17 — I spent an early part of today fishing through a sack of rubbish that had already been put out for collection. Prof R came down for breakfast, and through a mouthful of muesli tried to indicate to me that there was a problem with his mouth. Eventually I realized he was missing his lower partial denture. He had no idea where it had gone.

There was only one place it could have gone. And that was into the rubbish basket beside his washstand. Even then, it would have required him to have had the lid raised. The problem would have been more easily solved if I had not brought the bin down with me before breakfast, emptied it into the rubbish sack and put the sack out in the wheelie bin. But nevertheless, I did do that, and so I had to retrieve the rubbish sack. And after a degree of searching which could have been a great deal more unpleasant than it was, I found the teeth. As they were simply covered in coffee grounds, I washed them unceremoniously and gave them to Prof R.

My sister Stella has now said she will come in mid-October and stay three months instead of two. This will be an experiment neither of us is fully prepared for.

Alex, my senior son, rang me at lunchtime to flood me with relief. He loves the book. And jokes he has several scenarios already planned for potential film rights. How I love that boy.

September 18 — Tuesday. Gemma the dementia advisor came to visit me. More and more I feel warmed by these people who are here for me, not just for Prof R. Gemma was no exception. I have no idea what she does, but I can ring her if I am not coping with some aspect dementia-related and ask for advice. that is enough.

September 19 — Wednesday. V the carer has made a breakthrough with Prof R.

Today she got the whole 'seven ages of man' – childhood, teaching in France for a year (thus avoiding military service – he didn't tell her that bit), taking a play around Germany as a student, a stint on contract at the BBC; and the university career ending as Dean of Faculty. Although, when I asked, she said he left out his work in adult education and training the trainers, which I had found possibly the most interesting thing he did. The accuracy doesn't matter of course. It is significant he has found someone new to talk to about his life. Celebrate it, be grateful for it, as I do mine.

My sister Stella has bought her tickets and will now be arriving on 29th October, as first planned, because coming two weeks earlier would be $1000 more expensive. The 29th is a Monday. Today I discovered V the carer has another client on a Monday. We need more than just one carer.

September 20 — Thursday. Prof R took me by surprise at breakfast this morning by losing consciousness and falling sideways out of his chair. I was too far away to catch him as he launched himself headfirst to the floor, smashing his head on the metal rail of the dog's child gate as he landed. A sickening sight I replay in my head unless I am very careful.

Blood, quite a lot of it, on my hand when I checked his head. He woke quickly and clear-headed, very determined not to go to A&E, to which I agreed. But where to go? I called the GP line for emergencies thinking a GP might come to the house and was told to dial 999. I said thank you, but no, next suggestion please. And she said, "The Minor Injuries Unit". A lot more intelligent.

But first, quietly and slowly, with my help, Prof R had to pick himself up off the floor. Next, I had to call the garage where the car was having its annual service and ask them to return it. Which they did, in the space of 10 minutes, with the servicing done but no time for the MOT.

Prof R and I had a nice little 5-minute drive to the surgery, and his gash, which was jagged, was glued rather than stitched. With me holding the wound closed for the medic who did the job. We had only waited about 30 seconds to be seen. At A&E we would have waited several hours.

Now he is resting, and I am checking him every 30 minutes or so. The pain is minimal, the blood removed from the floor and the furnishings. It might be okay to relax.

I must rebook the MOT.

September 21 — Friday. Episode two of the denture story. At 6 am this morning, I investigated Prof R after too long a stay in the bathroom, to find his top dentures protruding from his pants pocket.

The bottom set, he indicated, were in his mouth. In the middle of the night, I had persuaded him to remove his half-inserted dentures from his mouth during an earlier toilet visit. A choke hazard we don't need.

This may be some kind of anxiety activity, although he is showing no signs of feeling stressed by his fall yesterday.

I, on the other hand, slept with racing dreams. This is not very restful.

September 23 — Sunday. When the unexpected happens, the stress levels climb. There were two attacks of vertigo yesterday in the late afternoon. At least, after an NHS online search, I have initially decided it is.

Prof R had come downstairs at 6 pm, looking normal to my eye, and sat down. There was no clue he was in trouble. Until I tried to tell him about a film he might like, the story of American film star Gloria Graham's last days in Liverpool. He managed to interrupt my flow with "I need to tell you something". There had been vertigo in bed when he got up and then a second attack when he entered the living room.

Was it the fall? Probably. Had he upended the balance of fluid in his ears? After a Google session on Parkinson's and vertigo, it was apparently not due to Parkinson's. I do know about Meniere's disease, because my first husband apparently had that, for a while at least. But this wasn't it.

It is thanks to Stella that I even know about vertigo as a condition – very unpleasant but eminently curable – rather than a phobia or a movie. She had told me how to deal with it. By a technique that involves turning his head to each side in a sequence of staged manoeuvres.

So I was able to calm him with the "vertigo-can't-kill-you" formula. Nothing to fear. It may also have been dehydration or the half-pill of levodopa he missed at 4 pm. For the rest of the evening and overnight, once he regained confidence, all was well.

—

On a wet Sunday what do we do? I do my domestic chores and watch politics and cooking programmes, and look after Prof R. Perhaps later, when he sleeps again, a film. It is even too wet to walk the dog. During the day I am afraid to read because I am in danger of nodding off, and one thing I don't want to do is sleep during the day. Night-time is for sleeping.

Prof R drifts on clouds of sleep and wakes to eat and sit and listen to whatever I can think of to talk about, and then takes himself back to bed to sleep some more. Sometimes I have to wake him for his medication and when I do, I often find him dreaming. This disturbed confused sleeping is hard even for Parkinson's medics to understand, but it is probably because, as one neurologist suspects, he has one of the other 'mimics' in this spectrum. One where dementia is the major player.

He has never been able to remember his dreams and perhaps it is just as well. His idle thoughts are a mysterious world I often try to enter. But they are sometimes a mystery to him too. Or seemingly irrelevant to the present situation or conversation. Although there is a lot he can discuss and a lot he can remember when prompted.

—

There's no doubt much to be learned from this end-of-life experience, and it isn't just the thought that a trip to Switzerland when my time comes would solve it.

Prof R's life has not been artificially extended by medical science. His cognitive and movement decline has been medicated, but he would be alive nevertheless. Paralyzed and comatose perhaps, but still needing care and resources. No blame can be levelled at our 'must-live-forever' generation for his situation.

My sister has her own plans in place for a 'quick exit' and so do some of our friends. I'm not yet in the go-quickly-into-the-night-light camp. I'd still rather take my time. It's a lot less scary than hanging yourself from a doorknob with a necktie like Robin Williams did.

Perhaps the 'I'm-where-God-wants-me-to be' brigade have the answer. They make it easy for themselves by not thinking too much at all. Clever of them.

—

Prof R stayed in bed until 4 pm. I fed him breakfast in bed at 1 pm followed by ice cream, always chocolate. At 4 pm I found him dressing, but he said he felt the fall had affected him. He wasn't exactly sure where he was or even who he was, although he could tell me his name. This condition does not necessarily require a fall.

Then he asked me to marry him. He had forgotten we were married. And I was strangely moved and pleased he would have wanted to marry me again. Or once, depending on your point of view.

I told my daughter, hoping she would not think me barmy to be so happy. She too thought it was lovely. But she did say I should have asked for another diamond. Given I didn't get one the first time, it would be nice.

It's very possible the shock of his fall has worsened his symptoms, but there is no point doing anything other than watch and wait. He has no headache and today no more vertigo. If indeed he is mildly concussed, it has to heal itself. Neither of us wants more MRI's unless absolutely necessary.

When I was putting the remains of his late lunch into the fridge, I saw the packet of rice crackers I had absent-mindedly put there yesterday. As we all know, rice crackers do not need to be in a fridge. I am very aware this is not necessarily a good sign, although I won't worry until I put the car keys in there, or anything else that isn't edible.

September 24 — Today is my 69th birthday and I shall be keeping it secret from Prof R. It's kinder. He has seen various cards arrive for me, but it doesn't seem to register with him. He knows, I think, but doesn't like to ask. His proposal of marriage yesterday was gift enough for me.

At lunchtime, while I was standing beside him as he sat at the table, he fainted again. This time, I had his head in my hands, washing his scalp with a wet wipe to avoid his wound.

These faints are horrific. All limbs flail when he regains consciousness. And he took a while to recover. Blood pressure readings are normal. But from now on he will sit at the table in the leather tub chair.

September 25 — Tuesday. Prof R now moves much more slowly and has had some more episodes of vertigo. Fortunately, without nausea. He feels the fall has changed something in his head. I do not disagree. We have an appointment with the GP but cannot see any urgent intervention being either forthcoming or useful. Hopefully he will soon feel better, if not actually *be* better.

At 8.30am a man arrived to deep clean the oven. He came laden with his own life story, and spent three hours telling me about it, but I was quite happy to listen. It was so much worse than anything I had experienced, it made me grateful. And I was delighted with the elderly oven, which now is a credit to me. Or at least, not an embarrassment.

The car was picked up again by my garage 'angel' and taken for its MOT.

I sent a text to Prof R's sister, telling her he is "somewhat wobbly", and it had the desired response. She and her husband turned up on our doorstep in the afternoon bearing mini Belgium chocolate éclairs. I fell on them. 'Oven man's' life story had exhausted me.

Doris and Brian left saying "call us anytime if you need us" and my note to self was "over my dead body". I like them – love them even – but I don't trust them. While they were here, a significant moment. Prof R needed to come downstairs on his stair lift, a first for them.

Siblings know us better than anyone when we reach our later life. No matter how much I love Prof R and no matter how long I have lived with him, his sister will always have known him for 60 years longer. She has the power to give him pleasure in their shared childhood memories. If she wants to. Memories of cockles. Gathering them on the Isle of Sheppey, where you could have them cooked for you in a large steamer pot before you took them home.

September 26 — Wednesday. This morning the Care Navigator came to visit me. (How I love that title.) She is empowered to obtain things like support frames for toilets with handles on them, and handholds for the back door.

This will be the first time we have properly entered the receiving end of the social welfare system and I, for one, am grateful. But she reminded me that the Kent County Council are just as grateful. They need me to continue caring for Prof R at home more than I need them.

Pilates again today and Prof R was not well enough to talk to V this time. I asked her to check on him in the loft every half hour to be sure he hadn't fallen.

Finally, the long-awaited GP appointment late afternoon and a doctor who took one look at Prof R's record and ordered blood and urine tests before I needed to ask for them. He hasn't been monitored since we left Wales. She has also ordered an ECG because his tremor was so bad, she couldn't measure his pulse. He was reassured by her about the temporary life of the vertigo, but I forgot to ask her to look in his ears. I feel he hardly hears me.

—

It's taken me a few days to notice that I don't want to go out at all when he is sleeping. He is so much more vulnerable and dependent on me. Perhaps it's not necessary for me to feel this way, but something stops me. And that will change how I do everything.

Seeing Prof R's face each time he fainted has made me lose any faith in his safety when I'm not with him. His eyes rolling, his mouth drooling, his head lolling and no obvious breath until he bangs into life, arms flailing. I never know when it might happen again or whether he will have vertigo on his feet instead of when he is lying down. Or whether his next faint will be his last, and I will need to resuscitate him.

It was a beautiful autumn day – 23 degrees – and I decided I must go out. So, for 40 minutes I went shopping at the delicatessen for cake and biscuits for Prof R and Italian coffee beans. Plus the things I had forgotten with my delivery order, potatoes, grapes and demerara sugar. And when I got home, I felt so much better.

Prof R needs much more help this week. Tonight we had a 'Laurel and Hardy' style two-hander comedy over the bathroom basin. First, I applied toothpaste to the brush, and once he got his hand to deliver it to his mouth, his tremor did the rest at breakneck speed. Frantic brushing and then the hazardous rinse, when what looked like half the contents of his daily food was splattered across the porcelain. The cup was in Prof R's shaky hand, creating stormy waters that flew everywhere. I became hysterical with laughter, but Prof R just ploughed on single-mindedly. Until I called a halt.

When asked if he was tired after that episode, he said "not especially". I, on the other hand, needed a glass of wine. He is less and less 'with me'.

September 29 — Saturday. The autumn warmth is clinging on. If I can get Prof R outside it's a blessing to get the sunshine on his skin for even just a few minutes. Yesterday we toddled arm-in-arm for 10 minutes in a cool breeze into the park and home again sharpish. But at least it was a walk. There are signs of a recovery of sorts.

This afternoon though, he gazed at me and said, when asked how he felt, that his head "felt empty".

A parcel arrived from Parkinson's UK with a suction-fix handle for the shower wall, and a table knife that resembled a machete – very unsettling – but it is designed to cut with a rocking motion and is so blunt I doubt it will do more than cut cheese. Also in the box were two silicone cup covers with holes for straws. Far better and easier to use we hope than the cheaper version we had bought from Amazon.

On Tuesday, the toilet frames will arrive. Then we can decide what other hand holds are needed. Each day is anything but Groundhog Day. If it were, things would be easier to manage. Or at least predict.

This afternoon he was so rocky, we again needed the stairlift to return upstairs after the tea and cake unbalanced him. I wondered at one point if I would have the strength to support him across the floor to reach the lift. Confidence – or lack of it – contributes to his lack of balance. He is becoming more anxious and asks me to check on him regularly, which I do. And will do now, as I can hear the floorboards creak as I write.

———

So, after barely being able to stand he has just successfully gone to the toilet and looks almost normal. Confidence returns. For both of us. But I won't risk going for a walk.

September 30 — Sunday. Prof R has forgotten the meaning of the word 'sage'. A final insult to him from his disease. I had been trying to tell him a new pun I was pleased with – sage mentality – and it drifted over his head and up into the clouds, even when I tried to explain it.

But he is a little better this morning otherwise, after forgetting his bedtime pill last night. I am now letting this accidental experiment take its course. Perhaps less is more. His tremor is always better in the early part of the day and he can feed himself reasonably easily.

But he can't keep up with my news from 'off'. Who has written and what news they bring. I remain eager to tell him and am only slightly deflated by his lack of response. He enjoys the engagement even if he misses a few beats.

Last night I dreamed he was healthy and his former self – not too long ago. I realise I have missed the intimacy. When I see his body now, I cannot recognize it. Although I still feel very attached to it. When I clean him, it's a new form of intimacy. One where we both giggle if he inadvertently farts in my face.

I seem to have broken his computer in my search for his photos of our house at Brookside (*in New Zealand*). Alex-the-computer-man will need to come back and see if he can retrieve the situation. There is a backup hard disk if all else fails. There will be no confession from me over the dinner table. Prof R would be distressed beyond measure – perhaps. But I have no intention of finding out.

October 1 — Is it bizarre to be excited about mobility aids? We have a shop in the nearby industrial centre, where we bought Prof R's wheelchair prematurely a year ago.

The vet is also there, so I was visiting to buy tic and flea and worming tablets for the dog. On my way home, I decided to see what they have in mobility aids. Prof R needs a walking stick.

It turns out, they have everything we might need and more. They are not just about wheels. Or sticks. Although I bought a lovely ergonomic folding stick for Prof R for under £12. They also have raised toilet seats that look just like normal toilet seats (they have lids) and there are more handrails and shower fittings and shower stools than I could shake Prof R's new stick at.

Plus, the most beautifully designed electric jug that sits on a cradle and tips without having to be lifted. Even though Prof R almost never makes his own tea, I want it. It is as desirable as a new handbag. Producing the same adrenalin pre-purchase buzz. Who would guess? Fortunately, it wasn't in stock.

When Prof R came down for lunch I couldn't wait to show him his new stick, but it was pre-meds, and he was shut down. So I waited patiently, and after three courses of lunch which concluded with carrot cake, he was ready to show some interest.

Surprise! He not only used it, he walked outside confidently and with a quiet pleasure. This I did not expect. In the past, he has been too proud to want any equipment of any kind. We had both felt almost everything was ugly. Not so. Now he has mellowed enough to join me in my appreciation of these designer tools to make his life easier.

—

Last night we finished off the box of chocolates we began the night before. I hate being given chocolates, so naturally, everyone brings them. I put them away and am quite safe from temptation as long as I don't break through the cellophane that protects them from me. But Prof R's life revolves now around an enjoyment of his food. So the chocolates are brought out. There is another box lurking in my office. That will be next.

Of note, the last two nights now there has been one less levodopa in Prof R's regime. Purely because he has forgotten to take his bedtime pill. I am letting this one run. There have been no more faints.

October 2 — Trapped at home waiting for the toilet frames to be delivered. They were unable to give me a 'window', so the dog doesn't get a walk until they have been.

Prof R had his usual schedule of pills last night and was dopey enough to need help on the toilet this morning. I cannot decide whether to cut out one of the overnight pills altogether. He is like a small child when he needs this help. I lie him down and turn him in the bed while I remove his wet pyjama trousers and wash him gently with a medical wet wipe. If asked, he can lift his bottom up to help me adjust his trousers. But he is only semi with me.

The afternoon is warm and fine, but Prof R cannot see or appreciate it. He is lost in his own world today. I am proud to show him I have powered up his two old laptops to find the missing photos, and it is hard to tell whether or not he is able to care. But later, when I asked if he was pleased, he said he thought it miraculous. So, the man is trapped inside the head, but how that feels is a mystery to me.

When I am pleased after achieving something – even cleaning – my first urge is to find something nice to eat and relax with a cup of tea. I know it's emotional eating and I have chewing gum on hand to still the craving, but oh how I want to reward myself this way. A digestive biscuit would do.

Boris Johnson's speech to the Conservative Fringe conference at lunchtime is so engaging I forgot to look for the holes in his arguments. I turn to see if Prof R is enjoying it, but he is gazing, not even into space, but within, and perhaps in danger of fainting again. So I leave Boris and tend to Prof R, helping him up to bed.

—

When I unpacked his old laptops, I admired how meticulously they had been placed in their bags with all the necessary wiring safely stowed. How methodical he always was and how clever with technology. Especially cameras and photographic computer programmes. Always a little anal perhaps. With everything. It was ridiculous to ever hope he would do something quickly. He couldn't jump from A to C to F even when the steps in between were non-essential.

And this, my friends, is how Prof R managed to avoid all housework. He would take an hour to do one room. Although his cooking was wonderful. As long as you were not starving. He is still meticulous in his micro world. The toothpaste and brushes used with care, if unintentionally violently at times, and the hair carefully parted on the left and combed slowly in front of the mirror. The wound still healing on his skull needs to be circumnavigated with care.

Beside the bed are nail clippers and files and an emery board – he prefers a metal one. If I need to cut his toenails for him there is always the right tool for every toenail. We have stopped going to the podiatrist as we seem to have solved our own problems. I with my gel inserts, and he with me to manage it for him.

His middle daughter Rachel rang and asked me if I was writing all this down. When I said yes, she suggested a blog. She felt it is of value to share the knowledge of my experience. She is not the first person to say this, but it doesn't serve me well to put myself out there every day, no matter what the mood. I have told her I want to have time to reflect on these experiences. There are any number of forums for public exchanges. I don't feel the need.

After dinner, at the end of a miserable day for Prof R, I suddenly suggested a walk. It was a beautiful balmy evening – 17 degrees at 7 pm. He said yes, so we did a turn around the block. He took his new stick to practice with it outdoors.

October 3 — Wednesday. How many people admit that caring for a loved one can make them angry? Especially with dementia. Sometimes, in the night, and last night was such a time, Prof R gets confused and gets up and down and cannot settle. Nor can he really process what I am saying to him. I do feel anger – or is it just powerlessness? – at such times. Pointless anger at the illness as much as the person. Anger that is grief in disguise.

And I don't express it openly to him. But I do feel it, and I understand why underpaid staff in care homes get tired and angry and are filmed shouting at a patient. Or are pressured so much by their manager, they become desperate enough to confine a demented patient to the bed, so the next patient will not be neglected.

They are immediately sacked of course, and rightly. And how horrified society is that anyone could do such things to someone powerless. Let them do just one shift in a care home. Then they will understand the professionalism needed. And possibly even be prepared to pay for it.

That is why I don't want to blog. Because I don't think snapshots tell the story of what it is like for people like Prof R and me. The desperation dissolves into love almost immediately when I see, from my side of the bed, him seated, the back of his head towards me, turning it left, and then right, as he wonders what it is he so desperately needs to do.

Why is the back of a loved ones' head so powerfully poignant? I think of his mother when I look at his head. How she must have felt. How his hair grows in whirls or sticks up on his crown. And the duck-bottomed hair at the nape which can never be cut properly.

—

I have just given him his breakfast in bed. But first, I had to help him put his teeth in. I will get better at this and he will gradually be less able to feel his mouth and where they should lodge. While I was gathering cereal onto the spoon, he stroked my hair. I said what he used to say when I stroked him – "purr purr" – and he smiled.

By 1pm he was still in bed and V the carer was due in half an hour to take over while I went to Pilates. My stress levels climbed with me to the first floor and then the second. I hate to wake him. But fortunately, he did it himself, was shoveled downstairs, and presented with lunch, a flatbread stuffed with chicken and rice and avocado.

If V had not been coming, I would have cancelled. But I'm glad I didn't. Today was one of the best Pilates classes I have attended. I came out lengthened, lightened and generally straightened out. And walked on air to the delicatessen.

At home, he was in bed and had barely spoken to V. Disconnected somehow – a few wires pulled out. Is this it? Or is it self-defence?

October 4 — Thursday. After such a bad day, the Parkinson's 'Bad Cop', Mr Parky, continued overnight until I almost begged for sleep.

But this morning, the 'Good Cop' turned up again at 10am, when I had to wake Prof R for his appointment for the ECG and blood tests. Prof R got up, had his breakfast, and allowed me to wash him in private and not so private places, so he wouldn't be smelling of sweat or anything else when he was on the nurse's couch.

Having left the house with the keys of the car, I noticed how strong he appeared to be. So when we reached the car I said, "would you prefer to walk?" and he said yes. Our luck held. No fainting at the sight of blood (his old phobia) nor a violent tremor that prevented the insertion of the needle. The ECG test said 'normal' on the screen.

The Good Mr Parky Cop stayed with us through the walk home and lunch. Now Prof R has gone to lie down, but whoever he is when he wakes up, our job today is done.

October 5 — I want Prof R to wake up. It's 6.30pm and he has been in bed all day. Well, half the day. The first half of the day he was lying on the floor of the bathroom. I had slept through his 6 am trip to the toilet, after a night of watching and waiting during other trips, and then he tripped literally at 6.30 am.

After three hours of believing we could successfully get him up, I had to admit defeat and call an ambulance. They took two hours to arrive, because it was not an emergency, so I was feeding him yoghurt and water and finally a coffee as he lay on his side, the bedspread pushed beneath him, and two dressing gowns on top. The floor is hard. And when he needed to pee, he was able to pee into a bottle for me.

The ambulance crew were, of course, wonderful and for the second time in as many days, Prof R had an ECG. The usual jokes about the number 3 bus. I was so grateful, and so relieved. Until I realized that until I manage this differently, I will never feel safe. The ambulance crew suggested a sensor mattress. Meanwhile, I want to tether myself to him in the night.

Literally 10 minutes after they left, a woman rang to say she was going to fix handles to our back door frame. Could she come in 10 minutes? I said of course, lovely, thank you. She took all of five minutes to arrive, and breezed in with her toolkit and two white metal monster handles that will have been pre-loved by someone who died. We're grateful.

Just now, I will go and see if I can wake him for his meal and a little glass of wine on a tray.

When he thanked me, after the ambulance crew had gone, I said "You need to know that I really want to do this." And he looked a little perplexed when my eyes filled with tears.

October 6 — Saturday. Prof R is being fed in bed. Yesterday he didn't get up and today he is also having his meals between sleeps. So, breakfast and coffee at 11.30 am and then I say, "Would you like anything else?" and almost always he will say yes, but today he said, "I'd like some more soup". That was a surprise. He got risotto from last night instead and was quite happy. Then I said, "Anything else you would like?" and he said, "Ice cream".

While he was eating, I told him about the equipment you can get to avoid injury in a fall. Knickers with pockets in the side for padding to put over your hips. We discussed how this could be expanded. Why stop at the hips? What about the head? The answer might be a shell suit that you could pump up after a fall to allow the person to pop back into an upright position. Rather like Enid Blyton's Wobbly Man, or Michelin Man. There is scope here for some real innovation. And he laughed.

October 7 — Sunday. He doesn't know for sure who I am, as I spoon muesli into his mouth mid-morning. So I ask him what he does know. He said he loves my hair. It's beautiful. And, when pressed, he thinks I am his lover and his wife? "Is the correct answer!" I reply. Which always makes us laugh.

It's been a good night, mainly because the fan in the shower room has malfunctioned. It began late yesterday and sounds like cats fighting, or a pig being slaughtered. After failing to find a switch for it in a remote cupboard that required me to move a chest of drawers, I decided this was actually a piece of good luck. My early warning alarm. As long as we turn off the bathroom light when we leave the room, so that eventually it stops.

And I was right. In the night, even though I sleep on a cliff edge, he often gets to the bathroom before I wake up. But now the blessed 'cats in sacks' in the wall wake me up. So I can supervise. I have no intention of having this intruder silenced until I get a mattress alert.

This flawed fan is so good, that when I came in the front door at 10.30 am after walking the dog, I could hear it at high decibels three floors up. He was up and had peed in the 15 minutes I was out with the dog. He had been sleeping like a baby before we left. But daylight hours are not quite so worrying. He can cope quite well.

He is beginning to wonder what is going on. Why is he sleeping so much? I tell him he is recovering from the fall, but he says, "Where do we go from here?" and I have to lie. "You'll recover from the shock and feel more alert." I will get him up today, even if he sleeps on the couch. Because while he knows he should be more alert, he does love to be fed by me in his bed.

Like him, I am beginning to think this is a turning point, this last fortnight and these two serious falls. He has lost something along the way. I'm still hoping it is temporary, but for how long can we go on?

There's no point making an issue of this decline. His vital signs are perfect, so it is his head that is leaving the room. No doctor on earth can really do anything about it, without serious side effects from some even more awful drug.

—

I wrote to his son yesterday with a smoothed out version of how things are drifting, so he won't panic but hopefully will wake up. I am sure he doesn't want to, and that's his decision. At my age though, I'm wise enough to know it is a decision he will more than likely regret.

October 8 — Now I know why people caring for someone don't have time to clean their houses. Or even finish a cup of tea.

This is a day of so many surprises I'm almost too exhausted to record all of them. Prof R began his day not being able to lower himself onto the toilet and not trusting me to help him. Only half in his head and probably less than half in his body. That might be a generous assessment.

In answer to my question "Why won't you trust me?", he said "I wouldn't trust God". Well, I can understand why he wouldn't trust God. He'd/she'd be no earthly use to anyone.

So, another pee in a bottle. He trusted me enough for that. And later a return to normal, except it's not normal. The shower fan is no longer giving me an early warning. It's finally lost the will to screech. He is up and down from short sleeps and not waiting for me, so I am up and down, trying to beat him to it. He manages, but usually I can rely on him to sleep more and perambulate less.

I ring the Friends and Family alert button suppliers and tell them I think I was too hasty cancelling it. Could they please reinstate the account and reactivate the sim? Whether Prof R knows what it is or how to use it or not, if it is hanging around his neck there must be a chance he may push it in a crisis. And if it isn't a crisis, it doesn't matter, because I am the only person that gets called.

The obvious outcome of all this is that I don't feel it is safe to go out. I call Gemma the Dementia advisor to ask her to look at a bed alarm I want to buy. She is marvellous, looks at the link, and says she thinks it will do the job. So, it is ordered.

Then I'm on the phone to the local Tailor Made Mobility shop to ask if they will deliver. What I want is a male urinal for bed or wherever, and a raised toilet seat. I also think we should have a perching stool for the shower, but they are all so expensive, I feel inclined to fall back on the State before Prof R falls back on the floor.

Mr Mobility didn't sound keen to deliver, although it's only three blocks. No doubt he will if pushed. I don't like the look of his bedpan. I'm going to get one somewhere else. Every time I get underway with one of these online searches I can hear Prof R on the move yet again.

In between, I got a call from a woman who calls herself an Admiral Nurse. They deal with dementia support for carers. Well, she may be admirable, but she was no use to me. I described the morning, the confusion, the inability to handle Prof R due to his Parkinson's with dementia and she said, "I can only advise on the dementia" and I thought "What are you saying, woman? These things come in a package; you can't cherry pick it". So I won't be bothering her.

—

It's only mid-afternoon and I can't believe it isn't midnight. Prof R is quite happy. I've been feeding and watering him with care. He's been downstairs once about an hour after lunch – surprise! – and had some cake and tea and almost immediately needed to go back up. I'm disappearing up my own fundament. It's not a learning curve, it's a bloody climbing wall and I'm short of equipment.

So next up, although I can hear noises off, I want to call the Care Navigator and ask about more wall rails. I don't care now if we look like a hospital on a low budget. I'm not about to get my own rails and then spend a month finding a guy who can be bothered to come and fit them. And I'm not about to get my own toolkit out thank you. Suddenly I really and truly don't have time to do it.

The dog is looking perplexed. No walk. Maybe tomorrow will be better. Maybe I'll need to hire someone to walk her. Maybe I can put her lead on and spin her around in the back garden.

The sun is shining. But I have a song on my mind, an adaptation of "Life can be a dream". "Life can be a bitch, sweetheart, hello hello again, de da de da. "

My alarm watch is telling me to give Prof R another pill.

October 9 — I'm feeling ridiculously self-satisfied. Mainly because I was ridiculously stressed earlier. The new bed sensor is on the bed and I didn't buy the wrong one it seems. The pager is in my pocket and Prof R is back in the bed. He doesn't mind, or doesn't hear, the crackling of the plastic under the blanket beneath the sheet. I could have put it under the mattress, but I don't trust it to work at his light weight.

It's beginning to feel like Christmas. The deliveries have been coming through the door today in multiples. The toilet seat (no lid – so Prof R thinks it's not a proper seat), the bed sensor of course, which sent me scurrying across to the hardware for batteries and a small Phillips screwdriver. Then there is the cup with the spout, and the 'man pan' – or more accurately, the urinal. The man pan has yet to be delivered.

The weather is heavenly. How sad Prof R cannot muster the energy to go outside and absorb some sunlight through his skin, instead of a vitamin D tablet. I sent an email to his girls – not too light, not too heavy – just to prepare them for the decline if he doesn't improve.

He sat in the cane chair while I fitted the sensor at 4 pm and when I asked him how he felt, he said "I feel dead". I have not told his girls this. But I assured him he wasn't and hopefully he might feel better later. All I can do is smile and hug and stroke his face and tell him I love him and that he is safe.

Only the last bit isn't true. No one is safe.

October 10 — Wednesday. An email from Julie.

> 'Dear V, dear Dad.
> I am so sorry that this is all so hard. Please let us know what we can do to support you practically (and of course emotionally). It is a huge thing for you to be trying to deal with more or less yourself V. Is it helpful for us to come down? To relieve you, or just to come and get some shopping in for you? Can he cope with us being there? Does it make it easier or harder? Let us know.
> Sending you so much love xxx'

On the face of it, a friendly, loving, helpful email. But so often I had asked them to visit more often, to sit with their dad, for him if not for me. Not just at the lunch table. I need them to 'own' this man. Not keep making these empty offers. My anger is a wild boomerang bouncing bomb. So I deflect it.

I need to send updates more often. Especially with photographs of Prof R on the floor waiting for the ambulance. I know it's hard for anyone to really know what it is like for him, day to day.

Julie is now coming down to see her father on Monday.

The eldest, Hannah, is coming down on Friday.

The middle daughter, Rachel, has asked if she can visit at the end of the month.

If I could fix their sadness about their relationship with him when they were children I would, but I can't. it is not my job.

—

Pilates today. It is so hard to drag myself to, but so brilliant for my body. V the carer is now to be called V2. It was Prof R's solution. As predicted, two V's was too hard for him to deal with. I think it is so appropriate – V1 and V2. Two flying bombs. Delivering care not explosives.

The bed alarm is wonderful. But didn't seem quite so wonderful when it went off while I was washing my hair in the bath before dinner.

October 11 — Prof R told me last night that he felt the first fall – where he cut his head – had robbed him of a good part of his mind. He feels he has lost a piece of what makes him who he is. These moments of clarity are both encouraging and also appalling. He is deteriorating so fast I sometimes cannot find the energy or the will to keep writing the diary. Although it will be my memento mori. My homage to him.

This morning he has been semi-awake (a nicer term than semi-conscious don't you think?) for an hour or so. I managed to help him to sit sufficiently to get his pills into him without choking. The new cup with the spout is now a godsend.

Yesterday evening I began to hate the alarm. He was up and down and up again and the last time, just before bed, when I was putting the dog out, I ignored it. When I came up a few minutes later he was back in bed and looking surprised. I said, "I was just putting the dog to bed", by way of explanation.

He looks for me now all the time. He wishes I were closer when I am downstairs. I explain that the only way that could happen was if he was able to get up and came down, or if his bed was in the living room. Which neither of us want.

I'm waiting for the grocery delivery man, and then, at 10 am, the Care Navigator. I am wondering if the rails, when fitted, will be used. Just now, Prof R can't get up. I struggle with the stupid urinal which is like a tank for spare petrol. Rubbish design. But he can't pee, and I give up.

The grocery man is at the door. Because I look frazzled, he asks me if I'm fed up with the replacement items and I say "Oh no, I'm not bothered by that. But my husband is in a tricky state upstairs, so I'm rather bothered by that."

Just before the Care Navigator was due, Prof R suddenly and miraculous rose from the semi-coma and entered the bathroom. The alarm told me sleeping beauty had been awakened. I was so thrilled. He did both pee and poo and was back in bed before she knocked. She measured parts of wall in the hall and hugged me and was off.

—

So now it is midday and Prof R was up and getting dressed at 11 am. The first time in almost a week. I have palpitations. I need more B vitamins. Or less, I'm not sure. I used to know how to calm them.

I helped him finish dressing and took him in triumph downstairs for his breakfast. He is now back in bed, but just this minute the alarm went off and I found him looking happy but not sure why he was getting up. Or not getting up as it happened. I have reset the alarm.

October 13 — Saturday. I've been too tired to write. The early mornings are strange. Prof R cannot wake up. Yesterday he peed into a cup. So much easier. Today I simply encouraged him to sit up long enough for me to give him his pills without choking him. And then he lay down again. The spout cup is so much better than straws. He doesn't have to make the effort to suck.

I've noticed that this man, meticulous in his self-care, has begun to wipe his penis with his flannel after peeing, forgetting that he really wants to reach for a neatly folded piece of toilet paper.

The false teeth are causing us both pain. They have metal claws with sharp ends to grip his existing teeth and are difficult to put in. But we can't leave them in overnight, as he used to do, because he can wake up with the bottom set in his hand, or in the bed.

His three wives didn't know he had false teeth when we first married him. He didn't take them out, for fear of horrifying us, and kept them in overnight. Until, some years ago with me, he developed a skin sensitivity – a rash – on the roof of his mouth and had to sleep without them.

—

The slipper bedpan was delivered yesterday. I'm very impressed with it, while hoping we will never need it, or at least, not for a long time. It has joined the dust under Prof R's side of the bed. Vacuuming our bedroom is something I am seldom able to do. It's noisy. And either he is asleep, or I am downstairs with him, or feeding him. I solve this problem by moving the dust around with a long-handled feather duster.

Hannah came down by train for lunch yesterday and sat with her dad while I raced to the chemist for the remainder of his prescription. I haven't really worked out just how much he remembers about her, his lovely daughter. But when she left, he agreed the visit was "magic".

My lunch downstairs, with her for company, created a frenetic burst of fresh energy in me. After she had left, I threw caution to the winds and ran off to the park with the dog to be blown around by the warm autumnal winds. If the alarm went off while we were gone, so be it. It didn't. I had underestimated the loss of Prof R's company. He's still present, with warmth and love and demands. But with little conversation.

Last night I was overtired and overstressed. I have to be careful when that happens. The alarm has created its own particular form of hell. I don't want to turn it off, but I'm going to have to change my attitude towards it. I must step away from the situation and breathe. As they say in all the best and worst self-help books. "You can control your thoughts." I know that. And I'm doing my best. I have remembered the technique. Choose a mantra and use it before sleep or whenever things overwhelm. As I lie down to sleep, I say "I choose love and I choose to be happy". It takes time, but over time, it works.

—

There was a little triumph in the day. One of the knots has fallen (or been pushed) out of a paling of the fence adjoining our semi-detached neighbour. They have a small son who may have helped it along. I found the perfect piece of almost sun-dried dog poo (provenance known) on the patio and made a little patch from it. It fitted perfectly, with the help of some smoothing and patting with the trowel. Perhaps the addition of a little straw would have made a proper girl guide job of it, but we'll see how it goes.

—

As if in answer to an atheist's prayer, today, Saturday, has been peaceful. Few alarms, lots of sleeping and eating. Breeeaaathe out. I have been lying on the bed next to him chatting or just dozing. I told him about Peter Jackson, the film director, who has been tasked with reconstructing WW1 archive film from the Imperial War Museum in London. He has used authentic colour and 3-D to bring the archive right into focus in our own time. It will be broadcast on the BBC so Prof R can see it.

His hands are beginning to look like my mother's before she died. Long lean fingers and loose rings.

Mid-afternoon peace is broken by a call from his sister. Can they visit? Of course. But when I tell Prof R, he doesn't want to see them. Fortunately, that will be easy to manage, now that he is virtually bedridden. We who are not bedridden sit outside for tea and cake. It's still glorious weather. Like summer.

Later, after they have gone, I race the one block between us and the park to catch the Carnival parade floats preparing for the evening's event. I'm surprised and shocked to see that all of them – perhaps 10 or more – are glass boxes filled with young women from all over Kent dressed as princesses and presumably Queens. Like little beehives on wheels, being towed by a variety of friends and family vehicles. The symbolism was a bit disturbing, but it was a wonderful photo opportunity.

The fireworks at 9 pm woke Prof R.

October 14 — Sunday. A dopey morning again, with me essentially force-feeding him his pills before helping him to eventually sit on the toilet, where he, after sitting there for an age, while I dressed, didn't pee. And was eventually helped back to his bed with no result. I've learned not to worry. If he pees, he pees, and he will when his body wakes up sufficiently.

1.00 pm. I have begun to worry in spite of myself and have had to wake him. Gently and quietly. The first words he says to me are "I need to pee". Which doesn't surprise me but does please me. And we manage it between us.

But he only manages muesli with grapes and a few mouthfuls of coffee before a last pee and back to sleep. Should I be reducing the levodopa? Or would that reduce his mobility? Overnight, because he woke so infrequently, the dosage was normal. Either way, halves or wholes, he sleeps. But now I am not afraid for a few hours at least.

The bed alarm goes off at 3 pm and that is a good sign. He is more awake and mobile. But when I ask him what he would like he says, "I want you". So I ask if he is hungry, and he's not sure. I forget about savoury and jump straight to sweet. "How about ice cream?"

He's had his ice cream now with sweet fruit cake mixed in and doesn't know if he wants anything else. He's not happy with his own performance, and pronounces "I feel like I am dying". I feel like he is dying too, but I say it is only his head that is misbehaving, reminding him that all his vital signs – heart, blood pressure, pulse – are top notch. He is having a sleepy day. "It doesn't seem to be worthwhile living like this", he says. Perhaps he is reading my mind after all. To comfort without lying – that is a line to walk with care.

I remind him that Julie is coming to visit tomorrow for lunch. "Who is Julie?" But with help he does remember.

We are both in a vacuum. Our own isolation pod, with oxygen and water and food and not much else. I don't know what to eat either. I am both hungry, and not hungry. Slightly nauseous and headachy. I eat boiled eggs and humus. And I don't feel like cheese. I never don't feel like cheese. This afternoon I made popcorn to make the dog happy too. I've not walked her today. If I think about the evening meal my mouth turns to dust.

The sky is very dark as the weather waits, trying to turn, but it is still warm. The bed alarm goes again. I resettle him after a pee without giving him his half pill at 4 pm. I want to see if it makes any difference.

It turns out it might. Soon after 4 pm and he's agitated. So much so, he is talking about wanting to kill himself. Although he is confused about what is really wrong with him. Questions. What is this for? Why are we here? And when I grabbed this bull by the horns to disempower it, and said, "How would you kill yourself"? he said he would throw himself downstairs. And I said, "You can't do that to me". Which he agreed.

After several sorties from his bed, I persuaded him to come downstairs. This I need to do more often, even if he doesn't want to. Then he can reattach himself to the real world. There was an early dinner, cobbled together in a rush.

He wanders into the kitchen while I am cooking. He's at risk of falling, which I tell him firmly. How can I cook and help him move safely? So I escort him back to his chair. Inside I'm as agitated as he is. Furious in fact, almost kicking a freezer drawer into submission when it sticks. He has a glass of wine and ice cream as usual. Now at 6.50 pm I have just settled him back in bed and promised to return in half an hour.

Twenty minutes later the alarm goes off and he is either looking for me or in the toilet. The evening turns into a marathon of my patience versus his inability to settle. I lay next to him in the bed for 10 minutes on one trip and waited till he went to sleep.

But 20 minutes after I crept away, he woke up. Now it is 9 pm and I'm so tired I'm going to bed too. I can hear him snoring as I climb the stairs. I'm not waking him for his bedtime pill.

This is a day to forget.

October 15 — I was nervous about Julie's visit. So to resolve that, I decided to be honest. When she walked through the door, I told her I wanted to understand. Why did they keep asking if it was okay for them to visit? In spite of my repeated invitations. At first, she said they didn't want to make it harder for me. But I said why? Why is it different to visiting their dad as if he were in a care home, or a hospital? It's not about intruding on me. Although I also said I understood that for them, it was more complicated. That I knew he could be a distant parent.

And so she told me how it had been for her. The absent father, who always seemed more like an uncle. Who left when she was a baby, and had serial relationships until she was a teenager, when he finally married his second wife. For the girls, and it seems for his son too, he was never able to be the sort of father they needed. So she, in self-defence, to avoid more hurt, had withdrawn. She still loved him very much, but it had become necessary for her to set boundaries.

The truth is somewhere in between of course. I know he made a second home for them wherever he was living. That in the early years, as pre-schoolers, they spent two nights a week with him and his partner Pam. That he taped bedtime stories for them to listen to when he wasn't with them. That he took them to classes on the weekends and on holiday in the summer. But of course, it isn't enough.

When she left, (before lunch, thoughtfully), she just said "Keep in touch". No change in the wind then. The arrow still points at me. I will not pressure them to visit.

Since lunch, he has been setting off the alarm every 10 minutes. When I asked if he had enjoyed Julie's visit and if he had remembered who she was, at first he said no. But when I expanded with prompts, he said "I haven't seen her for years". The girls have left their run too late.

—

The new urinal arrived and is a success. Well, until we try it. At least it has a penis-shaped entrance, which is encouraging. I have ordered a wedge bed cushion.

Prof R has had a proper bed bath with a warm flannel and water-free bath lotion. I also did his hair. It's the first full hair wash since he cut his scalp. After what felt like his tenth trip to the loo, I asked him if I could please go and wash my own hair without him setting off the alarm. He has given me the thumbs up. Last time, I had to leave the bath with a towel and wet hair to answer the infernal alarm.

It seems to me that as our world diminishes incrementally, the diary entries expand. The day is full of tiny events that collectively could floor me.

The lanyard with the yellow button he will probably forget to push is now around Prof R's neck. It's for the real emergencies, so I can leave the bed alarm to bleep for a while. It bleeped for too long tonight and he was needing a wipe. "But not quite yet." The waiting for him to finish seems like an age. Do I meditate? Or read? I can do better than this terrible impatience.

October 16 — Two words. Manual handling. I'm getting better, but the need is greater. He trusted me this morning to lower him onto the toilet and I didn't disappoint him. Carefully, carefully, cleaning him and putting clean pyjama pants on him in bed, while I bend my knees and not my back. But if he can't raise his bottom, it's impossible.

I have two hours later today to do whatever I like. No Pilates. I'm quite excited. But I need to go to the vet to get the dog's medications and to the mobility shop for another spout cup. Then I will try out the new café on the park.

Skin and bone. I've been trying to wake Prof R, but he is not responding. His breastbone protrudes from his chest in an alarming way.

V2 is not realising how things really are. "He seems to have lost ground since I began coming here." Surprise! All that drama we had over the past month, he taking to his bed almost totally, seems to have somewhat escaped her.

The difficulty is the short time she is here. If he is sleeping, she really can't assess him. I expect too much of her. I had hoped she would be proactive and full of knowledge I don't have. When she arrived today, I had reached the ice cream course for his lunch. All of it eaten in bed. I asked her to give him his ice cream, so I could go out, and she said, reluctantly, "If he is happy for me to do that". To which I, surprised and nonplussed, said "He'll have to be". Otherwise, why hire her? is the unspoken part of that conversation.

We've negotiated two extra hours on a Friday morning. She is too committed to do more. That will be enough anyway. Prof R's Attendance

Allowance will cover it but no more. We have to conserve this expense. Much more is to come, and by then I would prefer someone with a nursing background. V2 would be inclined to call an ambulance in any situation that's 'off book'.

When I got home yesterday, I felt exhausted rather than refreshed. I must learn to relax.

—

Peeing in a cup in the morning, when his head is elsewhere, has become the norm. He can stand at the handbasin in the bathroom, but it's a step too far to reach the toilet and sit down. We're good at this, but the urinal will be the only way to pee if he can't get out of bed.

By early afternoon his head had cleared and at 3.30 pm he came downstairs for the remainder of his lunch and some ice cream. A brief time of relative clarity, although, when asked how he felt, he said "lost". Me too. We sit in companionable silence.

Dinner, we decided, would be better enjoyed upstairs. So I fed him as usual, before having my own. Radio 3 is my latest brainwave. When I first met him, he always listened to music to go to sleep, a coping mechanism that helped him after his wife died. Now may be a good time to see if it still does.

Then I made the mistake of asking him if he would like a TV. He seldom watches it downstairs now, so I felt on safe ground. Wrong. He loves the idea. I'm just hoping he will forget about it. This man for whom a remote control is now an equally remote memory, is best without another reason to summon his wife. Although I've no objection if he summons V2.

October 17 — To wake him or not to wake him, that is the question. If the last levodopa I gave him was at 6 am – a half dose because of regular meds during the night – I am fretting by 10 am. I begin by washing his face, but that doesn't wake him. This mid-morning semi-coma requires a different approach. I can't just wait for the alarm to go off. I must be vigilant. He cannot necessarily get up even when he wakes. Today I was there when he woke and was able to persuade him to sit on the toilet. He was hungry but couldn't stay awake to finish his muesli and grapes. I promised to return when he is less tired, to give him a coffee and more grapes.

The dog got a 10-minute sprint to the park at 9 am. I'm lucky she is not the athlete I was warned she would be.

Surprise!! The nightmare of his disordered brain became clear at about 2 pm when I found two conjoined pills, side by side, half melted, in the spout of his drinking cup. He was more than two sandwiches short of a picnic. And he didn't want the sweet potato soup I had made him. If I can just keep him in bed for more than 20 minutes his head may settle and his toilet habits along with it.

I have emailed the Carer Support team to ask for a reassessment of our care needs. I can't wait until we/I see the GP on the 30th. I'm barely coping physically when his needs are greatest. And mentally, I am barking orders in an effort to get through. It could be a formula for despair, but it cannot be allowed to get to that point.

October 18 — Friday. We have lost V2. The job got too hard for her. Her training certification was not sufficient. Not that we knew that. What she actually *does* do is still a mystery to me. But I have asked her if she knows someone who actually *is* trained. I should apply for certification myself. I must be at least two-thirds qualified.

My sister Stella should be able to give me my master's course. She has been texting me all the things she thought V2 should have been able to do. And she was right. But things have moved fast in the last six weeks or so. Stella has also been asking me about the shower, and is not impressed I am bed-bathing Prof R. But I'm playing catch up still.

The Care Navigator, K, turns out to be my best resource. Unexpectedly, when asked, she can produce a shower chair. Not a stool Prof R could fall off, but one with arms and a back. It will be here in five days.

—

So now I have Stella arriving on 29th and I have no one to care for Prof R while I pick her up from the airport. But later I have the solution. A taxi. The combined cost of paying V2 and my train fare are equal to a door-to-door chauffeur service. No hassle, no bag carrying, no worrying about getting back here before V2 has to depart. No worry that she will not feed Prof R in bed. I am so relieved I can't believe it. To be happy that V2 has resigned. That is interesting.

The day continues fair and calm. No drama, no falls (at least by 8.30 pm) and some actual conversation with Prof R. He is alert and understands the issues with the carer. It's the first proper conversation we've had, and I know it will be rare in future. But a magical interlude to simply enjoy.

October 20 — Saturday. I've seen that look before. A direct and unfriendly stare. The first time was in the first year of our marriage. It is when he is feeling defensive.

Today he simply doesn't know me. At 7.15 am, when he should be asleep, and I was taking a bath and washing my hair, the alarm goes off. I go upstairs half-dressed and with a towel on my head. He doesn't answer my call through the bathroom door, so I pop my head around. Big mistake. Angry response. After another half hour of either angry looks or angry flailing, and not recognising me, he is back in bed and calms down. And when I bring up a cup of tea, he is mercifully asleep.

I gave him his breakfast at 9 am because he was awake again. I don't ask him if he knows me this time and I don't enter the bathroom. He happily eats all his breakfast, which is laced with St John's Wort and Slippery Elm. And drinks his re-warmed cup of tea. Before dozing off.

It's 10 am. Coffee time.

—

Feeding him his evening meal – stir fry vegetables and rice noodles – I said, "Tell me when you have had enough" and he said, "About 10 minutes ago." I should be pleased he can still be so sarcastic, but I'm not.

Earlier today he was nicer. When I said to him "Poor boy" he said, "Poor girl". He knows it isn't easy for both of us. But he cannot stop himself taking it out on me sometimes. I have begun, when pushed, to say "Wait till my sister gets here", like some frustrated stay-at-home parent longing for their spouse to return from work.

October 22 — Monday. Feeling less obsessed, calmer and happy after my little family visited yesterday. A perfect autumn day, a loving son and daughter-in-law, and two little girls with runny noses. I don't care. If we get their colds, we do.

I think some of this calmness comes from feeling that progress is being made. Things are happening, all is not lost. This morning a man from a company who "gives back" came to put the handles on the door of our shower room. We chatted loudly and long, and his drill whirred happily while Prof R slept on, oblivious. When he sleeps, he sleeps.

I have applied for the Social Services assessment for Prof R and a carer from a private company for me. We have too much in savings to qualify for any subsidised care. But that is an empowering thought. We can have real choice if we are paying, said the eternal optimist.

—

My sister looks forward eagerly to Prof R being on a hospital bed in the living room where he can be cared for more easily. As the person who just paid £8,000 for the stair lifts, I have a different view. But I'm not saying anything. I am just so glad she is coming.

I am also the person who wants to sleep in the same room as my husband. And the same bed. So he can reach out and I am there. Does no one understand how important that is to him? And to me? How frightened he would be if he was alone, with only a bed alarm for company?

This afternoon he's looking a bit puzzled so I say, "Do you know who I am" and he says, my name, triumphant. He thinks he is on safe ground. But when I am washing him with Nilaqua he says, "Are you my wife?" I laugh and say yes, and "I'm still learning how do this bed bathing lark. So bear with me."

—

I've swapped Radio 3 for Classic FM. It's so much friendlier, although the downside is the ads. While we had afternoon tea the most beautiful and familiar music began to play which made me want to cry. I had to wait till the end to hear what it was. *Finlandia* by Sibelius. It's dangerous to listen to beautiful music with Prof R. Although he is untouched fortunately.

As I kissed him and went off to make the evening meal I said, "Make sure you only kiss your wife" and he checked in with me again "You are my wife?" and we laughed. He has been instructed he is not to kiss my sister or any other caregiver he encounters.

October 23 — Tuesday. Trying to talk to my Sydney son, Douglas, but his signal keeps dropping out. We haven't spoken for weeks. I email but he's a receiver mostly. Not much transmission. What my father used to call a 'dead letter box', although the saying doesn't translate well to email and text.

Prof R was up at 12.30 am (levodopa), 4 am (levodopa), then downhill with 5 am, 6 am (at which point I gave him a rivastigmine) and 7 am when I gave him the levodopa.

He re-joined me in spirit eventually, and was awake at 7.45 for a cup of tea. I left a digestive biscuit on his side table. Usually, it would end up in the bedside drawer. But when I left the room to dress, he ate it. Another surprise. Usually, I will dunk biscuits or hand him small pieces.

A phone message to say the shower chair will be delivered on Thursday. Will I be in? I phone back to say I'm 'bound' to be in, which amuses them. Any time between 9 am and 6 pm they will knock on the door. Heaven help me if I am having a pee at the time. Or worse, Prof R is having a poo.

The hunt is on for a new carer. The first company I call, *Your Choice*, sound very efficient but charge £31 an hour. On the plus side, they do have male carers. But we could only afford to have them for three hours a week at that rate. I am trying to keep within Prof R's attendance allowance of £80 a week so that we are not in danger of having to touch more capital at this stage. Perhaps I am being over-cautious.

The second company, *Vanguard*, sounded as though they had set up in business last week under a railway arch, but on closer questioning, may be the one we settle for. They charge £19.50 per hour, which is still expensive but would give us an extra 1.5 hours a week. I could manage with that. They are to ring and make an appointment to visit, but only after I requested it. Otherwise, they would have sent someone 'sight unseen'. This poor standard of administration is not necessarily a reflection on the people who work for them.

So I tell myself.

—

Prof R lunches in bed, and the more I study him the more I think he does need the extra stimulus others will provide to help him want to exit the bedroom.

October 24 — Wednesday. What will happen when Prof R can no longer swallow his pills? This morning, he was difficult to wake and I was desperate to get his pills into him, so I got him to drink and swallow while lying propped up on a slope on his side. Less chance of a choke. The pills were staying lodged stubbornly in his mouth. He was chewing them. They're not meant to be chewed. I kept putting water into his mouth in the hope of washing them down. And then began to laugh. He sticks his tongue out to show me bits of pill casing in multi colours. I hope they don't burn his mouth.

It's time to order my own thyroxine prescription and my first instinct was to panic. I have registered for online, but they have never contacted me to set it up. Eventually the answer came to me – and now I have posted it. There is a little ancient post box set in the wall on the corner a hundred yards down the street. I can do this without leaving Prof R for more than 5 minutes. Just being out in the street made me feel exhilarated. Stella will be here when I need to pick them up. These problems will be solved when we have a new carer.

—

It's taken me almost two years but I am beginning to get used to the idea of a hospital bed in the living room. At first, the very thought made me feel physically sick. I made the care assessor laugh today when I told her that story. She had come to update herself on our ever-changing situation here. I am having to think about the future and what I will do. Our capital is diminished.

<hr/>

We had exited our New Zealand house in 2009 to return permanently to the UK, but I knew even then we needed to move nearer to the children. Nearer to everything. Here we lived in a village enslaved by the car. Without one, or without the health to drive one, you've had it.

Prof R was adamant he would not move. I understood he was tired, that the move from New Zealand had been a major one. But our finances were healthy. We had done well with the house sale. We had £150,000 in capital and a mortgage-free if modest cottage.

But I have a little weakness. It is, that when someone else wants something really badly, I tend to cave in. So instead of moving, we set about making the cottage into a real home. We bought some more land from a neighbour for a garden. Then extended the house. It cost a small fortune and the robber who made off with the bulk of it was our builder, who under-quoted, and was unperturbed about switching onto a daily rate once he had removed the end wall of the house. At the end of the process, I asked him what he would have done if we'd been unable to pay the over-run and he said, "I was worried that if I quoted you the real cost you wouldn't have hired me." How I've regretted not recording that conversation.

Eventually, the house owed us about £360,000. More in fact, but I stopped counting. And when, ultimately, we had to sell, and eventually actually *could* sell it, in 2017, time was running out for Prof R's health to allow it. We got £280,000 for the house. And spent all that to get the next one. Let that be a lesson to you. Fortunately, we still had our emergency fund.

***

We've had a good day. Prof R slept a lot, so that when he was awake, I had the energy and the patience to just be with him, feeding him, helping him clean his teeth, putting oil in his ears to soften the wax. All very chummy little things to do when passing the time on a sunny afternoon.

Now I'm trying to dry my hair and write this at the same time. His alarm is now wide awake and interrupting me constantly. When I go upstairs with my hair awry, he looks at me bemused. This does not increase my confidence, but it's beginning to affect it less.

He came down for dinner – such a treat for me. Even if it is more stressful. I ask him to stay seated while I'm in the kitchen and he says yes, and then I see him wander across the room without his stick. I don't want him to lose his confidence either, but I'm prepared to risk that to avoid calling 999.

October 25 — Thursday. Social Services phoned to book an initial assessment of Prof R's needs. It feels as though we are heard, even if that is the last we will hear for a long time. We have savings and need to be prepared to use them. There is a serious shortage of care in the community.

Prof R's sister who lives 10 minutes down the road and didn't visit for six months is now texting every day. I'm glad, but why now? Perhaps finally she knows he is not well enough to visit them. She thought I was just making excuses.

I have an obsession with 'nether regions'. Specifically, Prof R's nether regions and their freshness. A new larger bottle of Nilaqua arrived from Boots, the foaming kind, and Prof R stood obediently while I lathered him up. He is meticulous when peeing but there is something mysterious that happens which makes his pyjamas smell after only a few toilet trips. Pull ups will be next. I don't think he will mind. He is happy to be pampered and loved up.

1 pm. The shower seat has just been delivered. It is light and white and easy to manoeuvre. Who said NHS equipment was the cheapest and nastiest available? Not me. But I might leave it until tomorrow to test it. I'm rather tired.

Truly Loving Carers, third on our list, have rung to say that a) they are pleased to say they can provide care, and b) they have male carers. One in particular she is sure we would like. But c) they will confirm all that later today. They are also the best value for money, at £18.50 per hour. I am remarkably buoyed up about that.

———

In the night, at about 1 am, I started to worry about how much pension I will get when Prof R has gone. I was so worried I got up and made a cup of tea.

First thing this morning I went online and logged into Prof R's work pension account, to see if there was a calculation, but there wasn't. Each one is individual I suspect, and dependent on what criteria they are operating with when the time comes. I am going to guess about 40 percent.

If I want to rent or buy a tiny flat in London near the children, I will struggle to afford it without spending all my capital. Unless I am able to get a job. Or I rent this house out and use the income. But it's unlikely Prof R's children will want to wait for this part of their inheritance.

Now may not seem to be the right time to worry, but somehow my instincts tell me that it is. And my eldest son agrees. He has exchanged upbeat texts with me, and I feel much better.

October 26 — Friday. Prof R came down for dinner again last night and enjoyed it. He even watched half a documentary by Brian Cox on the universe. A safe topic.

But this morning at 7.45 am he was 'out of it' and hard to reach. I struggled to help him achieve a seat on the toilet, and we did. No peeing in a cup. At 10.30 am he was still fairly confused. But by lunchtime all was well.

I am practicing, when lifting him, holding my back straight and bending my legs. *(Skills picked up in London in 2002; for a freelance magazine article about a course run by Olympic weightlifter, Precious McKenzie.)*

—

At last, I have succeeded in securing what I hope will be a good carer for Prof R, a young man called Archie. Easy to remember, as the dog next door has the same name. We will meet him next Tuesday along with his employer, a woman called Claire from *Truly Loving Carers*.

If this much can be achieved while my sister is here, and beyond, we will feel much more secure. I have been assured that this is an agency you can call at fairly short notice. So much easier than V2, who was unable to be flexible at all. Even when it came to feeding Prof R his ice cream.

The hero of this story, Prof R, came down at 4 pm. A welcome departure; but not reliable. And here is where I have to admit how much I do rely on him being in his bed for reliable parts of the day. Or at least in a place where I will know if he gets up and moves. It is harder to manage this sometimes downstairs.

We looked at the photo album until his tremor reached take-off velocity, and I realised he was finding it all too much. And so was I. For him, it is sensory overload of one kind, and for me it is the same. The struggle to discover what he wants and how to help him achieve it. To find the right language.

He asked to go back upstairs, and when he got there, he asked me how long I had known the family. Momentarily, my place in his world had again dropped out of sight. When he retrieved me, he was so relieved and delighted I assured him it was worth the forgetting for the sheer joy of him remembering me again.

But truthfully, I had thought this; "He could remember his first wife in the album and his second wife but now he has forgotten the wife who has been with him the longest time."

As I left the bedroom to go downstairs to prepare dinner, I asked him not to get up again as I had things I needed to do. He said, "Why not?" and it was a reasonable question. Why shouldn't he get up? If we were not alone in the house, someone could be with him and he would be in less danger of a fall.

And I can hear the beep beep of his bed alarm one floor up. He has got it into his head that he can get up again, and he has. I can hear him moving around. I will go up and sneak a look to see if he gets back into bed safely without letting him know I am snooping. The double beep tells me he has landed safely.

Sometimes when I am as tired as I am now, I feel close to desperation. I can cope 99 percent of the time, but a few blips and I am off the radar.

October 27 — Saturday. Three-hourly wakeups overnight have inexplicably led to a good calm communicative breakfast at 9.30 am. He had his rivastigmine and morning levodopa at 6.00 am. Success today at any rate.

We talked about the sensory overload he had yesterday while looking at the photo album. He couldn't really describe the feeling, just that he desperately wanted to look at the whole album but simply couldn't deal with it. This is something we need to consider when my sister is here, and we want to take Prof R out in the wheelchair.

I will use his tremor as a coping litmus test.

And then he surprised me again. After another album session – this time in bed after lunch, which didn't seem to tire him – he was up and looking for his clothes. So I helped him dress and ride the rail downstairs. And then he set about looking to be entertained.

This is something I am not trained for. Spending awake time with a man who knows he would like to do something, but doesn't know what. Today though, his memory is switched to almost-good. He knew who all his wives were. He wanted to help me do something. But didn't want to go for a walk. It's as though he remembers that it was fun being downstairs with me once, but now he can't remember why. Neither do I.

I explain that what I do downstairs now is not very exciting. Managing the house, writing emails, this diary, dealing with the food, the dog or just chilling out reading or watching TV. (I didn't tell him I watch American sit-coms back-to-back).

All this is because we no longer go out. But we could if he wanted to. No doubt Stella would make him go out. I can't do that to him. It's cruel and shows no respect for him as a person.

It makes me so nervous now when he is downstairs, unless I can watch him constantly. I'm more afraid of another fall than he is, and he demonstrates his confidence by continually getting up and strolling around the room without his stick, unless I press it into his hand. Should

I be less vigilant? I've no idea. Except I know who has to dial 999.

When it was time to cook the meal, I asked him to please sit on the couch and not move. I put *Simon Reeve in the Mediterranean* on the TV and miraculously he stayed there watching until dinner time. We ate ludicrously early for us, 6 pm. But it didn't matter. He retired at 7 pm and the alarm went off just a few times. Why do I still get the muscle 'burn' given how often I climb the stairs?

October 28 — Sunday. There seems to be a correlation between a good day downstairs and a bad night upstairs. It wasn't every three hours last night, it became every 20 minutes until, at 4 am, I asked him to please stay in bed. That he didn't need the toilet, but I knew he was agitated. And then he calmed down. And we both slept.

I had decided to ignore the change back from daylight saving at 2 am. I was not going to mess up our routine with an hour change to the med schedule and our appetites.

And so I began the day still on summertime, until I realised my hybrid smart watch had changed itself overnight and I had been operating on wintertime after all. I didn't realise this until I saw the kitchen clock, which isn't smart.

I've decided it's time I behaved like other people do on a Sunday and stay in my pyjamas until 10 am. So I've done that, but it's only 9.20 am, and I have breakfasted, watched two episodes of *Hot in Cleveland*, had my coffee, got dressed, and taken Prof R's breakfast upstairs ready for him to wake. And written in this diary.

With so much time in hand, I'm going to finish washing the floor of the spare room for my sister, who is now in the air and on her way to Dubai. I'm wondering how I will be able to pay the taxi man while I cry all over her at the same time.

Meanwhile, I have achieved a degree of expertise in dental technology.

Prof R's bottom dentures have metal clasps, pointed and lethal looking and hurting him. I took to the main offender with a pair of pliers and the client is very pleased. Given these teeth would cost a fortune to replace if I made a mistake, I'm very relieved.

October 29 — Monday. 12.55 pm and I am waiting for Stella. Heart in mouth after a terrible night with Prof R and an almost as terrible morning trip to the toilet. He definitely seems to have bad nights after an evening downstairs.

Last night there was confusion once tiredness set in and the dinnertime levodopa had worn off. "How many times have I seen you in the last 5 years?"

I have to do better at communicating information to him. I'm spontaneous in my approach, eager to tell him things. But when there is too much 'incoming' he gets lost in the noise. I did it again last night, trying to tell him that his cousin Geoff had visited his sister Doris for lunch. He began to ask when the guests were expected, and I knew I had overshot the runway.

Overnight he was awake off and on, up and down, for about three hours from midnight. Until I wanted to cry, and might have felt better if I had. Prior to that, I had insomnia and used it to fix the upper stair lift at 11 pm. It needed a manual shift onto its charge point. This was a first for me, so I felt triumphant but still sleepless when I succeeded.

And this morning we had one of those episodes when he cannot follow my guidance in the bathroom — where to hold on, how to sit, until I physically moved him down into a sitting position to avoid disaster and apologised afterwards. He understood it was about safety, but not how to contribute.

It's been peaceful since then, with a nice break for his breakfast and a wash, and me happily polishing the living room floors and furniture and finding all the dirty corners in the kitchen. I think I am ready. Although I look awful, I know she won't look or feel much better after 30-something hours in the air.

I've just discovered the toilet cistern in her bedroom is leaking at the back.

October 31 — Wednesday. Our saviour flew in and was transported to us by taxi, so there has been no time to write in the diary.

Prof R remembered her, and the dog fell instantly in love. (It was not reciprocated). She and I have talked non-stop and interviewed the possible caregiver, Archie. He visited with the agency assessor, and I learned more about the realities of care in an hour than I could have believed.

They needed to do a mobility test with Prof R, and I got him out of bed to run through his paces. It made me feel his vulnerability acutely, to a degree that brought tears to the back of my eyes. But he did well.

And then the bad news. Again. If their client falls, they don't pick them up. Even if you are there to help. So, there will be no respite from the two-hour wait for an ambulance when they are in charge.

And who knew they cannot give a client medication from a pill dispenser? It has to be in its original packaging. Preferably blister pack and nothing older than a month.

And who knew that they would need 24 hours' notice if medication is to be dispensed?

But I think Archie is going to be good, despite these restrictions. He has said he will do any tasks required if Prof R is sleeping. He does not expect to sit on the couch and read for £20 an hour. And I'm hopeful Prof R will let himself be showered.

Stella has finally been able to get out today to explore the town alone. This can be the very best way to discover somewhere. We can wait for our time to go out together.

November 1 — Thursday. I am shell-shocked. Pro B's middle daughter Rachel visited today, and Prof R was ill enough to upset us both, which was bad enough. Then she asked if I'd had help with financial planning, and I said, "That was done long ago. Didn't Hannah tell you she has shared Power of Attorney with me for dad?" No, Hannah had not told her.

And so somehow began the apparent need to explain. The savings that were available for Prof R's care, her wondering if the government had the right to take money from the family home, once Prof R's savings had dried up. It was hard to know what she expected. Why the inquisition? She frightened the hell out of me.

The conversation, while upsetting, gave me an opportunity to do something else. A gift of sorts. I told her that she and her siblings would have priority when Prof R's funeral was being planned. They were his children. He belonged to them too. We both cried. And hopefully a bad day was made a little better for both of us.

But Stella asked me, when Rachel had left, if she thought I would have any relationship with them when Prof R has gone, and I said then, "No, I don't think so". (*Happily I was wrong.*)

At around midnight it struck me that I need to review my Will. So if I died unexpectedly before Prof R, only his half of the house could be accessed by Social Services for his care. My estate, and a small inheritance for all the children, would be safe. Thank you Rachel for shaking my little grey cells.

November 2 — Friday. Archie came and conquered. He is perfect for Prof R and for me. After an hour or so, settling him in, Stella and I went to the market. He will come three days next week for two hours each day. Problem solved. Prof R is very happy with the new arrangement.

But always, always, something new happening. Prof R did not come down for a meal today. I have to feed him first before Stella and I can eat.

And that includes ice cream and a chat. It can't be rushed. Or we will be interrupted by the insistent alarm.

I've learned to make a judgement about when to allow him to go to the toilet without my interference.

Saturday 3 — Stella cooked our meal. Pasta and a tomato and olive sauce. What a joy.

Sunday 4 — Letter to Prof R's eldest...

> *Dear Hannah,*
>
> *I just want to reassure you, as I told Rachel, that dad has savings available for spending on his care.*
>
> *Rachel asked me about Social Services being able to access the funds in the house. If I look after him here, and self-fund with perhaps Social Services adding funding later, they cannot take funds from the house.*
>
> *Or at least, that is my understanding!! I have read the relevant info on Social Services site and you may wish to as well.*
>
> *It's something I did worry about, but I am sure I can make his savings stretch.*
>
> *Lots of love*
>
> *V*
>
>
> *PS: Rachel had no idea you had joint Power of Attorney with me.*

Impossible to co-ordinate three daughters and a son if they do not co-ordinate themselves. I am keeping my plans for saving my half of the house for them if I die to myself. If the worst happens to me, let it be a pleasant surprise.

—

Prof R did well last night and managed to reach the toilet, with my help, this morning. It may be that I am improving my technique. I have slowed down to match his speed, whatever that may be. It is so much less stressful. But I can still move fast when I have to. It was inevitable that at some point the alarm would go off when I myself was on the toilet.

My exhausted sister is still asleep at 8.30 am. Normally she's up with the lark.

November 5 — Monday. The sort of day I would prefer to forget. Prof R woke late morning, confused and with muscles that refused to respond. He was desperate for the toilet, stood up, grabbed the handrail, but could or would not use the urinal or a cup. And I could not safely move him to the bathroom. So he became angry when I told him he must sit down.

It was all about his bowels. He needed to move them, and they were log-jammed. At one point I called for Stella to help, but she could not hear, and I could not trust Prof R not to get up the minute I left the room.

When he was finally able to move safely, about 30 minutes after having his pills, I helped him as he strained, and resorted to removing by hand (gloved of course) what he could not shift. We had two sessions like that during the middle of the day. And eventually he seemed comfortable. This has not happened before. And now I feel somewhat better qualified in personal care. Who knew what a gloved digit could do?

The rest of the day was calmer, and he seemed to forget the nightmare of the hours before. He has eaten and slept. And a few hours later, I found him emerging from the toilet, shocked but relieved, just like Rudyard Kipling at Mafeking. The torpedo had finally left the tube. (She says, mixing her metaphorical conflicts).

I made a fish pie, and it was a triumph, so all is not lost.

Tomorrow Archie is due to come for two hours. I will take Stella to Whitstable.

November 6 — I have no idea what to ask Archie to do while Prof R is sleeping. Today, I managed to come up with vacuuming the downstairs. But that's not clever. He could miss the alarm. Tomorrow what? Stella suggests cleaning the inside of the windows. To me, that just means everything off the windowsills and the job half done before he is summoned upstairs by the alarm.

Whitstable was a treat, but we overshot on the return deadline. Traffic and a custard pie were to blame. Archie gained 30 minutes on his logged time.

Tomorrow I am taking Stella to Macknade's Farm shop. She cooked both lunch and dinner. Luscious trays of roasted veg and bacon.

<hr>

October 17 2020 — A parade of carers, two by two, crossing the courtyard in front of my new cottage. Doing all the things for my neighbour that I did for Prof R. Four times a day, like penguins, masked and gowned. He too fell. But on the stairs. So, unlike Prof R, he will never get up.

<hr>

November 7 — I'm trying to keep up. Not enough sleep and Prof R at 9 am with muscles that refused to work, so that we spent an hour and a half waiting for him to be able to get to the toilet. But I am getting so much better at instructions and body support. I tuck myself behind him and put my arms around his waist. On these rare days, he still doesn't trust that necessary surrender required to lower himself onto the toilet.

The day has continued in this vein. Although he is up and down unaided, I'm not sure how much Prof R understands of what I say to him, and that is possibly related to his hearing. We tried a syringe kit, but it is so hard for him to cooperate with the head movements required. There seemed little point in continuing.

Stella took the dog out and pronounced her requiring training and a walk at the same time every day. "Preferably three times a day." The dog slipped the harness to prove her point, but was retrieved without incident, which is a major step forward.

But I felt overwhelmed by these new demands. How would that schedule be possible to manage? I feel bullied and stupidly upset. And when I tried to tell Prof R upstairs that I felt this way he was unable to understand a word I was saying. But when I just whispered in his ear that my sister was bullying me, he understood.

When I went downstairs, she apologised for upsetting me and I acknowledged she was also correct, and I should never have got a dog. Dog walkers cost £10 a time. It's out of the question. I have trained her well for indoors and the garden but that is not enough.

—

The financial issues still dog me (pun intended) as I wrestle with what changes I should make to my Will and whether I have the right things in place for us both.

Time will tell. A cousin frightened me by saying she knew of someone who had a joint account frozen. So I checked the situation here and it seems this is not the case. That it would be illegal to freeze assets that have passed to a surviving partner.

I hope this is right.

Clara, my Pilates teacher, hailed me in the supermarket. This is a first for me. I have deliberately not tried to make friends or network with anyone since I have been here. But I have to admit it was nice.

November 9 — Friday. Email from Katrina the Care Navigator: my saviour.

> *"If Prof R is not having accidents in the bed you may not need a waterproof sheet, but you could just lay a towel under him while washing. And use bed bath wipes as they can be easier to use than soap and water. I've attached a link.*
>
> *You can buy pressure-relief bed fleeces, but it may be best to speak to an occupational therapist or district nurse to ask for some expert advice as they may be able to provide you with a pressure-relieving mattress as well as advice on the best way to move him. You can call the district nursing team or the Kent Community Health Care Team on the number below. I have attached a leaflet on pressure sores which you might find helpful."*

Oh, the relief. Permission to continue caring for Prof R as I have been doing, without worrying that I am harming him in any way. Or not cleaning him safely. A fleece has been ordered because the Occupational Therapist said it wasn't her department.

Today Archie comes again for two hours and I will give him small caring tasks to do so that Prof R will view him more kindly. Hand washing perhaps, and combing hair. Little kindnesses that will help Prof R get used to being handled by someone other than me.

November 10 — Saturday. Prof R's sister Doris and her husband 'dropped in' unannounced early for coffee and did not leave until Archie arrived. Stevie held the fort while I climbed the stairs endlessly, attending to Prof R. When Doris later went up to see him, he remembered her, which was nice. She is the person he has known the longest. It would be sad if he didn't.

When Stella and I escaped finally, there was only time for a ciabatta sandwich at the Hot Tin Café and a brief encounter with a kind man as we explored the local church. He said "Welcome", and asked how far we had come. I said, "Two blocks", but put him out of his misery by telling him how far Stella had come.

Prof R knows me intermittently and his clues are in the way I speak to him and kiss him. Then he knows I am his wife and beams with pleasure. "Who loves you baby?" he said last night.

Stella is out walking the dog. It has been a terrible morning for me. Prof R had no muscle control and a determination to get up anyway. I have successfully got him to the toilet twice. The second time he immediately said he had to lie down. And refused to sit. But later, he could do it himself. It is horrendous when he cannot comprehend and cannot manage his body. He fights me. I come close to helpless tears when he does that.

I went to Boots while Stella sat with him as he slept, and bought; pull up men's waterproof pants, syrup of figs, eyedrops that can be sprayed on the lids, Anesol for his little haemorrhoids, spray that claims to dissolve wax in the ears, and something more palatable for lunch from the market.

November 11 — Sunday. Another morning of rigors but I managed it so much better, with medication taken safely lying propped up on his side, and a suggestion to remain in bed and rest. His bladder is fairly reliable so it's not necessary to panic about peeing.

Stella remarked how stressful the whole toilet thing is. If there was no need for it people would be much safer. But I have noticed that Prof R almost goes to the bathroom for something to do. Exercise for his limbs. So when we have an up-down day I don't despair as I used to. As long as his head is on straight, I leave him in peace. And I like catching sight of him through the door, opening the cabinet and carefully removing his large comb before meticulously doing his hair. It is very touching.

Eldest daughter Hannah text me, asking if it was okay to come to lunch. That was not expected, as I'd heard nothing all week, but it was welcome. Risotto is my default lunch menu for such occasions. She sat with him and fed him. And wasn't sure if he recognised her.

I gave her a copy of his Will and the portion of my Will that relates to her and her siblings. My fears around all of this were somewhat reduced when she said, in answer to my expression of regret about the up-front amount. "You must not think of that. You are up and down these stairs all day caring for dad and have enough to worry about."

And when I said I had to forward-plan, she added, "You need to have enough to manage your own life in the future." Perhaps she won't contest the Will at least. But even she has said her sister Julie is ruthless. No doubt she has the capability to apply that ruthlessness to other matters.

Stella talked to Hannah when I was busy, and tells me she used the time to dish up a big helping of 'this is how it is'. A forceful cheerleader type of exchange, but kindly she assures me. I hope so, or it could be counterproductive. But I'm glad someone is speaking for me. There are no witnesses here.

November 12 — Monday. Stella and I went to the museum while Archie received a lesson in building an Anderson Shelter from Prof R. I think Archie is going to be a success.

Food is steadily becoming more of an issue. Chicken cannot be chewed, beans – even with strings removed – stick in his teeth. Rice, unless sodden, cannot be cut up by his molars. It can be discouraging. Tonight I offered him rice pudding instead. He loved it. And then had ice cream as usual.

November 13 — A restless night from 4 am onwards that had me lying defeated in bed watching him roam or just sit, so that I put the fan heater on to stop him being chilled.

Rice pudding and ice cream at lunch when he grew tired of my home-made vegetable soup. Not exactly nutritious. But he loved his foot wash and massage.

He is becoming less connected and sees things sometimes which he reaches out for. Stella guessed what it might be and asked him what he was seeing. She suggested butterflies. He didn't say anything. The very word gave me butterflies. Does everyone see them when they are dying?

—

Two for the price of one today. The occupational therapist arrived at 11 am with a second woman, H, who turned out to be from Social Services. Surprise! Apparently that is deliberate, so we have no chance to prepare.

Prof R was about to have breakfast, so I took them both upstairs and we spent an hour talking about him in front of his face while he ate his cereal. I feel less able to remain unemotional, feel more exposed, when I see him through the eyes of others. It all seems so much sadder. But I was grateful for their visit and H seemed to think we might qualify for some financial help for Archie or his equivalent. We didn't discuss the future in front of Prof R.

In the afternoon, when Archie came, Stella and I went to Canterbury on the train. Her first visit there, and my first trip there by train. What a relief not to be trying to park and then taking the choked ring-road home at 'school run' time.

The new child gate for the kitchen door arrived while we were out, and Archie put it together for us. It has such an efficient lock I can struggle to open it, so a grandchild will be given the challenge on Friday. If she can't open it, it is £14.99 well spent. Although the bar at the bottom is a brilliant trip hazard. And potential head-splitter if it comes to that.

November 14 — Thursday. Suddenly mushroom scrambled eggs are too hard to chew. He says his teeth don't work. I try to whisk it in the blender, but it is too dry. Milk helps. Then he is able to eat it. But whether he enjoys it is another matter. I'm going to have to mash everything. Tonight it is fish which he can eat. So, fish and mash. He is going to get awfully sick of mash everything.

Brexit is coming to a head and I talk to him about it, whether or not it is clear he understands. I've bought him a lovely blue long-sleeved top to wear to replace the grey moth-eaten ones. Which were lovely when new but not now.

If I am even a little late giving him his pills, I've noticed that he has difficulty understanding me. So, when I ask if he wants ice cream he stares with incomprehension. I have started microwaving it for 10 seconds, so he doesn't get pain from the cold in the roof of his mouth.

It's bliss when he falls asleep again.

—

Today I'm feeling incredibly angry with Prof R's daughters. I've created expectations which are no longer appropriate. They expect me to feed them and nurture them whenever they are here. It is his 81st birthday on 2nd of December and stupidly I again said, "Come for lunch". My only concession being to ask one or all of them to make the cake. This was a big ask for me. I find it difficult to ask them for anything.

Of course, they still don't say "You mustn't cook. We will bring food", because they don't realise how difficult it is now for me to entertain, or perhaps feel I would be offended. They never will unless I enable them to. So I emailed suggesting lunch might be "too much for dad" and why don't they come for coffee and cake instead?

And of course, then Hannah rang me to see if I'm alright. That might be because I told her about the Occupational Therapist and the Social Worker, but I suspect the truth is she was shocked I was cancelling the lunch. How out of character!

But the whole truth is I also cancelled the lunch because I had asked the girls if they would mind me inviting his sister Doris and her husband for the after-lunch cake and coffee. Hannah had said, "As long as it's not too much for dad" and I could see that she was looking for a reason not to share her dad, but unwittingly she also gave me a reason not to include lunch.

So, it is solved. No lunch, no sister, just coffee and cake. But I'm still left defeated in my own eyes. As you are when no one has given you permission to say "no".

—

It is 8 pm and tonight Prof R is up down up down, and the alarm is constantly going off as I write this. And then he is back in bed. But I'm not going up-down-up-down anymore tonight. Only at times when he has been asleep for a while and I know he may need help or something to drink or eat.

Stella keeps badgering me to do less for the girls and more for myself. I find her judgment of them harsher than mine, but I also know she is right.

After dinner tonight I caught him looking at me slightly perplexed and I said, "Do you know who I am" and he said, "You're my wife" but he couldn't remember my name. I kiss him and tell him it's the right answer.

November 15 — Archie came and so did my daughter-in-law Ophelia with a baby granddaughter. What a joy they are. We went out for coffee after lunch while Archie looked after Prof R.

Archie is 21, it turns out, and he knows quite a lot about gaming. But I begin to think he may not know a lot about professional care. He is too inexperienced to be a fully-fledged carer of someone with high-level needs, and seems only reliable to feed and supervise and do the dishes if he has spare time.

Prof R's morning had been very rough. Lots of sleeping and little cognition. But he improved by the evening. I am frightened to weigh him.

Stella and I watched a Coen Brothers movie; me part-time as I traipsed up and down the stairs, as is my wont.

November 16 — Saturday. I know I am missing the small but significant changes from this diary because it is harder to make time to write.

Last night I gave Prof R fish in a child's mashed food of curry and chicken. The toddler food had been bought by accident and is designed to be squeezed out of a tube. He pronounced it tasty and ate it all. This feels like cheating, but at least it achieved the texture he needs.

Today he really wanted to try the bacon and egg pie I made for our lunch yesterday. So I cut it into tiny pieces and added fig chutney and he was able to eat a surprising amount, only picking out the skin on the egg surface.

I've begun to look for jellies and rice puddings as an alternative to the constant ice cream. I'm sure I could do more cooked fruit and perhaps custard. Pureed apple I use constantly for sweetening and texture.

The syrup of figs goes down after every meal and eventually will no doubt produce a result. His regularity seems to me about once every three days now. Fortunately, it no longer seems to concern him.

—

Market day today. It lifts my spirits to spend even 20 minutes cruising the stalls. More syrup of figs on the menu and we are also shopping for a small live tree for Christmas.

Prof R asked me if the dog was all right. Usually, he seems to forget her existence.

November 17 — Sunday. Too much couch time, Prof R sleeping too long and waking confused. He's not eating as he should and I'm not telling my sister, because she will say "Oh yes, that's what you can expect. He's on the final leg now." And I don't need to hear that.

Stella is avoiding most contact with Prof R now, but is full of advice, some of it very good, some of it may be her own guilt. She is not even walking the dog now. The novelty has worn off, once she realised she would have to run the schedule herself.

She has watched an entire film this afternoon and washed her linen, and I'm glad, as there isn't a lot else to do around here on a Sunday. I will miss her company, so it is just as well she is not too hands on. But I won't miss feeling upset when she is critical.

I'm quite afraid now he might not live until Christmas. He is not noticing that I have not put his teeth in for two days. I am feeding him such soft food there is no need. But I must keep his remaining teeth and gums rinsed with Corsodyl. It's easy to miss that step last thing at night.

November 18 — Prof R awoke much more himself after a night of two-hourly waking. He asked for his teeth. (Predictably) And with much encouragement they were put in without the usual wincing and complaining. The 'encouragement' was me saying "I cannot do this unless you help me. I am not a dental technician."

Today was also an Archie Day. Stella and I headed into a cold northerly gale and achieved the things we needed to do. Then we ate cake. The hail outside did not disturb us and I got a great shot of Stella with a black sky and bunting in the only patch of blue.

Archie says he hasn't given up on showering Prof R and will see if he can get a senior colleague to come and 'help' so he can demonstrate to Prof R that it is possible. I'm very pleased he is motivated to do this. Although clearly not already trained to do it himself.

November 19 — Prof R is sitting on the side of his bed at 9 am interacting with some imaginary objects and unable to do other than move his muscles incoherently. This time, although I knew he wanted to pee, I gave him his pills – the ones perhaps he should have had half an hour earlier – and just waited. When I felt it was worthwhile, I began to give him his breakfast. After 45 minutes he suddenly lined up all his nerve endings and got up to go to the bathroom – successfully this time.

Successful on two counts as it turned out. As I wiped him, I sang him a song. 'Easy peasy, poos and weesies' to the tune of *Lord Dismiss us with thy Blessing*, a favourite of mine since schooldays. It is hard to tell if it amuses him, but it makes me happier, which is half the battle.

So he slept. Coffee later, when he complained, kicking out with his legs, that he didn't know what was real and what wasn't, and he wanted to kill himself. I agreed it was awful, but said I loved him and he mustn't kill himself. These terrible reality moments fortunately pass.

Stella slept until 11 am. A catch-up day for her. I have sent her out to buy a cross-stitch pattern she likes so she can feel less imprisoned by the situation and the weather. It is 4 degrees C today. I have made chowder for lunch, her favourite, and it will be fish again tonight.

The phone rang and it was his pendant alarm telling me to contact him. Which I did. He had pushed the button by mistake, wondering what it was, and I told him not to worry, I was delighted to have tested it in the field, so to speak. We've agreed to leave it hanging by his side of the bed in case, in a real emergency, he remembers what it is for.

November 21 — Wednesday. Our luck ran out. Prof R fell in the bathroom at 7 am, even though I had medicated him at 6 am and watched him until he was able to move. This time I rang the ambulance straight away. And this time they came within the hour.

This could have looked like a good thing, but it meant Prof R's vital signs were still down. Low BP, very low heart rate, even though they observed him standing by the bed unaided after they had lifted him.

So we had to go to hospital. First I had to show the paramedics how to use the stairlifts. They looked at me perplexed when I asked how they would take someone downstairs without one. I had this unhelpful vision of a crossed arms two-hander under the bum that we used to do as kids. Then I had to race off to put some clothes on.

It was cold in the ambulance, and Prof R was in his pyjamas, half covered, but the paramedic didn't seem to notice. Until I asked if he could cover him. As the journey progressed, his readings improved, as they always did, and that continued after we arrived. In triage, a medic told me quietly not to let anyone stop me from giving Prof R his Parkinson's medications "no matter what anyone else tells you". Forewarned. So when I asked for a glass of water, I felt confident explaining why.

I hadn't taken the car because a) it can be a nightmare with parking fees if the stay is long, and b) Prof R needed my company in the ambulance. So the whole time we were there, I was wondering how we would get home.

At 12 pm, bloods done and approved, we were cleared to go, and Prof R wheeled to the exit. This after the ward staff had watched me struggle to help him down from the waist-high bed into a wheelchair. (Health and safety? I daren't ask). But two taxi companies I rang weren't interested in a one-way journey. In the end, it was Doris and Brian who saved us.

And while we waited for them, I bought cake and water for two people who'd had no breakfast inside them and very little to drink since leaving home. It was such a relief to be cleared for take-off, with a lift home in a warm car. Never underestimate the small comforts of life. And the ties of family, no matter how tenuous.

—

He's safe in bed, we've eaten, I'm shattered with fatigue but fine. Stella managed the dog and made the bed. This second major medical event neither shocked nor surprised me. How ordinary it now seemed to dial 999. But how annoying. I need to improve my response time to toilet visits in the early hours of the morning. It's not going to be enough to simply monitor.

November 22nd — The second ambulance crew had said what the first crew had said, "Get a key lock box put on the front of the house". Late this afternoon a man called Des came around and fitted one. Some of the challenges here are easy. Toileting is not.

Stella gave me a verbal bollocking today, saying I need to hire more help and in her view I will now need to spend all my time in the loft. Food should be put in thermos flasks etc etc. Any protest and I am deemed "over-reacting".

But by late afternoon she was back to normal, and when I went out to get the cash for Des, she didn't even go upstairs to check Prof R because the alarm didn't go off. But I gave her a hug and a new nick-name – the Face of Revlon – because she has lovely skin. I think she secretly likes it.

Prof R got agitated later when we were both with him, chitter chatter while changing the bed and giving him coffee and cake in his cane chair. I saw it coming, because I know the signs, but I waited until his silent rage took hold and then told him I understood. He should just say it was too noisy. We could leave the room if he found it stressful. And of course, he said to me, "I don't want you to leave the room".

—

There is no doubt that simply washing my hair is problematic now and I may have to get it washed professionally once a week instead of doing it myself. But it seems such a waste of care money.

I suspect a lot of Stella's rage at my not hiring more help is because it doesn't only restrict me in going out – she is also housebound. I may have funds in Prof R's savings, but I want to hang on to them until 24-hour assistance is needed. It will cost a fortune.

With that in mind, I have done as planned, changing my Will so that my half goes straight to all the children, by-passing Prof R, if I pre-decease him. It took courage to take that step – and a change to the ownership status of the house to Tenants in Common – but all the children would thank me. It's a temporary measure. And no one need ever know about it except me and my lawyer. None of the children will be told. It might be too tempting to push me under a bus!!

Prof R has no memory today of the trip to hospital yesterday.

November 23 — Black Friday in the shops. It's an Archie day, so we can do some Christmas shopping.

The patient had pills, a pee and went straight back to sleep this morning. This is the first time, with my blessing, that he has fired straight into the bathroom basin. Porcelain is porcelain, regardless of the location. And so much safer for Mr Woollyhead at 6.30 am. By 10.30 am he is able to sit on the correct porcelain to pee, but is still very woolly and has gone to sleep again. It feels strange to have free time.

His eyes are red and irritated and no amount of drops or Yellow Eye Ointment seem to have a lasting effect.

I want to cut his hair when I can catch him alert enough. I've been showing Stella photos from our previous house, and it's a sharp reminder of how much better Prof R was just two years ago, and even then, he was already very unwell.

Breaking new ground with Archie, asking him on his arrival to give Prof R his lunchtime pills. Archie, unprepared, ran to his car to get his protective gloves. I had no time to tell him I have a box of them in the bathroom, but he prefers to use his own. And even though I gave him the rivastigmine in a blister pack, next time I must give him the entire packet, so that he knows he has the right medication and can testify to that if necessary.

This day has been about sleep. Prof R still does not remember the hospital and only knows I am his wife. I daren't ask if he knows my name.

Tonight my eldest granddaughter Hester was rushed to hospital with pneumonia.

November 24 — Saturday. After a worrying night, Hester is reported to be progressing well at UCH. What a week of NHS for our little family.

And then we discovered that Archie, booked for today, didn't arrive, and had thought we wanted him tomorrow, Sunday. So the administrative side of this care company is not working well. Archie also tells me he is flying off to Australia in mid-December. It may be the right time to choose another care company. Although the best one is £10 more per hour.

I am now looking for a pressure cushion for Prof R. His bottom is looking hot and bothered. I put cream on it, but he spends a lot of the day sleeping sitting up. It was bound to become an issue.

Stella is bingeing on *The Last Man on Earth* on Prime. It's clever and hilarious and because I have already seen it, I can come and go with my little chores and care for Prof R without missing anything. I also hate to spend all that time on the couch. I become bored quite quickly if Prof R sleeps a long time. I'd rather be busy.

Prof R did not like his blitzed fish chowder, so I made him baked apple and ice cream. Sometimes in the evening I get tired and fed up when this happens. I try to explain to Prof R that I don't mean to upset him as well.

A text from Archie, who was at the office, saying did I want to cancel Sunday's booking? What didn't he understand? Given it was an incorrect booking, "Yes please Archie". And I am researching new care providers.

November 25 — Sunday. The dishwasher, which had broken, has now been fixed. By turning it off at the wall and counting to 10 before switching it on again. The error notice said E:19 and online NEFF said an E:19 required an engineer. So I had filled out a request form online for a repair. I am feeling quietly triumphant that this might no longer be necessary.

Hester is coming home from hospital today.

It's the first Christmas market. But it all seems like just too much trouble on a dark cold day. Stella slept in till 10.00 am and was woken by a man called James delivering our groceries. How I love the James's of this world who save me from the supermarket.

Prof R is still asleep at 11.am after waking at 2 am, 4 am, 5.30 am (pill) and then 8.15 am (more pills). He was a danger to himself going to the toilet. At the 2 am wake-up I got a fright when I heard the toilet flush and realised the bed alarm had not gone off. I have no idea why.

—

This evening Prof R had a flash of insight about his illness and I asked how it felt for him. He cried about his inability to make sense of where he was and why, and I could only lie down with him and hold him. He said it felt like childhood, when we don't really understand what is going on. But he knew what he had achieved and marvelled that he could reach the age of 70 (wishful thinking said I) and have such a rich past. The memories of which, I said, he could at least be grateful for, even if the present was not present and correct. The jigsaw has been thrown on the floor.

Stella said all the dementia patients go through this phase. I rather like to think Prof R is having his own particular experience, not just a textbook version.

November 26 — Monday. The brainstorm seemed to tire him immensely and he slept too soundly overnight, so that I had to break through his subconscious to give him a levodopa at 4 am. He was unable to get up, and whispered "help" and I knew he needed to pee. The urinal has proved its worth again. At 8 am he was still semi-conscious and unable to move safely to the bathroom, but this time was able to stand and hold the rail by the bed as he peed into the urinal, before falling back into a deep sleep.

But by midday the mattress alarm went, and he was a different person. Alert and ready to face the day, including his breakfast.

Archie came this afternoon and Stella and I braved the rain to walk to Sainsbury's, just out of curiosity. I haven't been yet because it's quite a long way and requires a car to bring everything home. Nobly we succumbed to a cream tea halfway back. I felt so much better after the rare experience of a long walk.

Now I have washed my hair and Stella has answered his alarm. I'm not sure how I will shower and even dare to use the toilet once she has gone. I fear another fall in the bathroom.

Hester has recovered and will be back at school tomorrow. It is hard to believe.

November 27 — Tuesday. "How long and how legally have we been married?". This after asking who I was, although at least he thought I was his wife. For some reason, for the first time, I feel really hurt. And sad.

He agreed without a murmur to having the pull-ups on in the evening. This is a relief.

Helen from Social Services says we can have what is called a Kent Card rather than a bank account for Direct Payments towards care costs. So I have agreed to go ahead. It's not a lot, but it will be welcome. *(Although, as it turned out, how we were paid wouldn't be an issue.)*

—

Food is my biggest challenge. He can't live on ice cream and jelly and cake alone. I have at least one meal rejected each day. At lunchtime it was a vegetable frittata cut up very tiny, but still his tongue finds a fault and spits something out. So it was soup and bread for dinner. Let him eat cake perhaps. But it does matter.

Overnight now he sleeps soundly and only wakes once, so he is having one less levodopa on a regular basis. This may be a good thing and reduce the hallucinations, although they are benign.

He had another clarity moment at about 8 pm, so that time of day seems to be significant. It feels like Groundhog Day for me, but I am pleased that he is pleased to feel he has a handle on it, even though the handle doesn't appear to have a door. (What did we say before we had Groundhog Day? *Déjà vu* doesn't do it. It's more immediate and repetitive than that.)

Stella is watching at least two films a day. I get to watch part of them.

November 29 — Thursday. Prof R drinks like a baby calf from his juice bottle. The juice bottle is designed for children to take to school, so it is the perfect size for the bedside. I have been shown by Archie how to wet Prof R's bottom lip to get him to suck fluid when he is comatose. This has been a revelation.

Yesterday Stella and I went out for lunch while Archie did his two-hour stint. I took her to the Taverna, which is Mexican but does a burger called Jumping Jack which I was drawn to like a wasp to beer. Stella had the fajitas. We were like two 20-year-olds, but without the alcohol.

But when we got home, I spent the next two hours on the run for Prof R. It was so exhausting, I wished I had lain on the couch during Archie's visit rather than go out. It took wine, home-made vegetable soup and a long bout of *Olive Kitteridge Part 2* to restore me.

No matter how tired I am, escaping into an excellent film is nearly always the total cure. That should tell me something. But it's nothing I didn't already know. That it is incredibly boring to care for someone 24/7 who only eats and sleeps and drinks and occasionally says thank you or smiles at me or wants a kiss.

Yesterday, at least, he did know who I was.

—

Earlier today he finally managed to poo, after several aborted 'mining' events yesterday. What a relief it always is. I have given him stewed prunes in syrup on his cereal this morning and he loves it.

Stella has gone to the health store to get other essential supplies. When she has gone back home, my trips out will go back to being chore trips. Playtime leaves no time for essentials.

Just now I raced upstairs after hearing pounding on what sounded like furniture. Prof R said he had been drumming his feet. And that he felt desperate and was going crazy. I calmed him and suggested he sleep to let the chemicals sort themselves out.

Doris and Brian came for coffee and cake at 4pm. They brought the cake. It was chocolate and Prof R had three pieces while each of them paid homage to him in his bed. They seem to have decided not to be offended that they are not invited on Sunday, his actual birthday. For his present, they bought three tubs of exotic ice cream. It is a brilliant present. I'm not even going to try giving him a gift. He will be happy with a card.

I have dragged home a Christmas tree in my wheelie bag from Tesco. It even has the lights already on it, run by little batteries. How perfect.

—

The podiatrist, Liz, made her house call. His ever thickening toenails had finally beaten me. I had forgotten to tell her Prof R was two floors up. But she is forgiving. He struggled with the treatment, crying out in distress, but she was totally unfazed. There are many more difficult patients on her client list, and she has empathy with all of them.

—

He is playing games with me. I turned off his light tonight and he turned it on again. When I asked why he said, "Because you turned it off". And when I said, "You are bullying me" he said, "Why are you here?", to which I replied "Because I am stupid" at which point he told me, as usual, how lovely and beautiful I am, which is his way of saying sorry.

When I left the room, I turned to ask if he was all right. He said, "No. Half of me is left." A joke! Later, when I was settling him after the toilet he simply said "sorry" and I pretended not to know what he was sorry for. And kissed him.

I hope he isn't going to make the job unrewarding by trying to make me dislike him. I am devoted to keeping him safe and as happy as possible, but I am also vulnerable if he isn't kind to me.

December 1 — Saturday. In an angry mood over breakfast Prof R wanted a gun or a knife. When I asked why he said, "So I can kill someone". That is the first time he has directed his anger towards others, rather than himself. I'm shaken and glad he is neither strong enough nor 'weaponised', as the Americans would say.

Stella is disgusted and thinks he is performing, and a care home would sort him out. He's getting his cake and coffee and being pampered. I've had to stand up for him and say, "His illness makes him harder to love, but I do. And caring for loved ones is what people do". Stella shows her concern by being angry too. You would think she would understand Prof R.

Hope is coming for lunch today and it will be such a ray of sunlight.

December 2 — Sunday. Prof R's 81st birthday. Already I've had a call from his eldest Hannah asking, yet again, what time they should come. She is naturally full of sentiment and my job will be to give her a reality check and tell her to just enjoy her dad as much as she can.

Last night he was wandering, after sleeping too much in the afternoon while Archie was here. He was confused, aware of his illness and yet not aware enough to process it. Depression is probably setting in and St John's Wort can only do so much. I will need to monitor this.

He is losing interest in food. Savoury has gone first. He is spitting it out. Cake and ice cream and the morning cereal and fruit are still acceptable. I told Hannah he is preferring sweet to savoury and she, flipping the coin, said "Oh, is birthday cake the wrong thing?". Clearly, she is tired. Rachel has made a Victoria sponge and it will be perfect.

With Stella here, I have someone who can see how his girls fail to connect with all this. She cannot understand why they are not texting each week at least. It's because they just have one switch – which is either on or off.

A birthday email has arrived from his son in New Zealand, so my 'heads up' to him has borne fruit, even if Prof R's parenting style hasn't.

Stella will go into hiding while they are here, and I agree. It is the only sensible thing she can do if she is not to be drawn into the sort of family dynamic that is this family.

If only I could open the door, greet them with a kiss, then hand them the matches for the candles and go off to a café. But it may be the last time we have this ritual so it will be poignant.

December 3 — Monday. The birthday boy managed to surface from slumber for his daughters for a short while yesterday. It was a blessing. He opened his presents and his cards and held court in the loft bedroom, awake or asleep, for the entire afternoon. I left them to it as much as possible. It will be the last birthday they are able to really share with their father, even if he is still with us for the next one.

I recorded the candle ceremony on my phone. History is weighing heavily on me.

Stella disappeared into her room as planned. This meant she couldn't even cross the floor to the toilet because the floors in this house squeak and her cover would be blown. But it was the best thing she could have done. We wanted the day to be about Prof R and his girls. And it was.

They did admire Stella's gift to him – hand-knitted socks that looked stunning on Prof R's feet.

The daughter who had asked what he needed, actually brought what he needed – pyjamas. The others appeared to have grabbed whatever chocolate thing they could find. It doesn't matter. He has a chocolate advent calendar, and he can have a little dwarf Santa every night before bed. (*That was the intention. In fact, he could no longer eat chocolate, because it made him choke, so I ate every single one.*)

—

Today I awoke too early. So by lunchtime I am tired. I had the forms to sign for Kent Social Services and I am still unsure of what I am signing up for, in terms of legal, time-consuming stress-making requirements. They will do a financial assessment of Prof R and will get a surprise when they discover he has no savings in his own name, (for tax purposes), but that we are not trying to escape from our obligations.

Archie comes at 1.30 pm and Prof R is still out of this world, clutching the air for invisible things and difficult to reach for pill times. He has his pull-ups on so there is no stress from that department.

December 4 — Tuesday. Yesterday became very difficult with Prof R after Archie went home. He was confused and angry, trying to use the toilet and having difficulty. And then even worse, bursting into anguished sobs. The only moment that lightened the situation was when he began throwing the toilet rolls around the bathroom. We both laughed then.

On reflection, I have been thinking about where scissors and other sharp objects are located in the loft. Could he be a real danger? I have no idea.

December 6 — Thursday. Yesterday, Archie's first full day in charge and our first day away in London. A triumph. The weather, the trains, coffee and sandwiches with my three darlings at the Tate, and at last, the view from the 10th floor of the new extension at Tate Modern. We only managed to 'cherry-pick' the South Bank and cross the Millennium Bridge in both directions, so that Stella could say she had.

On the way home, when we changed trains, I jumped out of the first one and mindlessly darted straight across the platform into the train opposite, thinking to myself that it was Platform 4, when it wasn't. The doors closed behind me and Stella was left on the platform with the guard, who seemed to take pleasure in separating two women travelling together.

I laughed all the way to the next stop (I have done this once before elsewhere) and came back on the other side to Bromley South without too much delay. Seeing no Stella on the correct platform, or at least not where I expected to see her, I presumed she had made the connection that I had missed, and I jumped on the next train.

But when I got home, no Stella. Mild panic set in. Archie totally lost it and suggested the police, before she put her key in the lock. We had been on the same train, she at the far end of the platform. Laughter and relief all around.

An aside. On the station at Bromley South, when I was checking for the correct platform, a woman who looked in her 40s offered me a seat in the waiting room. It was a salutary experience. So, I do look old. And yet I have never felt better or more alive than I did yesterday.

—

But joy soon evaporated. Archie had made a pig's ear of helping Prof R on the toilet. Two of the toilets were blocked with an entire packet of wet wipes, handed to Prof R in succession by Archie in the hope that eventually he could clean himself.

And Archie said, "I'm not sure how clean he will be". Archie had not understood it was his job to wipe a bottom. Or that he should not stuff wet wipes down a toilet. I feel so much less confident about him now, that I have asked for a review of Prof R's care level.

Today, after I have pulled more fistfuls of wet wipes out of the toilet bowls, I will also book an assessment with the agency I had first called – *Your Choice* – who charge £30 an hour but may send someone with real qualifications.

In the middle of the night, Prof R spent several studied moments rearranging the objects on his bedside table. His favourites are there. A Swiss army knife (small!), a folding comb, his torch, his glasses – he needs to keep checking they are there.

December 7 — Friday. Prof R came downstairs. I had found him wandering in the bedroom and putting on his shoes, so I grabbed the opportunity to suggest a proper excursion. It is the first time in almost two months, and I couldn't believe how happy it made me. To have his company downstairs, where we can see him, and not be abandoning him to the top floor.

He coped quite well with all the attention and managed lunch, sitting at the head of the table in his leather chair. He had previously told me he couldn't remember what the rest of the house looked like, but I suspect he does most of the time. He registered no surprise.

Upstairs again, he keeps telling me I am beautiful, and I know it is partly because he is anxious to please me now he is so dependent on me. I am the only one who is prepared to excavate his back passage. This makes me quite an asset.

—

Today Archie comes again, just for the afternoon. I will ask him to flush the toilet frequently, and help Prof R rather than just watch him struggle to clean himself in the event of a bowel movement. I find I am angry at the incompetence of the company he works for and sorry for him.

Prof R is comatose again this morning, in spite of a totally different night to the usual three-hourly waking and half-dose juggling of levodopa.

Last night he only surfaced once at 4 am and I made sure he had his medication as well as a pee. That is the longest I can remember him sleeping in almost three years.

He manages not to use his pull-ups, regardless of the time between pees, but I notice his prostate is probably making peeing less regular with more 'dry time' on his loo visits. It is prominent now, but the GP assures us it is quite usual in older men and not a problem that needs any attention.

—

I will be quizzed on the phone next week by Social Welfare as to Prof R's financial situation. I was expecting this, and have the paperwork ready. I have many times been grateful that I dealt with all the messy small investments a year ago. Now it will be straightforward.

It's raining today, so while Archie is here we may just go to the local museum. Stella would love another trip to Whitstable, but Archie leaves soon and so far we have no replacement.

Your Choice will visit for a care quality assessment next week. For Prof R, there have been fewer angry moods. He hasn't said "I want to kill" lately.

December 10 — It's becoming harder to find time to write. Even with Stella's help. Or perhaps it's just that I'd rather spend my spare time with her. We talk, watch films, eat candy cane (that has to stop) and play with the dog. I feel the days dwindling ever faster towards her departure.

I managed to decide *not* to cook a turkey this Christmas. My visiting family were 'upscaling' to roast vegetables from our original hamper idea, and I knew it was my fault, suggesting a turkey. So I have curbed my enthusiasm and feel a lot better for it. We will have a hamper (brought by them) and a salad (made by us) and a tray of festive roast veggies. More and more I am learning how to peg back on expectations.

Prof R meanwhile becomes more emotionally and physically dependent. I have to be careful not to use this knowledge to control some of his behaviour, but when he is demanding and needy, I find myself saying, "I am going downstairs now if you continue like this" and he begs me not to. I have to find a way forward that avoids these negative tactics. I feel my fear rising in advance of Stella's departure.

December 11 — Tuesday. *Your Choice* Agency Day.

These in-depth endless assessments are exhausting. At some point, after hours of questioning, my tears threatened to surface. They 'escaped from custody' when I was trying to describe a typical action of self-care that I witness. Prof R combing his hair in the bathroom in the middle of the night. Somehow its poignancy in the retelling caught me unawares. I hate having this vulnerability laid bare. It undermines my coping mechanisms. Mostly I am in a 'calm enough' place even when things are very challenging.

This morning I had to step back from Prof R in the bathroom when he baulked at sitting on the toilet at 6.30 am. I kept saying "sit down, sit down" until eventually he did. I cannot and will not try to make him do it physically. He naturally resists. But if I fear a fall, I have to. At times like these my refusal to fail him is my only protection against giving up.

—

Forewarned is forearmed. I have now been told by someone-who-knows that three callouts for an ambulance can put us under scrutiny. I have become anarchic in my determination to beat these authoritarian systems. If there is another fall, and Prof R is not injured, I will go next door for help or down to the men at the hardware store to borrow some muscle to lift him.

Another fear surfaced when the *Your Choice* agency owner warned me that we need a health and welfare LPA as well as the financial one we have. Otherwise, she says, Prof R's health management can be taken out of my hands. Why did our last lawyer, who witnessed our financial LPA, not advise us of this?

She has referred me to a lawyer she knows, who will visit, and I have an appointment for a home visit next Monday. It will cost £650. Extortion. Twice as much as the usual £300 fee. How many people can afford that? It should be a basic human right, like a Do Not Resuscitate certificate.

Fortunately, my role as Prof R's permitted health manager/guardian has been recognised by every health provider for three years now. Even so, it will take up to three months for this second Authority to be registered with the courts. I hope we won't find we need it before then.

———

Stella made another lovely meal. I have been racing all day, not because of Prof R but on his behalf. The evening was his time to drain what was left of my energy. I'm not pleased when I hear myself begging him not to get up yet again. It feels like a failure reasoning with a man who can only half respond.

December 14 — The gaps in this diary are an indication of the week we have had.

A deluge of water through the ceiling downstairs, the legacy of Archie and the packs of wet wipes. A drainage expert took over from the plumber to clear the pipes. The access point is in the loft, behind a chest of drawers. He took one look at the stairs before he sweated and strained to drag his machinery up two flights. There was some doubt whether he would survive the climb. Prof R was tucked up in bed asleep, and slept on, while the equivalent of a jumbo jet revved it's engines within feet of his head.

The new rule now is that all wet wipes, regardless of their contents, go in their own little metal bins in each bathroom. As I discovered, to my embarrassment, we should have been doing all along. Because 'flushable' does not mean 'flushable'.

And Archie has been 'let go'. The whole company of people at his agency have been let go because they kept letting us down – and Archie. Who never got the support he needed to shower or care professionally for the Prof.

The new person, Netty, from *Your Choice*, will start on 20th December from 10 am till 1 pm. The agency calls their staff PA's. I approve of that. All care workers deserve a professional title. But I am unable to take Stella anywhere until then, so we go out in shifts.

—

Social Welfare interviewed me at length on the phone about our finances and said, "You have been awarded £93 a week, but because of your income and savings you will need to pay us back the full amount." They would not begin to contribute until our costs exceeded £500 a week. She seemed perplexed when I pointed out there was therefore no reason for them to pay me anything at all at this stage. So thank you, I must turn down their generous offer.

They will keep Prof R's details on record in case we qualify for help at a future time, which I assume we will. Care could cost up to £1000 a week, and many more adaptations will happen to our house and sleeping arrangements before we see out the time for Prof R.

—

His oldest friend, Nigel, who now lives in Bath, sent us a Christmas card that was so devoid of mention or awareness about his friend's illness, that I sent him the 81st birthday video in an attempt to wake him up. I have been trying to tell Nigel how things are for two years. He wrote back, saying he was 'moved'. Even though neither he nor Prof R ever made much effort to connect without the help of their wives, they were each other's enduring friend from university days. And when they were with each other, time fell away. I loved watching them together.

—

When I go out to do chores, Stella watches and manages Prof R if he wakes. I am sure she is exasperated by the situation. She feels he manipulates me, but if she is right, that is survival. Wouldn't anyone, in such a weakened and vulnerable state?

She is now on a video call to her daughter and grandson. From the stairs I can hear her tell them what she thinks of the state we are in here – the untrained dog, the difficult patient, the overworked carer. She is terribly homesick I know, and will be glad to go in two weeks. Out of jail free. It will make her appreciate her single life.

—

The lawyer comes to do the health and welfare LPA on Monday. I will be surprised if she can get enough cognitive understanding from Prof R to follow through with it legally.

My revised Will has been signed by a friendly neighbour (after Citizens Advice said they could not oblige) and is in the post, along with the letter severing the joint ownership of this house and converting it to Tenants in Common. I can breathe again on that front at least.

December 17 — As predicted, the visiting lawyer could get little sense out of Prof R other than the names of various wild animals. He had just dropped off into a deep sleep after a restless morning when she arrived, and he didn't appreciate being disturbed. I was relieved he didn't say 'hippopotamus' as she might have been offended.

He had begun the interview more sensibly, but lost interest when she tried to find out how many children he had by holding up her fingers one by one. She didn't realise how much that might piss Prof R off. So he retaliated with the list of animals, which began with a camel, moved through ostrich, chicken, turkey etc. She was only mildly bemused and will come back on Wednesday. Ethics do not appear to enter her field of vision.

The most disconcerting thing for me was that she asked him a two-part question about who he wanted to manage his health care. "Would you like your wife to manage your health decisions ("yes" says he) or your wife and your children." Also "yes". Not exactly encouraging grounds on which to proceed.

—

Yesterday Hope and her partner Simon came for lunch. He is a lawyer, so I quizzed him about health and the law, as it is his specialist subject. But even he does not know his way around the entire health and social welfare system. No one does.

Prof R said yesterday "Darling, I'm sorry I'm not a better partner." And then later "Thank you for your love." But today he can't remember my name.

December 18 — Tuesday. I have written to the lawyer from the LPA legal firm and cancelled the process. Prof R has been asleep all morning, with my needing to get his pills into him while he is semi-conscious or hallucinating. Probably both. He hasn't had a day like this for a long time, but today is the sort of day that confirms for me that ethically we have left this process too late.

The dog has had her booster shot this morning and the vet, Andrei, tells me she has floating patella, or to those of us not in the know, her kneecaps, on both back legs. He suggests early surgery, but I have been googling this issue and will await developments. Eager veterinary surgeons seeking more business will have to wait.

The current wisdom is that more exercise should help strengthen her legs and we can return to the vet if she seems in pain or has a limp.

So far, she has no symptoms, which is probably why she has remained undiagnosed. But I have emailed the breeder, Lucy, with the bad news.

This afternoon G the plumber is finally returning, this time to mend the detached tarpaulin on the shed roof, which continues to creep further east across the surface in each big blow.

—

G did not come. He's a master at this tactic and I am captive to it.

Prof R did become alert at around 4 pm. And seems to have been awake ever since. His delayed bowel movement annoys him, and he panics if it doesn't arrive on time to his demanding schedule. Rather like the 16.45 train from St Pancras.

So I am tired and briefly doubting my ability to 'man up' once more. The best answer is to hire people for several hours each day so I can recharge my batteries. Constant attention to Prof R leaves me with no time for anything else. And my empathy button is jamming.

We have missed the Christmas food delivery slots, but it doesn't matter. While there are still two mobile adults in the house it really isn't an issue. I worry about silly things like running out of Prof R's pull-ups. The shops will only shut for two days but we have developed a siege mentality along with the rest of the Western world. It's nuts.

I have ordered a bank draft in NZ$ to give Stella for her air fare. Reluctantly she has accepted. It has been a ridiculous state of affairs with her borrowing the fare at seriously insane rates of interest. Our relationship will be returned to a level playing field. When she had paid her fare, I felt captive to her opinion. But I've been grateful for her company nevertheless. And I try to take on board the relevant things she observes, even when it upsets me. She is thrilled when I am angry with Prof R because she sees it as progress. She is more certain in her view he should be in care. I hope that won't be necessary, but I am less certain every day.

Tonight he said, after his third visit to the toilet in 10 minutes, "I shouldn't be here." I know he means "on the planet". I feel it is my fault that he feels like this. I am panicking about him moving around when he is not taking enough care. I tell him a trip to hospital is the worst thing that can happen. I might have to stop saying that because he is not fazed by it.

About getting up he says "I can't stop it" so I say "I know. Don't worry. Just do it carefully." And he was a lot more careful coming back to bed the next time.

December 22 — Saturday. I'm feeling rested. Even though Prof R was up in the night, he is sleeping more during the day. I have a chance to go shopping or just chill on the couch. It makes a difference.

G the plumber finally did come yesterday, after a second SOS from me, to put a new temporary tarpaulin on the shed roof. He informs me that some of the roof is rotten.

—

Last night Prof R became agitated after his meal. As always when he cannot settle, I suggested he come downstairs. This is proving a more useful tactic every time he agrees to do it. But there was a condition. He must not to try to go to the toilet while he was there, if at all possible, as he had already been several times.

The minute he landed in his leather tub chair he was making moves in the direction of the bathroom. To distract him, I asked him to stay where he was, and put on the latest David Attenborough documentary series, *Dynasties*. The episode was about chimpanzees and the music was loud. It almost drowns out David's commentary, but Prof R remained focused on the screen for almost an hour. This has not happened in months. We will try to do more of this when Stella has gone.

Because I am rested, I have more energy to spend time with him. When he returned upstairs, I took my Christmas presents up with me and wrapped them on the bed, showing him what I had bought everyone. I've also been to Tesco and bought a ridiculous number of bagged sweets, most of them for my niece and her son. Stella and I have demolished one already.

Prof R is eating well, and I am finding new ways to make good food that he can also swallow and chew without his dentures. Chicken soup he can eat. Chicken he cannot. He seems to have almost let go of his desire for his dentures. Instead, he combs his hair a lot.

Stacey next door tells me that she is sure she and her husband or son could easily help us lift Prof R if he falls again. She is trained in manual handling and says she has no compunction about being able to use her skills successfully, unlike every agency carer we know. How refreshing. Now all we can hope for is that if he falls, it will be on the weekend when they are home.

Suddenly, even Stella has stopped saying Prof R should be in a home or brought downstairs to sleep on a hospital bed in the living room. I know we are right to feel any move like that is a long way off.

My youngest son, Douglas, texted to say he has moved into his new flat in Sydney. And can I send our address so he can post a Christmas present? Just ask me once darling and I will obey.

—

December 29 — Stella has gone. I was so busy it didn't hit me until dinner time. I looked at her photo – the one I took of her from the top of Tate Modern – and cried over the mash. There were wonderful times and not so wonderful times. Times when she scared me by what she said to various assessors and health people when I wasn't in the room. She was always quite happy to tell me the whole horror of it. Tough talking is her forte.

So the house is quiet, and I am busy doing all the stuff that I put off, like descaling the coffee machine and washing the bedspread. Meals have lost their gloss. Cooking for one and a half is not rewarding. Cooking with, and for, Stella was.

Our Christmas Day was one of the happiest I can remember, in spite of everything. Alex and Ophelia arrived with enough food for a Drop-In centre, in an enormous hamper. I felt truly nurtured, even when the inevitable subject of my care job with Prof R being "too big" for me surfaced. At such times I have learned to say, "Doing it at home is half the cost". That seems to shut discussion down nicely.

My eldest granddaughter Hester gave me my first real hug from her when I caught her looking sad, and asked her if she would like one. She is growing so quickly in her confidence and maturity. It was lovely to feel I am getting to know her more at last.

Her younger sister was just being herself, getting on with things. Prof R was being Prof R, and didn't come down. I took him his presents and hoped he really did know that it was Christmas Day.

—

I have asked for more hours from *Your Choice* and will have six next week. Netty said on Thursday that Prof R complained of having a sore tailbone. She told her manager who now insists I contact the Kent District and Community Nursing Team. She's covering her tracks. Stella, texting from Abu Dhabi, agreed. She felt they are going beyond their brief, given Netty did not examine Prof R and he has no sign of redness there. Nevertheless, I rang the Community Nurse yesterday and left a message, just so that I can say I have. These people continue to intimidate me. I ought to get over it, but I will listen and take their advice when appropriate.

I have changed Prof R's sitting position and remove the large support wedge between meals. Netty's tip about almond oil for his scalp seems to work. I take the oil from the top of my almond butter. It's organic, so why waste it?

Today I am trying not to be bored by the repetition of his care and the smallness of his responses to me. Empathy and love rescue me. Frustration can make me a worse person than I want to be. For two months I have had Stella to return to downstairs. Now the real challenge begins. She has taken bets that he will be beyond this life by mid-summer. She believes she has a gift with predicting these things. A gift it is not.

I have managed not to eat any sweets. Although after dinner I may steal another candy cane from the tree.

December 30 — I actually stole two candy canes from the tree and a small dark chocolate sample bar.

At 9 pm Prof R went wandering and the alarm did not go off. I heard footsteps upstairs and could not fathom the cause. Did we have an intruder? A rat perhaps, a large one that could make the floorboards creak. Or did Stella do a U-turn in Abu Dhabi?

None of the above, was the answer. I found Prof R in my office, in the dark, looking at the window; not necessarily out of the window. He had come down from the loft unattended and unaided without falling. I never react but simply say, "Hello, did you feel like exploring"? As he said, "It's a long time since I walked downstairs." Why did I feel guilty about that?

When he is physically on form, he can do these things, but if I had found him halfway down the flight he might have taken fright, lost focus, and fallen. So I'm glad I didn't. I made no fuss, except to say that I would prefer to be with him if he wanted to do that again.

The mystery of the absent alarm may have been due to the way I had placed the receiver, upside down, at the head of the bed, so that the flashing light did not disturb Prof R. It did work on other occasions but for some reason the signal was blocked. Now it is right side up with a flannel over it to mask the light.

This morning I have been doing more admin. Collecting the phone contacts of important health people into safe places on my phone, changing my diary to 2019 — but being sure to note the dates of Prof R's last falls in the new one. I always save my old diaries, but it is so much safer to have those details to hand. I never know what questions may be asked and I count every day without a fall a victory. His last was on 21ˢᵗ November.

Stella has returned safely to Dunedin. Now asleep hopefully, and recovering from the impossibly long trip. Also safely extracted from her compression stockings presumably (no mean feat) because her daughter tells me she had taken a shower.

I'm back to normal business here, talking to the dog and keeping my house and papers in order as well as my husband. He needs his fingernails cut again.

December 31 — The alarm proves its worth. At 9 am I find Prof R with his pyjama trousers down sitting on the side of the bed, having presumably fallen back down into a sitting position. He needs the toilet, and halfway there I find I need to bark instructions to stop him lowering himself to the floor before we get there. His body resists me when he is like this, so I have to be 'commanding'. It works, but it is hard work. And a loud voice is not only unattractive, it feels like bullying.

New Year's Eve and another crisis averted. But at least today our neighbours would probably be home to help me if he does fall. The ambulance service has asked that we not call them except in a dire emergency as they will be overwhelmed by NY revellers.

At lunchtime my daughter Hope rang from France to say Happy New Year – and then sprang a brilliant surprise; news that she is six weeks pregnant. I was with Prof R while I spoke to her, and when I shed a few happy tears he reached out to hug me. I assured him they were happy tears, and when I told him why he said, "Well done".

To celebrate New Year's Eve and Hope's baby, I ate the entire pack of Jaffa sweets sent to me from NZ. And I felt great.

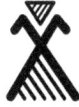

Winter–Spring 2019

JANUARY 1 — Three hours of Netty this morning, of which I managed to remain out for half, before returning to walk the dog. Nothing is open on New Years' Day. Except I found my café at the Quay miraculously serving coffee and pastries.

I felt so much better for my walk that I decided the £33 an hour for public holiday time was probably worth it.... until Netty had left. Prof R has been up and down at least half a dozen times in the two hours since. I am feeling as ragged as though she had never been here. The stimulation of her conversation disrupts him for the day. And yet it is very good for his 'little grey cells'.

The little Christmas tree has been undressed and is now sitting out on the patio waiting for summer and inevitable death from lack of water.

January 2 — Yesterday afternoon into early evening Prof R drilled a groove to the toilet about every 30 minutes. I ate my dinner in shifts. And at 3 am he started again, and was too dopey to rise safely at 7 am, so took his pills propped up like a rag doll.

When he is like that I get as close to tears as is good for me. So I'm spring cleaning. Why people leave it till spring is beyond me. The winter days are short and dark. What better time to get in behind the undisturbed parts of the house? It makes me feel the 'at-home' days are not wasted.

Prof R's bottom has a dry patch that the most expensive cream on the market won't shift, so I am trying the tried-and-true chickweed cream. He used to recoil from me when I put it on my eczema. It stinks and it's an awful charcoal colour, but it works.

Netty asked Prof R yesterday if he had any pain anywhere and he said, "just emotional". So, good news and bad news, and in spite of appearances, still a great deal of insight.

January 3 — Thursday. I've had my last three-hour break for the next week. But I made the most of it. All supplies are in, almond oil for Prof R's head, a new cream for his bottom, more pull-ups, his medications, a book from the library for me and tea and a jam pastry for morning tea.

Now I have just sat for some time next to his bed to dissuade him from a third trip to the bathroom. It's worked. And he has gone to sleep finally.

The new coffee machine has arrived, and I have set it up ready to go for the morning.

G the plumber came at 1.30 pm and pronounced the cistern very sick and needing more work. But he has staunched the leak so I can remove the metal dish that needed emptying every day.

We talked about his son, who is home schooled. He had come with his dad on the last visit, but reportedly couldn't remember us until G said to him, by way of a memory jog, "You know, the house with the two old ladies". So, it's official. I am declared old at 69. The boy, to his credit, apparently replied, "Oh yes, the two posh ladies" so he is in my good books at least.

But the implication is that only old people live like this. With wooden bookcases and cabinets and nice art on the walls. He makes me feel like a museum piece, but I must remember to tell him that when I was in my

WINTER–SPRING 2019   197

20s, my homes were nothing like this. My taste has evolved, along with my belongings. Even Alex and Ophelia have started painting their walls with colour. Minimalism is dead. It comes to us all.

—

When I first met Prof R, I thought his furniture – a lot of it – was horrible and kitset. A 70s museum piece. He didn't seem to care much what things looked like, as long as they were functional. The nice pieces it turned out were mostly bought with his second wife. Or inherited from his grandparents. Those, he treasured.

But he did eventually buy himself a beautiful Rosewood desk in Battersea for £1200 and I was pleased he had. Everyone should have one divine piece of furniture. My pieces are not expensive, I prefer second hand. So, I am rustic rather than a museum piece.

January 4 — Friday. Tonight's dinner – a meat sauce that I blended, on my second attempt to feed him, to disguise the texture – has just been flushed down the toilet. Another in a long line of failed experiments. But lunch – scrambled egg softened in mash – was a success. Mustn't be downhearted, as they say.

Eating my solitary meal downstairs gave me little pleasure. I would prefer to eat with Prof R, but it would hardly be conducive to a pleasant digestion. How does anyone get used to just cooking essentially for one and having to cook separately for another? It could be likened to being a single parent of a very young child. That is the nearest I can imagine.

It takes practice, cooking for one. Unless it's a simple fish and veggies or salad each night. I have ordered a cooked chicken this week from the delivery man. At least that will simplify my choices. But Prof R continues to be a challenge. I want to tempt his palette.

The day drags, even when I seek out neglected tasks, like sorting out a drawer. Not enough exercise outdoors is good for no one. Including the dog, who seems to be feeling quite ill after having her worming tablet this morning. I watched *Mamma Mia, Here I Go Again*, and realised how tragic I was to even consider wasting my time on it.

January 4 — Now, in the middle of watching *Women on the Edge of a Nervous Breakdown*, I am rung by Prof R's sister Doris. I had been silly enough to tell her that the Parkinson's nurse has made yet another appointment for Prof R to attend their clinic, when I have already advised them that he is not well enough to do so and needs a home visit.

Doris is, as always, full of advice. I should ring for a home GP visit. And then ask the GP to advise the Parkinson's Nurse that Prof R is not able to attend the clinic. My advising them myself is apparently not the correct procedure. Too efficient presumably.

Then she said, "They could then advise a hospital bed with a ripple mattress for the pressure points" at which moment, close to tears, I felt I would explode with suppressed anger. "The last thing I want in here is a hospital bed for months on end when there is no immediate need for one."

Doris means well always. It makes her feel useful to share her extensive knowledge of the system, gained over many years as a primary NHS beneficiary. But at times, such as when she insists I am entitled to an allowance, as her brother's carer, even though I have told her several times that I'm not, because I receive a state pension, I wonder how much longer I can stand her 'advice'.

I feel like picking Prof R up and absconding with him to a place where the so-called health provider busy bodies cannot find us. People have died in their own beds since time began. Or at least since beds began. The over-medicalisation of everything and the inefficiency of the interference makes caring for a loved one so much harder and more frightening. Far from being supportive, they make us lose trust in the system.

I've not met a single person yet, no matter how kind, who really makes me feel safe to share honestly whatever may be happening with Prof R. Even my lovely dementia and care navigator people are unsafe confidants, because they too are bound by regulation. Although Stacey next door might qualify as a safe one, given she seemed unperturbed about the prospect of helping me lift Prof R off the floor.

It had been a good day until the call from Doris. And remains a good day overall. No dramas, a happy patient and tasks done as required. Including my first exercise in three months. I'm tackling the 5 Tibetan Poses again and can see how poorly I perform them after such a long break.

My 'first trimester' daughter says she feels better today and went to yoga. I cannot wait to see their baby.

January 6 — Sunday. Depending on which of my own pressure points is being pushed, I swing between wanting to run away with Prof R, or wanting to run away without him. Mostly the former.

It's been a rough morning, masked initially by a reassuring few hours of peace while I presumed he was sleeping. But when I went up to check, he had gone beyond his used-by time, and had rigours. It infuriates me when I get it wrong, because it is almost impossible to get it right. Twice today a pill has ended up left behind in the spout of the cup. That's a record. I always discover them when I refill the cup, but it has the potential to be a real problem.

I have just asked him not to get up so I can go and have some lunch. He is now setting off the alarm for the second time since I began this diary entry. Telling him we cannot go on like this without help gets his agreement but not his cooperation.

And when I said to him, "Darling, unless you can stay in bed when I need you to …. (and now, as I write, he is off again) …. we are going to have difficulty managing on our own at home. What is the solution?" and he says, "Put me in a box", knowing it's the last thing I want. So he is aware enough to say that, but unable to follow a request to stay put long enough for me to have lunch.

—

Finally the bowels have moved, and the bladder; there is no other reason to rise. Except for exercise on a less precarious day. What a mysterious thing this dementia is.

January 7 — Finally, in the night, he stayed in bed when I asked him not to wander. He understood. "When he sleeps, you sleep" was the parting advice of a midwife when I left the maternity home with my first born. I so often think of it. So wise, and yet it was such a simple thing she said.

And I am following her advice. When Prof R is resting in the afternoon, I rest, and often now, up in the bedroom beside him with a book. In the morning, if he's sleeping, I'm busy in the house, but afternoons can be his. If I am calm it is easier for him to be calm.

Stella read several books while she was here, and I am going to take a leaf out of them. Reading in the daytime always used to put me to sleep, so I have avoided it, but not now. Now, it's the TV that puts me to sleep.

Yesterday was so hard, so awful, that today was necessary respite. Prof R has slept a lot. I've just been lying next to him on the bed reading, and just knowing I am there comforts him.

Bedtime for me is now at around 8.30 pm, so that I am there if he is up and down, rather than being annoyed by the alarm downstairs. Why did it take me so long to just stop resisting and accept the change to our lives?

Prof R can't hear the church bellringers practising, although it is quite loud on the breeze. I'm wondering if he has lost his upper register, as he can hear my voice, which is quite low. They don't usually practice on a Monday. For two years it has been a Wednesday night.

January 8 — Tuesday. Prof R the Bastard is back; the man who is restless from 5.30 am and keeps threatening to rise, so I cannot sleep, until I ask him to please stop, and stay in bed. And then he throws the covers off in a pique.

If there was no danger of a fall, I would cheerfully leave him to it. I'm a prisoner of this one fear and I'm still struggling to separate Prof R from his disease. Because the way he responds to the disease can often be a larger version of the Prof R I know – selfish and petulant.

At these times it can be hard to remember that I love him. It's a relief when those feelings return.

—

Prof R agreed to come downstairs for lunch. Whenever I find him wandering – often around my side of the bed, perhaps checking his shirts which hang in the alcove – I suggest he come down. Because clearly he has the energy to be on the move.

I fed him soup and ice cream on the couch, and he picked two pieces of corn out of the soup, claiming them to be too hard for him to eat. Several dozen other pieces of corn from the chowder went down undetected.

We had a photo album session. As much for me as for him, we go down the straight memory lanes of Otago or revisit the beaches of the Bay of Islands. Both of us looked so much better then. Me slimmer, him fatter. And it was only six years ago.

—

What I call his 'fake bladder' strikes again in the afternoon. I will not be going up every 10 minutes to respond to the alarm.

My daughter texted to say she and Simon are going to have an early scan to see if they can detect the baby yet. She feels that will make it real. I know exactly what she means.

January 10 — Thursday. Netty the PA is here, and I feel almost too tired to go out. After being inside for a week, this is not a good way to feel. But Prof R has done everything he could possibly do this morning before she even arrived. So much so (including clearing his bowels) that I ate my breakfast on the run and have yet to have a coffee. But strangely I don't feel like coffee either.

We need more affordable hours of care, i.e., not from an agency. I can't afford to increase Netty's hours, and it rankles that there will be little correlation between her pay and the agency rates.

So yesterday, a new freelancing angel, named Tina, came for an interview and will be more than satisfactory. We will begin with a Wednesday afternoon and see how it goes. She has worked in the care field all her working life and is possibly more qualified than Netty, although perhaps less proscribed by regulation – I hope.

I will build her hours up to supplement Netty's visits.

—

I shouted back at Prof R this morning. I had read about 'mirroring'. It sometimes works. It was about 5 or 6 am. He had lost his temper with me trying to resettle him. When he does that, asserts his authority to roam at will, I can feel helpless. Even if I understand his wish for autonomy.

Hope and Simon have a baby that is 9mm long and has a heartbeat. It's incredible. What a joy to have something so wonderful to look forward to when Prof R's life is ebbing away. I feel so sad always, without realising it. The tears come out in funny places.

—

Again, I am less than refreshed and oddly stressed by the three hours of care today. When I should have been desperate to get out the door. But it is 3 degrees outside and who is going to wander the streets in that temperature? So I came home an hour early and made Prof R a bread and butter pudding, using eggs and cream and dates. It is totally delicious.

I have asked the agency to reduce Netty's hours from three to two on one of the two weekly sessions. I have been marching to their schedule, rather than my own. Mornings would not be my first choice. 1 pm is too late to arrive home and be ready for Prof R's lunch as well as my own.

January 11 — I've been awake since around 3 am but am neither really tired nor distressed by it. I am on red alert. It is so much easier when I am not heavily asleep. The fact that Prof R fell out of bed at 10 pm may have had something to do with it.

He fell onto the bedside stool – a blessing even though he cut his hand. He was able to get up with my help, but I was very shaken. I found plasters and added a bandage to keep them on. And he slept until 3 am. I can anticipate the restlessness that precedes semi-waking and can get his medication into his reluctant mouth before he eventually wakes properly a bit later.

Now we need a side rail – just a short one so he can still get out of bed once seated.

There have, for me, been three cups of tea, one biscuit and a slice of cheese over this time and I am still hungry at 8 am. Off to have breakfast.

—

A critical irritated email from Stella. She says I should be having at least 9 hours care by now and increasing blah blah blah. In truth, Tina is going to be the one to save me I think because she will initially at least be flexible. She has said, "Call me if you just feel the need to get out." She will be living two blocks away and doesn't drive, which makes me hopeful she will be a success and I can employ her at least three days, and later more.

She has experience of "seeing people off" and says end of life care does not faze her.

January 12 — Saturday. Any setback, even if it is relatively minor, diminishes Prof R a little. Yesterday he slept almost constantly, after his encounter with the bedside stool. Incredibly, there are no bruises on his face where he struck it. Only the bloody wound on his hand, which is now healing well.

I've ordered a short rail for the bed and hope it won't hinder him from getting up, when he is able and needs to. If necessary, it will be easy to remove for daytime.

But I also need the bed alarm to go off at night if he is trying to get up. Only experience will tell us whether this is going to work. The price of the rail was right –£55 – so it is not a terrible expense if it is no good.

As I fed him at lunchtime today, I asked if he was still hungry. He said, "only for information" so I said, "ask me". He said, "I would like to know more about these wounds on my head." So again, I explained there is only one and it was several months ago and has healed. It was no one's fault. An accident that happened because he fainted.

Then he said, "I don't know how I'm going to cope", and there followed a discussion about aging and the illnesses we will all get, me included. I also say, "You are already coping, and very well." It seemed to satisfy him.

He remembers who Billy Connolly is so I could tell him Billy's joke about the man who had given his name to Parkinson's; "I wish he had kept it to himself!" Although apparently it had a much worse name before he rediscovered it. "Shaking Palsy."

January 13 — Sunday. I first learned to love Prof R – when we still lived 12,000 miles apart – by sleeping with his photo next to my heart. After he declared his love for me, when we hardly knew each other, I wanted to catch up. And a photo was all I had.

I have always believed we can choose to love someone. Or not. Depending on the circumstances and whatever crime they may or may not have committed. I ignored his crimes as he ignored mine, so eventually, it worked out fine.

Now I am fierce in how I feel about him. Both fiercely loving and fiercely angry with myself when it is all going pear-shaped. But he is teaching me patience, so there is less frustration for both of us. But this morning, after he had wakened every 45 minutes or so since about 2 am, I was back in fierce frustrated mode.

It's not so bad when I have insomnia, or am sleeping lightly. Then I am reading my book or making tea for much of those small hours, so his waking was less damaging to my health. In the hours before 2 am, my dreams were all about losing custody – being deemed unfit to 'parent' in the dream. Not hard to interpret as a fear of being deemed unfit to care for my husband.

—

There has been another flurry of spring cleaning. I notice that I am more energetic when I have slept poorly. So perhaps heavy sleeping brings on lethargy during the day too. Yesterday was a torpid day, although there is no such thing here in reality, and I watched two films and dozed and possibly ate too much. Just humus, but my sister tells me it is very fattening.

After dinner tonight – chicken which was soft enough for him to eat – I asked him what he was thinking about and he said, "my brain". And when I asked if he remembered my name, he did. So that was better than a few weeks ago, which I reminded him of. Progress.

January 14 — Prof R complained of a bruised feeling on his tailbone this morning which prompted a flurry of research from me and a phone call to our local mobility company. Darren, the manager, was incredible and talked me through all the products available – not just his own – so that I was informed but still not decided.

There are several options, the cheapest of which may be an inflatable pad for the bed. In the meantime, I am not allowing him to recline when he is resting. It seems mean. But I cannot persuade him to sit at upright, and any leaning back beyond 90 degrees causes the skin to slide across the bone. 'Shear' is the correct word.

—

It's not a good day for him mentally and that makes talk difficult. I suggested I read to him from his work diaries, and he liked the idea, but they are totally monosyllabic; dates and times, and meaningless to anyone who did not attend the meetings or write the paper with the deadline. There is no glimpse of the personal. And for Prof R those events will be impossible to place.

I'm very tired today after a disturbed night and dreams to match. I struggle to be patient when he gets up again a few minutes after I leave the room.

The Care Navigator, K, when asked, was not able to advise me on pressure relief equipment but she did refer me to several helpful sites. Who knew rubber rings can make things worse? What it comes down to is that we need to get the Community Nurse to visit and advise us before buying any equipment that may or may not help.

This afternoon, feeling somewhat stonewalled, I reappraised the bed wedge and have decided to use it without pillows, to attain as straight a position as possible for Prof R. He has a 'Parkinson's curve' on his upper spine which does not help. But we have agreed that the wedge with just a bolster cushion at his neck is the best we can do.

Netty is not coming tomorrow because she has a cold, and I'd rather she didn't come when unwell. Her agency manager continues to impress me very little. After being quite unperturbed that she could only provide a replacement PA on one day last week, suddenly this week, on learning that I have a private person for Wednesday afternoon, is bending over backwards to tell me she will be trying to give me more hours as soon as possible. Translated, that means she anticipates Netty's other client will no longer need their services, 'all being well'. If she thinks I am going to offload Tina as soon as Netty's other client has died, she will be sorely disappointed.

More and more I resent the fact that the over-priced private agencies of this world are not equipped to advise us on care, such as pressure points, other than to refer us to the local health authority. The upshot is, that Netty is brilliant at stimulating Prof R's mind but not at preserving his body.

Prof R wasn't hungry at dinner but finally felt like his fish pie and ice cream at 9.30 pm.

January 15 — Tuesday. The big Brexit vote today. This drama is a blessing for me, being exciting and mentally stimulating, but not so good for Theresa May.

Prof R is comatose this morning having slept through from 1.30 am until 7.30 am. A long time without levodopa but as always, I wonder if it matters. We both needed the uninterrupted sleep. And he is wearing his pull-ups.

Strangely, I feel relieved that I don't have to prepare for Netty this morning. I may need these people, but I don't always want them. No matter how nice they are.

Later, Prof R was still asleep. Woken by me for coffee through a straw and pill, but unable to get up. By 1.30 pm I woke him again because he had slept long enough. Breakfast and lunch and pills, all in a row, restored him enough to walk to the toilet, where I changed his sodden pull-ups that he had no idea he had filled.

—

The bed rail arrived and is installed, although it is perhaps a bit too long for Prof R to climb out past easily when he needs to. A work in progress. But it is nice to see him tucked up safely in bed when he is so often half out of it with legs dangling in the air. They become heavier to lift when he is unable to help.

January 17 — Thursday. A terrible night followed by my desperate urgency to escape as soon as Netty arrived at 10 am. So often a broken night seems to leave me primed for action. But not in the small hours, when exhaustion makes everything so much harder. And once, in the night, when he seemed unable use his leg muscles to help me lift him back into bed, I ended up begging him, "I can't do it on my own".

I have circumnavigated the agency manager and achieved a shift swap, despite her bullying, from Thursday's to Friday's. I even dared to ask for the afternoon when she suggested 10.45 am. A triumph, although Netty will not always be able to do three hours on Friday afternoons. Which is another triumph, as two hours are enough, and every hour down is £31 up.

I am booked to begin Pilates again next Wednesday. Teacher Chloe is so kind and welcoming it makes me feel far more motivated than I really am.

Today, determined to learn how to use my respite time effectively, I had lunch out. It felt quite decadent. A poached egg on mashed avocado and sourdough bread. I will do this again.

—

Delighted by a notice from the publisher to say I have sold a copy of my book. Given how low my expectations of sales are, the pleasure is magnified far beyond its true importance.

January 18 — Friday. Chronic boredom has driven me to clean out my filing cabinet and shred those files I feel able to let go of. It's surprising how the archival eye prevents me from doing a total clear-out. I have kept my accounts from 2000-2005 because I want to be able to remind myself of the freelance work I did in those first years in London. It would be easy to feel I had thrown away 'my brilliant career' at UK customs in February 2000.

Just now, achieving something other than cleaning, cooking or tending to Prof R each day seems to be necessary for mental health. Prof R is now sleeping and eating or being groomed – and that's if I am lucky and all is well.

The dog doesn't appear to be losing weight and neither do I. The housebound are challenged, even if busy in the domestic sense.

January 20 — For the second time in a week I have managed to shower and wash my hair early without Prof R's alarm going off. This a small step for anyone else – massive for me.

He is in the eye perhaps of a storm of some kind, but he sleeps more reliably. Perhaps, also, he is being less driven by his confusion and is more placid with his illness. Less up and down for part of the day, although that can still happen in the small hours of the morning.

Yesterday I managed the entire 5th Netflix series of *Grace and Frankie* – which I had been waiting months for – simply because Prof R slept between meals. At first, I felt desperate that I wasn't doing something more constructive, until I remembered that if I take to the couch in the afternoon I am able to be more patient and loving with him in the evening. Cleaning out my filing cabinet can be tackled at another time of day.

—

Breakthrough. Feeding him in his cane chair instead of the bed has been a remarkably simple solution to the pressure marks on his tail. This advice has come from the man in the mobility shop. He has my undying gratitude. I will tell him so.

And it is so much more companionable and 'normal'. The food is becoming more cunning. Yesterday a salmon fillet in creamed rice, because he cannot eat plain rice, or even risotto.

In an exercise in self-discipline, I made my own risotto earlier in the day.

Meals are taken in companionable silence. Unless I can think of an anecdote or event that he will understand and appreciate. But there is joy in his unexpected moments of humour. As I knelt at his feet changing his pants and trousers, he said "I think you really enjoy doing that".

January 21 ('Blue Monday' apparently) — The sun is shining, there are no blues in this house, just interminable time. Even the plumber is another week late. And I haven't the energy to summon him yet again.

The dog is being exercised on the stairs. It's the recommended treatment for her floating kneecaps and stops her declining through lack of walks.

My sister is in hibernation, 12,000 miles away, not answering my texts. Her daughter says she is okay. I will not 'chase' her, as has been my usual pattern. I should not feed that particular wolf.

Mid-morning, I began to try and wake Prof R again. He'd last had medication at 7 am. But he wouldn't wake up. Barring firing a gun or ringing a bell. So, I let him sleep and kept reheating his coffee, confident he would soon need the toilet. But he didn't, even though I sat in the room and read for a while, he did not wake until after midday.

This is not a good shift in his sleeping behaviour. Even when seated in his cane chair, he needed a lot of encouragement to eat, or even open his eyes. But I just kept telling him he had to, so he did. And he enjoyed his coffee afterwards.

In between, we did his grooming – almond oil in the hair, a hot flannel on his face and clean socks. All designed to keep him awake and feeling nurtured.

—

When he had returned to bed, I took myself and his alarm pager (in my pocket) across to the hardware store to get replacement batteries for one of the bathroom scales. My intention was to weigh the dog, but she was not heavy enough or cooperative enough to activate the digital scale. We shall have to wait until we visit the vet.

The walk to the shop, in the sunshine, no wind to spoil it, without a handbag weighing me down or a dog pulling on a lead, reminded me that I must do this short walk, 100 yards or so either way down our street, at least once a day. My spirits have totally recovered from the stifling first part of the morning. So much so, I have opened my office window, despite the chill. It was -3C this morning and so much nicer for that.

January 22 — Everything hurts today. Not Prof R this time, but me. Probably because I had one of my downstairs 3 am 'burning of the oil' nights with the consumption of tea and cheese. But also, because Mr Sleepy became Mr Jack-in-the-Box this afternoon. To divert my irritation at the insistent alarm, I changed the cover on the duvet. And fed him cake. He's still active but I've left him to it. In these moods he is safe unaided.

Netty came this morning. I tried to discuss with her my need to plan the process ahead, and whether she and her team could advise me as things change. Because she is able to say so little, legally speaking, it's frustrating. But she did say she would flag up to me (and her manager) anything she felt needed a different approach. Which is a two-edged sword.

Her previous client has just died, and she feels the loss of what she called the 'bubble they were living in'. I feel like that here, now.

(*Revisiting this now, in a Covid-19 bubble, the feeling is not dissimilar*)

A beautiful sunny cold day which I used to ramble through town in a deliberate and careful way. The mundane is my delight. The unexpected discovery of slippery elm tablets in the Apothecary, with its exotic perfumed products and shelves of huge jars filled with herbs. I've always had to buy them online.

I also came home with the first packet of pork scratchings I have bought in years – and scoffed them this afternoon. Ah, the joy of comfort food. Feeling hungry, when it cannot be real hunger, is stressful in itself.

—

My daughter Hope has had her first visit to the midwife and has been pronounced fit and healthy. She is pleased she will have the same midwife right through to the birth, and can have her baby in the maternity wing, rather than in a hospital ward.

I remember being introduced to the on-duty midwife whenever I arrived to give birth. She or he would go off duty and be replaced by others as the labour wore on. It never bothered me unless they were short-tempered. And some were.

January 24 — Thursday. Tina arrived yesterday, and after waiting while I briefed her for 30 minutes, nervously admitted she has got a job at a care home for 21 hours a week, so cannot guarantee Wednesdays. I wish she had told me earlier.

But instead of sending a 'knee-jerk' email to the agency immediately to see if Netty was still available on a Wednesday, I drew breath and raced off to my Pilates class. After which, (rusty joints, squeaky limbs) I dropped into my local café for a hot chocolate and messaged Netty's manager. She is available, and will come on Wednesday afternoon instead of Tuesday morning. An unexpected result. Perfect.

—

A minor domestic triumph this morning, when Prof R, eyes open but no one at home, gave me the courage to have a bath and wash my hair at

9.15 am. I had been dressed, made up and ready for the postie at 8.15 am, but I am becoming more adventurous about self-care and where to fit it in.

Downtime is still couch time. Midnight red-eye-time watching episodes of *Call My Agent* on Netflix in subtitles. It's the perfect fix for the wife of a restless husband who will keep me awake anyway.

When Prof R finally surfaced after 11 am he was in his 'I will put my slippers on' mode. No matter if I try to say he doesn't really need them. His socks only leave his feet to be changed. This morning I have put his syrup of figs into his morning water to reduce the choking he has from dryness. It works. And seems preferable to trying to keep a fruit juice carton fresh by the bed.

While eating his breakfast, sitting in the cane chair, he begins to complain about discomfort where his bones are pressing against his skin. It is not surprising. I cannot understand how his breastbone stays inside, given it is making a tent on his chest. It hurts me to see it. (Note to self: bring this up with the community nurse).

As he was resettling in his bed, I said, as usual "Are you okay?" and he replied, unusually, "Yes, and what about you? Are you okay?" So unexpected, so kind. Perhaps I was looking a bit tired. I blamed the Pilates.

January 25 — Yesterday, while looking for a book Prof R might like to be read from, I found a group of letters he had written to a friend while he was working in France in 1960. I've begun reading them to him. I'm probably enjoying them more than he is.

January 26 — Saturday. Another fall in the bathroom at 10.30 am, just as I was halfway up the second staircase answering the alarm. Lying on his side, his pants mostly down, clearly about to pee but either missing his balance or having a faint.

214 THE MAN WITH THE COLANDER IN HIS HEAD

This time, as it was a weekend, I went straight next door for help. Stacey and her eldest boy came and lifted him off the floor and onto the bed, Stacey issuing instructions. She mentioned she was about to go on a specialist course for falls on Tuesday.

Two ibuprofens later and he was up having his breakfast and finishing the task he had set out on, to have a pee. No ambulance, no broken bones, and by early afternoon, when he awoke from a long sleep, he had forgotten the fall.

In deep gratitude, I have ordered flowers for Stacey to say thank you. It seems inadequate, given the stress they have saved us both. This time I will not be telling the agency or Netty. I don't trust their reporting system and the likely outcome that they insist on a doctor's visit. Covering their backs is not my main area of concern.

So now we start the count again from zero to the next fall. I tell him we should aim to have zero falls in 2019. He agrees, after mentioning a little vertigo. I'm not surprised. He was mildly concussed after the bad fall last year and has probably got similar symptoms. Or not. Maybe the vertigo caused his fall. Either way, we are back on high alert.

—

I have ordered some shampoo caps that work by being heated in the microwave before 'washing' the patient's hair; a bulk supply of 10 so that we are not running out of anything in the short term.

The jolt from the fall has definitely given Prof R a recurrence of his vertigo symptoms. The fluid in his ears has been displaced again. So now I am saying to him that he must not leave the bed unless someone is with him. I have moved the mattress alarm up closer to his pillows, so that when he moves down the bed to the 'escape hatch' in the side rail it should go off before he stands up. We shall see. I have lost my faith in the alarm once again, after so many weeks of feeling we were on top of this.

He is eating fairly well, and so am I, having had a stove-top chicken stew on the go, freezing it overnight and starting again the following day. It's alchemy, adding something new each day so that it never actually runs out. Why didn't I think of this earlier? Probably because it would horrify anyone else. "What? Refreezing after re-cooking? That's so dangerous." Poppycock, as my parents might have said. Logic tells me I am handling it safely. It also means I can eat in his room with just a bowl and a spoon. So much better than feeling hungry and irritated if I am late getting my own meal.

January 27 — Desperate times, desperate measures. After 24 hours analysing the problem of falls, there is only one solution. To keep him in bed with a second rail. One that drops down for easy exit. I have ordered one that not only drops down, but extends if necessary. Today I have put one of the cane chairs in the gap at the bottom half of the bed to prevent Prof R getting up without an escort.

In the morning, it worked well. I came up regularly until I found him awake. He also stayed seated in the cane chair when I asked him to, while I fetched lunch and ice cream.

But in the afternoon, it was 'all change'. He wanted to get up earlier than I expected, but he didn't sit up and activate the alarm. So that when I did go up, he was puce-faced and had been ringing the hand bell for goodness knows how long. I don't hear it unless I am in the hall. These events make me sick with misery.

So how to keep him safe while I bring food? When I sat him in the cane chair, I blocked his exit with my own chair, and asked him to stay there while I fetched afternoon tea. I returned to find the cane chair empty, mine pushed aside, and him back on the toilet. Why was he there? Just because he could, that's why.

Now the bed alarm has been put under his pillow and I have asked him to sit up if he wants to alert me. He may or may not remember to do that, just as he couldn't remember to stay in the cane chair. Sometimes all is logical, sometimes not.

I have rigged up two trouser belts to act as a seatbelt for the cane chair. He likes it. No doubt my lovely carers will tell me it is unsafe to use it. He might end up on the floor carrying his chair on his back like a tortoise. I will see what Tina says tomorrow. On the plus side, I used one of the shower cap shampoos on Prof R and it worked a treat.

January 28 — Monday. A difficult afternoon yesterday was followed by a very difficult night.

Prof R was very restless, yet unreliable in his head and on his feet. The pillow positioning of the alarm has helped enormously. I can reach him when he is just about to place his feet on the floor.

But overnight I had to 'loudmouth' us both through one of the toilet visits just to keep him on his feet and both of us off the floor. The loud voice definitely has 'cut through' and can help him focus.

At midnight I lay in bed watching him peeling off his socks, lying on his back. His flexibility was impressive. Later he mentioned he could probably manage some food if it was forthcoming. I said, "What time do you think it is?" He said "8 pm".

—

This morning he is eyes open; brain only half engaged. I am checking frequently and offering water and coffee. So far, he is only taking the water. Laced with Syrup of Figs to make it slip down his throat without choking, while I raise him with my left arm beneath his back.

11 am. He's had most of a cup of coffee in bed, but had trouble following my instructions to suck on the straw. Although he can talk to me, after a fashion. He keeps trying unsuccessfully to get up and I tell him to relax, it isn't safe to get up and he must stay where he is. He has his night pants on and can pee if he needs to.

4 pm and Tina has been and gone. Prof R slept blissfully through her visit and has awoken able to communicate and walk with me on one arm and his walking stick in the other. He has eaten a meal and dessert. Plus, a fruit smoothie for kids in a cute pouch. He is much happier, and so am I. The effects of the fall seem to have passed.

January 29 — From the ridiculous to the sublime and back to the ridiculous. Always expect to be surprised, and then you will hopefully be less horrified.

The new bed rail arrived and required serious installation, it being better and more versatile than the one already in situ. So, much puffing and panting and sweating to put the ties under the mattress, across the bed and out the other side of this super king bed. 'Super-latives' were expressed.

Prof R had slept most of the night with only one wake-up, and then slept all morning. I was waking him for pills, coffee, liquid, until early afternoon when I got him up for food in his chair. He was with me, but not with me. Dazed and unresponsive. Nothing suited. The saved breakfast muesli and fruit, rejected after a few mouthfuls. A meal replacement strawberry drink was okay. Coffee was okay. And then ice cream was okay.

And then we spent the best part of an hour trying to expectorate the mucus that accumulates in his throat. Perhaps he should be eating only dairy free. I feel so sorry for him. He never learned how to 'hoik' like a nice street boy could. So I'm hooking it out from the front of his tongue with finger and tissues and in between he tries to swill it out. Eventually, both exhausted, we called it a day.

Five minutes after he was settled back in bed the alarm went off. He was outside the blankets but not sure why. So, he was settled back down, with the request he go to sleep.

The next time the alarm went off, I was halfway through preparing spinach and half a fish pie for my dinner. Me, the born optimist, confident about the new rail, walked upstairs rather than ran, and arrived just in time to find him poised, seated on the footboard of the bed, about to launch himself, looking for an exit. This man is either unable to move a muscle or faster than a whippet.

The optimist took a hit. It is times like these that I seriously wonder, yet again, how I will continue to keep him safe. No matter what I say or how often I stress safety, there will always come the time when he acts spontaneously, without thought. Angie tells me that In care homes they just get the paramedics in regularly to pick them up off the floor.

I have retracted the new rail, which can extend, so that there is now a gap between the two rails at the side of the bed, where he can see a safe exit. And hopefully choose it. Now I must simply run up as usual. Or add the cane chair at the new exit to slow him up.

I'm now off to warm up his leftovers to put with ....

(7.10 pm And the alarm went off. A toilet trip.)

.... As I was saying, dinner for Prof R was cottage pie, which he rejected, so I took the mash off the top of the left-over fish pie, added cream and gave him that.

Therefore, for my dinner, I have the rejected cottage pie, mashed to a grey pulp, mixed with water and looking like a prison meal, plus the underside of the fish pie. A mixture of beef and salmon. Sitting on a bed of spinach. Could anything be more tasty?

January 30 — Wednesday. The whippet got away again just after 11 am. The alarm still sometimes does not trigger when it should. I ran upstairs to find him already sitting on the toilet. This is very clever of him, to be sitting and not lying on the floor, but it makes my heart race more than is good for me.

I have returned to putting the cane chair in the gap and hope he will not head for the tail of the bed next time.

Netty comes at 1 pm so I can go to Pilates and post a birthday present – and go to Tesco's. She will need to be very alert.

January 31 — I took the risk and had a shower this morning, even though Prof R is restless, with his eyes open, having taken a non-productive trip to the toilet. But I didn't push my luck and wash my hair. It is my first shower since Sunday. Don't tell anyone.

Netty and Prof R had a lovely afternoon yesterday apparently. After he and I had that nervy morning. I'm really delighted he enjoys the visits of his two women so much. For a largely anti-social man, this is a bonus. Netty is good, and understands my fears regarding his safe mobility. I am beginning to sound her out about the suitability of our loft bedroom for a hospital bed. She says, "Don't worry about that now, he is okay at the moment and you have enough to deal with."

Pilates was painful and enjoyable in one. I needed two ibuprofens on my return home. But I'm certain I gain at least a centimetre in height after each session. Or perhaps I begin to look ahead rather than at the floor or Prof R's wobbly feet.

—

Another breakfast has been rejected. This time, I tried creamed rice instead of oats with the usual prunes, grapes, supplements, kefir, and a rather naughty maple syrup. But his palette has changed. It may be the fruit, or disliking the supplement flavours.

So instead, I gave him a fruit smoothie. No one can object to those. He asked me why I needed to go downstairs. Probably because his carers spend the entire three hours sitting with him. They have no need to do anything else. Other than fetch the food I have prepared. So in compensation, I groomed his feet. I don't ask them to do that, or clean his fingernails, or wash his "underlings" (our name for his 'jewels'). Or put cream on his buttocks or check for rashes. (Although Netty sometimes does).

I have succeeded in curing an angry red rash on the back of his head which he scratched almost to bleeding. It was on the site of a pink birthmark under his hair, so the skin may be more sensitive.

The repositioned alarm is still not 100 percent reliable. If I run the very second the pager goes off, I can just about catch him before he moves towards the bathroom. Good exercise you might think. Good for the heart but bad for the nerves.

Just now he rang his hand bell. He wanted me to do the impossible and put out the sun. The hanging blind above his head leaves a gap that reflects on the wall and somehow disturbs him. He is reasonable about it, and understands I cannot fix the side of the blind to the frame. The sun will move.

—

I can hear Prof R's right hand beating on the bedclothes. I know it's his right hand because that is the worse one and it beats like a drum when he is stressed.

We've just been trying to make the bed alarm perform better. It is not providing enough safety. Just now I ran from the first floor up and he was already hanging onto the bathroom door wobbling and dangerous. Even though it is under his pillow, the alarm seems to be slow responding until his bottom is about to leave the bed. And Prof R cannot help us with this. He will get up and never be able to think about whether he should wait. And he is dizzy today.

I'm trying something new. Pushing the alarm reset button even though it supposedly resets itself when Prof R lies down. He's just tested it again, although I didn't know that and thought he was getting up. It seemed to set off a second or so earlier. But I was only down one floor. The next time he exits we will see.

My nerves are stretched almost to their limit. How long before he has to have a hospital bed with rails?

It's nearly 4 pm and I have been on the run with him all afternoon. Food first, and then, to keep him company and avoid total frustration, I did the grocery delivery order and tested one of the shampoo caps on my hair – all while he was sitting on the toilet. It certainly helps to pass the time.

The shampoo cap is definitely hugely better than a dry shampoo, although there is a little stickiness from the lack of a rinse. The contents of the cap read like the inventory of a chemical lab.

4.10 pm and he has just got up again. He was on his feet before I got there. I am now afraid to go downstairs.

February 1 — Rabbits! Pinch and a punch...

Friday. And a new day. Yesterday is one to be forgotten. All downhill until after 10 pm, and eventual tears from me. Fatigue yes, but also afraid to go to the toilet, or even leave the bedroom. Although there was a hiatus when he slept, and I managed to eat my evening meal.

I have written to my Care Navigator for more advice on how to avoid disaster in the loft. An accident waiting to happen, and yet not an accident, as it is predictable.

Netty helped me analyse spaces for a hospital bed. Two flights of stairs may be at least one too many. But do I have to take what is offered? Can I install our own version that the medical people find acceptable for nursing?

I went to the library and discovered that Market Town has a literary festival this month. I intend to go to at least one event. Will Self or Jo Brand perhaps.

A quieter evening, perhaps because Prof R managed to move his bowels at lunchtime. It seems to make a difference.

February 2 — It's become the norm to give Prof R his breakfast-time pills semi-conscious. His head is turned to the side, raised by pillows. He can respond just enough, with eyes still closed, to do it safely. Our definition of safety does not match the speech therapist's.

From 4 am I have been waiting for him to get up for a pee, because he was restless, and appeared to be ready to launch an assault. Mind the gap! Legs bang against the rails, covers are thrown partly off, and then the momentum dies. I'm relieved, because it gives me time to kick-start my own day.

After lunch I persuaded Prof R to stand on the scales. 53 kg. I knew his weight loss was shocking, but not quite so much. I remember weighing that when I was about 26. He begins to look more and more like his paternal grandfather, the butcher. Whose face we used to laugh at, so long and cadaverous was it. Like my favourite joke... a horse walked into a bar...

February 3 — It only takes one mistake, but today I got away with it. I forgot to take the pager from under my pillow and put it in my pyjama pocket when I went downstairs early to make myself a cup of tea and feed the dog. Fortunately, I noticed its absence, and ran up to retrieve it, because at 8 am the alarm went off. He is not usually alert at this time. Although he had woken at 7.30 am already and had his pills. And equally fortunately, I had not decided to sneak in a shower.

I notice I'm a bit shaky this morning, probably from the sudden awakening at 7.30 am. My system is on high alert. All limbs buzzing. A morning run would fix it, but fortunately I have an excuse not to go out.

February 4 — Monday. His daughter Julie is giving Prof R his breakfast. She has come down by train for the morning and has caught him at the right time. It's so nice to see him smile at her.

We had a restless night and an insecure attempt to get up early in the morning. I had to persuade him to return to bed after we were stalled, immobile, between the bed and the bathroom door. If he is at all alert, when I say, "It's all right, you can pee in those pants", he says "Why would I want to do that?"

I am picking Julie's brains as well as everyone else's to think of clever ways to keep a safe structure in place. When she and I went up to feed him he was already in the bathroom. The alarm had not gone off at all.

He is beginning to eat less. Today it was breakfast and a late lunch. No dinner, just some fruit smoothie squeezed into his mouth from the tube. He likes it very much. But says he is not hungry for anything else.

February 5 — Tuesday. The zimmer frame has been delivered and is standing guard over the rail gap while Prof R sleeps on after his mid-morning coffee through a straw. It looks impressive, so the hope is that it will *be* impressive. If it is, we can postpone a move to the lower floor.

—

The Pension Service informs me that my weekly pension will go up to £131.84 a week in April. It feels like riches, undeserved, although of course it is subsidised from my New Zealand taxes. I have begun to think about the fact that in the foreseeable future I will be living on that amount, plus whatever portion of Prof R's work pension they choose to give me. A windfall, gratefully received, no matter how small it is.

The belt will be tightened on food and utilities. Clothing won't be a problem. I need very few clothes. But I will want to spend money on train tickets, going up to London.

(*At this point, dear reader, I had not even considered I might get a single household increase in my state pension. That surprise came later.*)

—

After a late lunch we went on a tour of the first floor. Exploring a possible move down. Once we've made the mental shift, we are both excited about a change of scene, which says more about our situation than the event. But nevertheless, it will be refreshing and allows Prof R to explore more of the house without needing to use the stair lift. Much safer for him when I am running one flight not two.

We tested the zimmer frame in the new space to see if he could use it to stand up from the higher guest bed. It worked. He would not need the wall rail. And we practised the path to the toilet and how the frame would be used, or not. Like two children, exploring a new house, as though we had never been there before.

Tonight he ate a fish pie at last. It's a mini pie designed for toddlers, and it's perfect. With cream added of course. Ice cream followed, so I am hopeful of a more restful night. He didn't get up last night, but he shook all through the small hours until I asked him – or more accurately, his body – to stop. And amazingly, it did.

Hope has sent me a photo of her almost-bump. A gentle curve that is beautiful. It is such a special experience for a mother when her daughter becomes pregnant. I had known it would be lovely, but I underestimated the emotions it would bring.

February 6 — Wednesday. We're in a little happy place, anticipating our big adventure. Proof, when living in ever-decreasing circles, that everyone needs something to look forward to, even just little things.

The plumber G has finally been, the toilet fixed and cleaned. Tomorrow a riser seat should arrive for the guest room toilet, soon to be renamed as our bedroom. Then we can move whenever we wish. Joking, I suggest we pretend we have two flats, and move between the two if we wish. Depending on what takes our fancy. (I don't mention how unlikely that will be.)

The zimmer is a success, so even the loft is not quite the burden it has been. I can climb the stairs with a normal heart rate. (*Reader, this was short-lived*)

Today, being Wednesday, I went to Pilates and stretched myself in ways I never have before. Or perhaps I am just better at it. I'm now convinced I come out not only taller, but with longer limbs. That 'walking on air' feeling doesn't last for long, but it's worth the hour of hard work.

Today it was followed by a walk to the Quay, fruit bread pudding slice and a cup of tea. Afternoon tea is a good idea for me. It meant I could feed Prof R before I went out. And he's eating well today. Mash and sardine for lunch (with cream of course) and fish again for tea.

And he is smiling more.

—

The Quality Care Commission are reviewing the agency and rang for my views. I found myself in some difficulty. How to say they are almost too rule-bound, so that I am intimidated by them? How to say they don't provide any advice, just report on any perceived health or safety issues? And then bully me to contact the GP, or the Community Nurse, to cover themselves and their insurance policy; even if my knowledge of him tells me it's unnecessary. How to say they charge far too much and should jolly well be good at the price? Well, I actually did say that last bit, and she laughed.

But of course, I also praised Netty to the skies and gave examples of her creative ways to stimulate Prof R intellectually. But how to say, "Did you know she isn't a trained carer at all, more a companion and educator? And has only been with them 18 months, although they told me it was two years."

February 8 — Friday. We have moved. Prof R is tucked up in our new bed, the toilet riser has been fitted, and only one rail seems necessary. The bed is very high. I have tripped over the zimmer frame several times already but will just have to learn to avoid it. One of my toes has turned black.

It's a huge relief to be only one floor up. Earlier today I was unsure if we would make the move until tomorrow. Several blasts of the bed alarm acted as the best incentive I could possibly have to get us both out of the loft.

He's still in a fairly happy space and eating well. He seems calm. And stimulated by the move. Tonight he appeared reluctant to get back into bed, and when I asked what he would like to do he said, "If we had a TV in here, I could watch it." This from a man who has shown no interest in the television for some time.

So I said, "Of course you can watch TV. Any time you want to. Would you like to come downstairs?" There would be no space for a TV in our cosy room if we wanted one. Not even fixed to the ceiling. So I took him downstairs and we watched a film he probably couldn't understand until he became tired, and I brought him back to our 'new' room. So much better for him to leave his bed than be 'enabled' not to.

It was an up and down sort of evening all round.

February 9 — Saturday. My children bring me joy. The Sydney boy rang this morning at 8 am and the little family of Alex and Ophelia came for lunch. The girls are in good form and so is the dog. They feed her crackers and she throws up on the floor. It's an improvement on the dog eating the tires off a toy car.

Prof R and I had a remarkably good night, but he's been tired today and slept a great deal, waking only for food and a pee. It meant I could spend more time with the family. Bliss.

But tonight, he has been over my side of the bed again. I can hear him from downstairs when he is active without actually leaving the bed or setting off the alarm.

I found my book, my pen my special coaster from mid-Canterbury all on his side of the bed. Missing are my notebook and my bookmark. I'm not happy. But when I asked why he was on my side of the bed, he said he didn't know it was my side of the bed and didn't even know I slept there. More guilt.

When I am there, of course, he does know it. I had notes I wanted to refer to in the notebook and the invasion looms larger than it should. Which says more about my state of mind than his.

He's now ringing his handbell and I feel like telling him to fuck off. But I won't.

February 10 — Sunday. If Prof R's head is awake before his legs, both of us have a miserable time. He cannot be allowed to go to the toilet, and he gets agitated. Even though he agrees his legs are not ready to hold his weight. And he knows, or seems to, that he can pee in his pull-ups.

He does still empathise at times. If my head is in my hands, perhaps only because I am tired, he reaches out and strokes me. And keeps telling me how beautiful I am, proving beauty is in the eye of the beholder.

But when I ask him to stay in bed so I can make him a coffee, the bed alarm will sound before I have finished grinding the beans and I am left grinding my teeth.

And so it was today, when his legs woke up. And I can understand he would rather pee in the toilet than in his pull-ups. Who wouldn't? So I helped him and put him back to bed and knew I could forget about coffee until later because he would go to sleep.

—

It turns out someone else nearby uses a hand bell. Twice yesterday, when I heard one and thought it was Prof R, it wasn't. Whoever is using it must be very nearby, in a neighbouring house. Calling their cat?

The walls are not particularly soundproof. The good thing about that is, I am constrained from reaching my top notes when I feel particularly powerless in the face of Prof R's determination to throw himself off the bed.

—

I found my notebook inside the library book, along with the bookmark. I am comforted by having my small possessions restored to me. And in the night, I found that I could safely carry a cup of tea back to my bed even though, because I'm now almost against the wall, I have to climb over the tailboard. But I can reach across and put the cup on the radiator before I make the hazardous journey.

Climbing out of bed is not so straightforward. I need to be on my hands and knees, or I get cast on my bottom with my legs dangling over the tailboard and not enough strength in my arms to complete the move. This is an unwelcome sign of advancing age.

More progress. We've discovered a new technique for removing the mucus from Prof R's mouth. It lodges in the roof. Who knew? But he pointed it out for me wordlessly, and when I investigated with a tissue, success. Not exactly mining for gold but fairly satisfactory nevertheless.

—

He is very dopey this morning, after the almost violent insistence on visiting the loo very early on. Now he sleeps again, having to be woken to have his breakfast rather late – 11.30 am.

We're not cleaning his teeth often enough, mainly because he is often so tired after eating. It is not something I can insist on. But we must do better. Oral health is one of the major problems of care, so I've been told. Neglected people in care homes have been discovered with their dentures embedded in their gums.

After his lunch, when I thought he was settled, he decided to get up. So we took a turn around the first floor and discovered how few spaces the zimmer frame will fit through. It doesn't really matter, as he can take my arm for the narrow bits. A three-legged zimmer would have been better perhaps. But at least he has a frame to stand up in when he leaves the bed.

—

He keeps getting up. I have told him I am next door, in my office writing my diary, and he said, "Have you found it yet?" Meaning my missing notebook. So that is one short-term memory he still has in his 'open' file. I had to confess I had, but didn't tell him it was in the library book all along.

When I talk to him about our 19th wedding anniversary on the 18th, he looks bemused. I think memories of being married to me – or anybody else – are mostly obscured.

I want to go back to the living room to continue watching *The Seagull*, although Chekov seems terribly dated in its entire obsession with jealousy and human emotion with little intelligence involved.

February 11 — Monday. My respect for *The Seagull* has been revised somewhat, having finally watched it to the end. But it is still just a black comedy, rather than a tragedy. Perhaps that says more about me than the play. I also laughed at *Les Misérables*.

—

Once again, Prof R cannot fit his head to his legs this morning. It's a mystery why the connection between the medication and his alert state of mind is so obscure. He had levodopa at 6 am but was still too dopey at 9.30 am (is the clue in the name?) to have the legs to walk, although he had set the alarm off trying. So I gave him another levodopa and his rivastigmine and we're still waiting, at nearly 10.30 am, for his head to clear more.

When I gave him his coffee through a straw, he began to chew the straw instead of sucking it. This is the second time this has happened. Red flags are going up all around us. But he woke properly at 11.30 am and ate his breakfast and ice cream and jelly.

Tina came at 1.30 pm. It was her first sight of the new location. Because of her care home work, she is able to give me a steer about equipment, like portable hoists, and how much space they are likely to take up. And whether a hospital bed would fit in the little children's living room. Netty had thought yes, Tina is not so sure.

And when I talk about months in a hospital bed, she says, "Or it could be years". I feel we are coming to an impasse with where we can go next.

This afternoon I sent an email to our agency manager, asking if developing an ongoing care plan is one of the services they offer. I need to see if there is a way forward for us in the spaces we have here. Timing cannot be planned for, but contingencies can.

While Tina was here, I had a bath and washed my hair. Finally, I have realised it is worthwhile paying someone so I can do this without stress. I've noticed that any sort of bell or buzzer, be it the dishwasher or the washing machine, makes me jump.

Prof R is happy tonight, well fed, well kissed and hopefully not fearful.

I have eaten more of the pasta bake left over from Saturday, with Stilton cheese to dress it up. As long as food is home cooked, I don't care if it's the same thing dished up every day.

—

When I shared pieces of the diary with my niece so she can see what we are up to, she says, "You sound like you are at the end of your tether." She isn't registering any dry wit. I'd no idea that's how I may appear to others, although I am honest about anger or tiredness or frustration. It would be lying to say all is calm, all is bright. How could it be? I think my tether has a bit more length to spare.

February 12 — Tuesday. I should be more grateful. Our nights are relatively undisturbed, if short. Midnight to 5.40 am is good. But another pee trip at 6.40 am is irritating, until he says, settling on the toilet, "Thank you darling".

He is sound asleep at 8 am and I'm dressed and made up and ready for breakfast. I cannot imagine lying in bed late, and wouldn't want to now. The habit is set in concrete, and the body isn't far behind.

Mr Parky slept and slept with a pee at 11.30 am and no appetite until 3 pm, when he awoke legless. It took some waiting time and a very urgent bladder to succeed in getting him to the toilet. But once he is awake, he is Prof R again and able to eat in a mild feeding frenzy of sorts that includes breakfast, lunch, smoothie dessert and a chocolate Complan drink.

We now remove phlegm from his mouth regularly throughout the meal or any time he detects he is log-jammed. It works, it's easy and I think it may just be a phase, as he was much better in the night. He is cooperative, happy and calm today. It makes me feel this solo care project is manageable after all.

—

I find myself sometimes daydreaming when I'm feeding him. Often I think of the young Prof R, and the photos and papers of his I have been putting in safe places for his daughters to find. Time is a mystery to us all, but we never stop trying to understand it.

Sometimes I expect too much of him, which ironically can also be too little. He was up and halfway to the toilet on the zimmer when I came up tonight. Clearly the alarm has slipped down the mattress again. So while he was on the toilet, I went beneath the sheets to move the mattress pad back up to the top under his pillows. When I turned around, he was up, off the toilet, pulling up his clothes without holding onto any support. And of course, I was startled, whereas I should have simply congratulated him on being in such good form.

Note to self: must do better. Meantime, I have used white tack to secure the pad a little better to the mattress.

February 13 — Today my niece wrote again accusing me of neglecting Prof R. Elder Abuse she called it. With capitals. Her verdict: I must immediately put him in a care home. I re-read the diary entry I sent her and can see I mention not being able to clean his teeth and the rare scent of his sweat that day, notable because it is unusual. The black humour which makes his daughters "laugh out loud" is passing her by.

She assumes I am not cleaning him or changing his clothes. And because, that day, he didn't eat breakfast until 11 am, and went back to sleep before coffee, she also accused me of not feeding him properly. To avoid any credible denial from me, she implied my mental health was in question. Try coming up with a defence for that at 12,000 miles. Although I did say his daughters receive the same updates and appreciate them, because the occasional humour makes the truth easier to digest.

She also didn't get the joke about him asking for a TV. If she had been here with her mother, she would have laughed like a drain. Come to think of it, most of this stuff Stella could have explained to her. But perhaps she wasn't asked.

This sort of misunderstanding is bizarrely helpful. I need to be careful the diary is not open to misinterpretation. Not playing for laughs too much by just focussing on the parts where it's all going pear-shaped. It never hurts to be reminded of my own need to edit.

I shared her email with Netty, just because I needed to share it with someone. It has shaken my self-belief, because there is always self-doubt when caring for anyone. And there are no witnesses. I consider a camera in the bedroom. A silent witness. But then there is no privacy either.

Netty said, "When did she last visit?" The answer of course is, "Never". I have to trust she would tell me if she thought his care had shortcomings. And she offered to try to persuade him to clean his teeth!

—

We had shallow sleep last night. One of those nights when Prof R is half awake from around 2 am and makes attempts to get up by throwing off the bedclothes and then replacing them again.

A woman from the agency has replied to my request for more advice. Kay, from their office, will visit on 1st March to observe Netty and look at the ongoing situation for me. I need unbiased views, which I don't get from some members of my family.

The agency cannot send me anyone on a Monday afternoon yet, except over the lunch hours, which does not suit.

Today is also Sydney son's 36th birthday.

February 14 (Valentines' Day) — Netty told me yesterday she had suggested Prof R give me a Valentine's card. He quite correctly told her, "We don't usually bother". But she persuaded him to write in a card she had bought. I haven't opened it yet. I'm waiting for him to wake up more.

I managed a shower at 7 am and by the time I was dressed, with my face painted, he was waking. Perfect timing. We'd had a rough night after an exhausting evening yesterday. That's when I do feel less confident about the future. I still feel sick when I think of my niece's email. She hasn't responded to my olive branch reply. Another wolf I seem to feel obligated to feed.

(A friend of mine calls makeup 'slap'. I never tire of that expression. Although she is the only person I have heard using it. When I googled its origin it said, "Cockney rhyming slang for makeup – particularly heavily applied".)

—

I discovered I had put my trousers on back to front after the shower. My excuse to self being that they are jeggings, with no zip. Having now put them on the right way around, I think they were more comfortable back to front.

As Prof R used to say, this day, like the curate's egg, was good in parts. Doris and Brian arrived carrying chocolate cake and more ice cream – so much ice cream I had trouble finding space for it in the freezer. We all paid court to Prof R, seated in his bed, and it was a delightful couple of hours of good company.

From there, the egg turned. He has been up and down all afternoon, save a blissful hour in the middle when I tried to doze. He is still up and down early evening, and I can't even be bothered having a meal. I have snacked. I'm too tired to care. I will eat rubbish probably and have a glass of wine when he eventually settles.

February 15 — In the end, I had cheese and crackers for dinner last night. Prof R didn't settle until close to 9 pm, and most of it was solved when he managed to pass a motion at around 9.30 pm. I wish we didn't have to go through this whenever he is literally full of shit.

No reply from 12,000 miles away to my olive branch emails letting them know about future care planning here. They are only supportive when I am doing what they want. And that is, putting Prof R in a care home. And their disapproval has me struggling with guilt. 'Could do better' is their verdict, and where there is a grain of truth, they have baked half a dozen loaves of hot air.

—

Speaking of guilt, I have remembered to buy safety corners for the furniture in our new bedroom. Plus, I have finally managed to talk to someone at the Community and District Nurses office and they have registered Prof R, and referred him for assessment for a visit. It turned out I had been ringing the wrong number; given to me by various people who should know better.

I used to be able to live in the present until this year. Now I can't avoid looking forward and it's hard not to be afraid. But the community nurse turned up unannounced in the late afternoon and cheered me enormously. She arrived looking like someone from the *Sound of Music*. Friendly round face and two blond plaits, bearing gifts of barrier cream and offers of help.

She pronounced Prof R's skin to be excellent. So is his circulation. She showed me how to check by pressing on the flesh of his big toe and noting if the colour returns quickly. I showed her his breastbone as I worry about its prominence and his weight loss. She looked with interest at the breastbone without offering an opinion, but she did offer to refer us to a dietitian who could provide special supplement foods to boost his intake.

———

Netty is a hit with Prof R and has him not only eating out of her hand but cleaning his teeth. While she was here, I walked with my Fitbit over 8000 steps along the Creek and through the wharf boatyards. It was a beautiful day. Unbelievable for this time of year. My head needed it as much as my feet.

Prof R has no memory of his sister and her husband visiting on Thursday morning.

February 16 — It's already Saturday – 1.30 am and I'm awake because the library book I am reading is not a good one for my current state of mind. It's about a man who has lost his son to drugs. Not exactly what the doctor ordered.

Prof R is struggling to wake, possibly because his 9.30 am rivastigmine pill popped out on his tongue an hour or so after I gave it to him. It may not be funny, but it looks very comical after surviving for that length of time on the roof of his mouth.

He woke twice in the night at midnight and 4 am, so I gave him levodopa then. If he sleeps right through, I follow the instructions of the neurologist and leave him till morning. I've noted before, it now seems to make little difference. He was virtually comatose until well after midday, in spite of my attempts to help him drink water and coffee. He cannot suck on a straw when he is in this state.

Doris and Brian returned this afternoon with bendy straws and new rice desserts to tempt Prof R. We talked around him while he slept; about life, and my lack of legal protection as a carer. It worries them and me. They are familiar with the problems carers can face at home. My niece has done me a back-handed favour by alerting me to my vulnerability. And I feel safer now that the Community and District nurses are visiting.

Later, when Doris and Brian had gone, and Prof R was once more in the toilet, I asked him if he would like to clean his teeth. And he said no, and became cross. But when I tried a little gentle persuasion, which involved mentioning the expectations of the medical people who need pleasing, he changed his mind.

While this discussion was going on, the vegetables I had put on the stove to steam began to burn. I have a good nose and know a too-far-gone burn when I smell it. But I'm hoping to retrieve enough from the top for his dinner.

—

Now we are having a chat about television. I'd rather hoped he'd forgotten that debate. Does he really want one? Perhaps. A lot of thought would be needed to have a screen accessible to him while he lies in bed. He cannot sit in bed for long periods or risk skin problems.

A lovely surprise later when he said, "This room is like a prison". Why is this a positive sign? Because he has never said that before. Usually, when invited downstairs, he would say "Why? Who's down there?" It's possible our new room, being so much smaller, has caused this feeling of confinement, and if so, I'm pleased. Because I would love to get him to spend more time outside it. We shall see.

The half-scorched potatoes were delicious, reminding me of the ones I used to retrieve from the embers of a dying campfire when I was a child.

February 17 — In the small hours, during a pee stop, not always the best time to make a decision, I decided that I should send my niece an acknowledgment that she had given me a wake-up call; a realisation that sole carers are at risk; they have few witnesses. And that I am grateful for those I do have.

I'm not looking for redemption from her. Or am I? She used a very blunt stick to hit a soft target. But I did feel I had to acknowledge she had helped me be much more aware of the pitfalls around me.

(Note to self: never feel you must respond to silence. If the relationship is in a hole, stop digging.)

And so onward. No response either from her or any contact from Stella. I can live with this. Or more accurately, I can live without their support. It's not ideal, but there are bigger issues to worry about.

—

The first bigger issue to worry about was that I could not wake Prof R properly again this morning. It was after 11 am before I could get him to sit up and take his pills, and at first he wanted to take them out of his mouth. It isn't possible, or safe, to feed them to him only half awake.

The problem, apart from sleepiness, was our old enemy mucus, which once discovered, we managed to get rid of. It was the colour of the ice cream he had before bedtime. I think it might have to be a different sort of supper – lemon and honey drink springs to mind. And more advice from the experts. Although the dietitian said dairy is not necessarily a cause.

There's not much humour to be found in our daily situation just now. When Prof R is properly awake, he does smile and laugh. But so much of the day is hard work for both of us. Food has been a marathon of hit and miss most of the afternoon. We decamped down to the living room for the more successful menu; jelly, mash and avocado with cheese, followed by chocolate cake watered down. Breakfast cereal had already been rejected upstairs, then a mango yoghurt only half eaten.

Again, the problem was mucus; causing a blockage. I have now perfected pulling it slowly out of his mouth, rolling it out on the tissue in a continuous stream. Like making candyfloss. I'm surprised he has room for anything else.

All the advice is to increase fluids, drink in small sips, and not raise the chin when drinking to avoid choking. Prof R coughs almost every time he drinks. Except when we use the toddler feeder cup or have a sugary juice in the water. Even if dairy should not be an issue, it may have to go, or at least be reduced.

—

When we were downstairs, I tried to talk to him about what still interests him most. Not politics he said. Or the news. And not Brexit. He seems to have forgotten what it is. He could not tell me the name of the PM.

I asked if perhaps he still found animals and plants interesting. And he nodded. But the last time I took him down to watch David Attenborough with the chimpanzees, he stared at the screen without obvious connection.

When he was tired, and back upstairs washed and bedded, I asked him if I could have a bath and wash my hair. It's possible to do this at his best times of day. Today he has done as promised, stayed put. So I'm clean.

—

Something ordinary but nice happened. The Legal Deposit people have asked for five copies of my book. One for each of the Legal Deposit Libraries – The Bodleian; Cambridge University; The National Libraries of Scotland and Wales; and Trinity College, Dublin. I had no idea I was legally obliged to lodge it with all of them, and had only sent one to the British Library. I shudder to think of the underground storage bunkers full of everyone's books, terrible or otherwise, that will probably never see the light of day.

—

Supper for Prof R was toddler fish pie and strawberry ice cream. Yes, dairy, but I will find some coconut ice cream to replace it. I'm going to more closely record food intake from here on in, so we can track what needs supplementing. Today was a good day in the end. He was happy to clean his teeth and we talked about the animals who have been escaping from Belfast Zoo.

He said, "I love you deeply" when I left him. Ditto darling. "You're *my* boy" I remind him.

February 18 — Our 19ᵗʰ wedding anniversary. We have two cards. One Netty helped Prof R write for me on which he has put row upon row of Xs. It will be one to keep. The other card is from his sister, who never forgets our anniversary.

To celebrate, I cut Prof R's hair and washed it with a shampoo cap. He brunched on cereal, creamed rice with tomato and fruit puree, strawberry ice cream and coffee. And when he was resting, I had quark and humus with crackers, because I couldn't be bothered cooking anything else.

A padded metal-framed folding office chair arrived for Prof R's side of the bed. It is perfect, and will give the zimmer more room to move. Tight spaces require clever solutions; but overall, we feel a lot safer now there is less room for Prof R to measure his length.

—

Hope sent me a photo of her baby scan. They all look the same of course, but it's a miracle nevertheless. Three months and all seems well. Finally I can tell anyone who cares. And no doubt a few who do not. I've sent a message to Stella. This baby is going to be fun.

—

Prof R seems more alert in many ways. It would be easy to think his cognition has improved, although I know that cannot be the case. We are making the most now of every moment we have together. I had worried I might withdraw to protect myself from the inevitable, but that has not happened. We are closer than we have ever been. I'm not afraid to love him.

And in that spirit, I approached the evening with optimism. Poor Prof R was on a different page. He sat in the folding canvas director's chair — which until now he had reliably remained in, it being harder to exit than the cane chair — and then suddenly decided to get up, halfway through my food preparation. So that I raced upstairs mid-prepping.

In the event, nothing suited Goldilocks, not even the spout drinking cups, which were declared too difficult. I was determined not to be beaten and put a straw down the spout. It seemed to work for him. In the end he managed to eat yoghurt with orange jelly and honey. Not exactly a meal, but followed by a Complan milkshake it was nutritional enough.

In spite of our exhaustion, we made ourselves clean his teeth. He doesn't fight it now. Although it's fraught with mucus extraction and flying water.

Finally, him safely settled, I said, sweaty and tired, "Right, now you rest, and I'll bugger off." And he said, "Don't bugger off." And I realised he thought I meant I was leaving. An immediate promise that I was only going downstairs clarified that.

But much later, after more ups and downs, he lost more of the plot and asked, "Do you think of yourself as my wife?" I was lying in bed beside him, so I replied, "I'm in bed with you, so that's the clue." We joke about everything. Nothing is off limits.

He's always relieved when he rediscovers that I am his wife after all. Because in the daytime, he still forgets we share a bed.

February 19 — Stacey next door knocked on my door at 3 pm because she was worried that I had left the milk on the doorstep. The trouble with milk deliveries is that I cancel them so often I sometimes forget when I haven't.

How nice to have a neighbour who would check on me if I fell down the stairs, or got stuck in the tiny space between our bed and the window – a distinct possibility if I'm silly enough to try to retrieve anything from under the bed.

It's been an almost 'normal' day. So 'nothing to see here'. But still it's a struggle to get him to eat more. If all else fails, the default is chocolate cake and ice cream. It has a guaranteed success rate. I'm afraid to weigh him again.

The agency wrote to say Netty can now do Monday afternoons. This is a real bonus. So I will have 12 hours of her help now, and Tina for 3 hours on any spare day each week that she is available. It might just be enough downtime for me.

The weather is beautiful. I spent a few minutes in the garden this afternoon letting the sunshine soak into me. I need to do this more often.

A huge relief when he ate his meal – mash, crushed sausage, beans and cream – and strawberry ice cream this evening. He seems less frail when he is eating properly.

I asked him what he used to have for school dinners at Haberdasher Aske's school. He said, "Minced meat and mash potato". And what was dessert? Him: "Custard" Me:" But you hate custard". Him: "I didn't have it."

February 20 — Netty comes today. We had a peaceful night, with, for me, strange dreams. Prof R doesn't remember his.

I was dreaming about someone who was my boss when I was 23, newly married, and he was 52. He was witty and we had such fun, I fell into a kind of love for him. Not exactly Hayley Mills and that ghastly chap Bolton, more a kind-uncle-hero-worship crush. And it lasted all the time I knew him, although I didn't see him often in later years.

So the dreams were nice, and every time I woke up, I was aware I was dreaming of him and promptly went back to sleep and dreamed of him some more. Nothing inappropriate, just friendly and warm. I guess I needed a nice dream.

Prof R has been sleepy and eaten very little today. Even Netty was beaten by his lack of appetite. I've just spent an hour or so feeding him little yoghurt pots – one chocolate coconut and the other an apricot fool. Now he is supposed to be resting but I can hear him clattering about in the next room. It may end up being a busy night.

Later, after I blitzed his rejected lunch in the blender, Prof R ate it all, and followed it with ice cream. Result. Plus his brother-in-law fixed the broken handle on the bedroom door.

Neither Netty nor I could get him to clean his teeth today.

February 21 — I should never go back to bed if I have been woken by Prof R after 6 am.

This morning, I was tired in that way I only recall feeling when the children were babies. Bone tired. So I went back to bed, and at 8.30 am I woke to Prof R coughing up his phlegm and me feeling as though I had been in a nightclub all night.

Food log: 10.30 am coffee and raspberry yoghurt. He could not eat the muesli. I will try blending it in the food processor.

When I clean his feet, I am amazed at how the skin on humans sheds, regardless of the environment. He is lathered in Germolene and reclad in socks. He doesn't want bare feet. Never has. They are very sensitive.

Tina comes today. It will allow me to have my own feet done. They hurt so much I hobble. If my feet could talk, they would be swearing. There isn't a cream to be had that stops this happening. Or at least, not one I am using. And walking on all those tiny seed corns seems to throw out every other muscle in my body.

—

Prof R's memory can be much worse in the evening. It took me by surprise tonight. He really didn't remember that I had just left the room. He also didn't remember that I always come when he gets up and his bed alarm goes off. I was upset at first, sad that I was invisible to him. But that's not what it is. He hasn't forgotten me yet and he always tells me he loves me.

When I mention Tina, he can't remember her. But when pushed, he says crossly, "All I remember is a little round head popping through a hole". Poor Tina. It's not an inaccurate description.

Food log: finally he ate a proper evening meal and two desserts.

Then we were up and down until 8.30 pm because his body was signalling he needed a bowel movement. And he finally did.

While we were chatting in bed before sleep, he said "We would love to see more of you." I said, "Who's we?" and it turned out the 'we' was a royal one. "You see more of me than anyone else". And he grinned.

February 23 — Saturday. Prof R kept me awake last night because I was waiting for him to wake. But he didn't until 4.30 am. And now he is sleeping again for too long, as he did yesterday. And waking him to have his pills is fraught with danger if he does not swallow them safely. Often found hours later, stuck to the roof of his mouth and spilling their contents on his tongue.

Yesterday he ate a lot – after not waking properly until after 1 pm. All I had managed to give him by then was half a cup of coffee. He can't suck on a straw in this twilight zone – it has to be by spout.

By the time Netty arrived, I was feeling very worried. But once awake, he kept her busy for three hours; eating, toilet, teeth cleaning (which he did not refuse this time) and generally managing his body in one way or the other. And of course, his mind. She's very good at that.

While she did that, I walked. Across the old swing bridge, along the creek edge and into the meadows. They are lying ploughed and fallow at the moment. Not as pretty as they will be. And when I came home, at around 3 pm, I bathed and washed my hair before Netty left.

In the evening Prof R ate well for me too. And we talked about the events of the day. I was able to tell him about the flypast held today for the ten American airmen who had crashed and died in Sheffield 75 years ago, during the war. Into a woodland instead of landing safely in an open park, because they had seen a young boy standing in the way. The boy, now in his 80s, has thought about them every day since.

These times of 'normal' are such a welcome respite. I will read him the online news of the day more often. When he is in the right frame of mind. There are fewer dramas now, fewer opportunities for falls or other disasters. The new room has created a womb of sorts. We feel safe within it, and from below, I can hear when he stirs, long before the alarm goes off.

—

I spoke too soon about our new 'womb'. Prof R went to sleep on his feet after the toilet and only my loud and constant voice kept us upright until we got back to safety. But he did manage to stay awake long enough in his chair to eat his muesli. Although he couldn't manage his coffee.

2.00 pm. He's woken for coffee and tastes some food before suddenly feeling desperate. Throwing himself around on the bed. I asked if a cuddle would help, and he said yes. It's amazing he doesn't feel like this more often. He is overtired from yesterday. I've made a cup of tea for me and a plate of ice cream for him, and will sit with him and read my book.

February 24 — I drip fed Prof R through the afternoon yesterday, finding little tempting titbits and failing sometimes to feed him anything that resembled a vegetable. The toddler foods are surprisingly awful without a great deal of alchemy to make them edible. I wonder how many parents actually taste them?

Later, a chicken carcass, which has completed its lifecycle on the stove this week with a fresh load of veg, was eaten by both of us. The chicken shreds to a consistency that he has no trouble swallowing.

We both ate chocolate cake.

I sent Stella the photo taken by Netty for his memory book. Stella wrote back "He seems to have rallied since he came down from the loft", I didn't disabuse her. Photos almost always lie, and I'm glad of it. The lighting has hidden his sunken cheeks. I could have said to her "Not bad for a man who is the victim of Elder Abuse" (with the capitals) but she's not responsible for her daughter.

—

I watched a film called *The Tree* about an 88-year-old woman who took a road trip back home so she could die under the same tree her best friend had been killed falling from. On the way she dispensed wisdom and money to those fortunate (?) enough to cross her do-gooder path. I kept waiting for it to mean something.

Our Sunday has been; making food, eating, sleeping (Prof R), cleaning his teeth, bathing the dog, doing the recycling, reading upstairs on the bed with Prof R (dangerous, as I fall asleep) and doing it all over again in the evening (except bathing the dog). The chicken casserole is almost exhausted. And so is Prof R this evening. I'm having to wake him to eat.

Last Friday, Netty told me, with real pleasure, that Prof R had wanted to hold her hand. I smiled and said, "How lovely". I didn't have the heart to tell her that it gave me a pang. She's a caring intelligent person and I'm surprised she didn't guess that I'm still his wife, and I don't want him to hold hands with another woman.

February 25 — Prof R had both toothache and hot sweats in the night. The sweats have happened occasionally, and I change his clothes, but the toothache is predictable and caused by hard brushing a tooth that was flagged up by his dentist as a possible problem.

Corsodyl mouth wash and ibuprofen have hopefully held it at bay. But his cough is lingering and probably needs looking at, so I will request a home visit from the GP. This will be interesting.

———

Proof again this morning that regular meds through the night make no difference now to his morning state. Last night it was regular four-hourly intervals, just because he happened to wake. But this morning, he could barely function until lunchtime, as seems usual at the moment. All I could succeed with were pills and coffee through a straw.

His tooth seems better, but he has a fat eye, which I've been treating with yellow eye ointment. Something else for the doctor to look at. Because Prof R's cough is hardly bothering him today. I shan't be telling the doctor that, in case they cancel. I want to see how well this home visit system works.

Small pleasures — At least five reasons to be pleased today:

I succeeded in booking a GP home visit. The doctor will visit tomorrow afternoon, between 1-3 pm.

The car was taken to the garage and given a new battery. Contrary to expectations, when it was returned there was a parking space right outside the front door.

Prof R's sore tooth is no longer bothering him.

G the plumber came this afternoon, also contrary to expectations, to sort out the cistern that broke again this morning.

The sixth reason to be pleased is that today was the warmest February day on record, with a maximum temperature of over 20 degrees C.

February 26 — I've been reading a biography by Viv Albertine in which she lays bare the whole complex and sometimes sordid business of sibling rivalry. She had a much more turbulent childhood than we did, but it's made me think about my own situation. Why my sister has withdrawn because of her daughter's conflict with me.

This sibling relationship, which should be our closest, is fatally flawed, because neither party is neutral. Both are programmed by nature to compete for the prime spot in the nest. Even when the parents are dead. The most attention, the most love, the best presents, the most successful marriage, the cleverest children, and so it goes on.

Prof R told me a story about a memory he has of his sister. She took his copy of *Black Beauty*, which he prized above all others and had been given to him by his favourite aunt. And she tore the covers off it. And predictably, when he flew into a rage, he was punished by his parents. I don't think he ever recovered. Childhood is like that. Injustices loom large and are imprinted for life.

—

The doctor didn't come. So much is sadly predictable. Instead, he rang, as expected, to triage Prof R. He asked if Prof R was having trouble breathing, or had a temperature, or there was blood in his mucus. I couldn't lie. No, no and no.

So I'm to call again if I am worried, as they do home visits every day. He also offered to pre-prescribe antibiotics if I was worried. Frankly, if Prof R needs antibiotics, he needs a visit. And if he is gasping for breath, I'll be calling the ambulance. I hope that wasn't a kneejerk reaction I will come to regret.

He's been woken at about 11.30 am for breakfast, followed with some persuasion by the first course of lunch.

His head is covered with cradle cap again. While he was sitting on the toilet, I gave him the almond oil treatment, but I'm convinced it merely makes all those little yellow platelets lie down and become invisible. He's gone to bed oily, on his sleeping towel. Later we will use the shampoo cap, which seems to contain so many conditioners and moisturisers that the little yellow flat-caps will be afraid to raise their heads.

I had to wake him after 4 pm because he has slept too long. He woke enough to have his levodopa and his top was damp with sweat. This only happens sometimes, and usually at night. I've left him tucked up. I don't want him to get cold, which he might if I change him now.

February 27 — All change. Prof R woke at a normal time – 8.00 am. And later, woke again at a 'normal' time for coffee and some breakfast – 9.15 am. Not at all normal for him, and he soon tired. But at least his pills were administered when he was vertical under his own steam, rather than my sweat.

There is nothing normal about this life. I used to think it was our own special normal, a new normal each day, but now I feel totally out of kilter with the rest of the world – or at least, those who are not caring for someone who will not recover. It's sadder when you take the blinkers off.

Food is the biggest change. I am eating a totally different diet now, to chime with Prof R's needs. The interminable stove-top chicken and veggies; the salmon (which is delicious) but nevertheless teamed with something much simpler than before. Either a portion of Prof R's mash or some grains pre-prepared. The tomatoes we used to consume every day (and I ate like sweets) are now rotting in their packets. Prof R cannot eat tomatoes at all, and I am simplifying my meals in ways that doesn't use them, unless I am making a meat sauce for several days' meals.

Tonight I'm defrosting a Charlie Bingham fish pie for one. Prof R is having salmon and mash for lunch, but we will both have fish pie for dinner. It's enough for both of us as I do a green vegetable as well.

Netty comes today and I am off to Pilates. I couldn't be less motivated, so I'm sure to enjoy it.

—

This morning there was a news item about a breakthrough in Parkinson's research. Typically, and ironically, I heard Prof R begin to make a move just as the item began. So I missed most of it. But apparently they have done a six-year trial of a drug that is injected into the brain. My respect goes to the volunteers who have given themselves over to the scientists for this dangerous project. It is apparently a success, (*which was later proven to be temporary*) but all these breakthroughs seem to relate to Parkinson's movement disorders. More and more I feel Prof R's brand of Parkinson's is outside the realm of most of the others.

February 28 — 6.00 am. A bad night. A little waking nightmare, just made for two, that nobody else can share. The sort of night when I remember why I longed for a night nurse when these nights were more frequent. Fortunately, we have far fewer nights like this now, of unproductive trips to the toilet and untold lowering and lifting of pyjamas and pull-ups and legs lifted back into bed. Best forgotten.

When Netty came yesterday and I went to Pilates, it was a session so demanding for me that I felt sick. But the weather was beautiful, and I was out. Prof R was having fun with Netty talking about the past and making a scrapbook. At least, I hope he thinks it is fun. It must be nice to do something different with someone different for a few hours a week.

Our early unseasonal summer should end today with normal weather resuming. The purists didn't allow themselves to enjoy the little heatwave, proclaiming it a portent of climate doom. It is the last day of February, so I shall be looking forward to more of the same, very soon.

—

Prof R has continued to be up and down during the morning. He's had coffee, a body wash, a clean top, his nails cleaned and the yellow eye ointment in his troubled eye.

The alarm gets out of sync and can lose its signal. I came upstairs in answer to the pager and found Prof R in the hall by his office, wandering around, apparently perfectly safely, but not using any handholds. He had tossed aside the zimmer. The bed alarm signal had taken probably two or three minutes to reach the pager.

So I suggested breakfast in my office, which seemed like a good idea to both of us, until he pegged out after the first mouthful, declaring he had to lie down. I'm having my own coffee in my office in anticipation of another call from his bed.

Doris and Brian popped in while he was sleeping, and gave me the tonic of good company and conversation. When they are good, they are very, very good, but when they are bad ...

The afternoon has been constant, and I have succeeded in getting him to eat a lunch of avocado and creamed rice, cake and ice cream and a chocolate Complan drink. Now of course he has phlegm from front to back and is having trouble swallowing. So he drinks as much water as possible to disperse it.

Then I said, "Can I get you anything else?" That is a loaded question, and his reply was, "Some fish". I suspect that response might almost be automatic. But happily, I had salmon and five-veg mash and I put it all together with cream and manuka honey and carried it proudly upstairs. Where he decided he didn't want that after all, and also, he couldn't swallow it. The texture was too difficult.

So downstairs went I, and put the meal in the mini food processor and smashed it to a pulp. And then added water. And then heated it up again, but not before his bed alarm went off as I was halfway through the process.

It's really hard to know what he does and doesn't understand. We can have such good conversations. He says he doesn't connect the bed alarm with my having to come up to help him. So I said who did he think it was for? And made a joke about a servant hidden in the fake panelling. But then I had to explain the joke, which rather spoilt the effect.

There was another attempt to eat the salmon but 'Goldilocks' still had a problem, the dreaded phlegm. By now I was running on empty and asked for time out. More accurately, I begged for it. He understood the concept, but driven by something neither of us could fathom, it was not to be.

The salmon will be reheated later. I will find something I can face eating first, because as usual, I am hungry. But I am grateful these days are fewer and further between than they were.

Eventually, it turned out to be a positive feeding day. The salmon was eaten and three desserts. And for an encore, he had to spit out the deeply coloured syrup of figs to rid himself of some phlegm. It went everywhere, being rather too prolific to be contained in a tissue.

The end of a perfect day.

March 1 — The first day of spring. I feel amazing. While Netty was here this afternoon I had a bath and washed my hair. What a luxury.

Kay from the agency came to observe both Netty and Prof R as part of the agency's self-assessment. I had asked for advice about how well the house will cope with necessary changes as Prof R's illness advances. She agreed that the obvious place for the (dreaded) hospital bed will be the ground floor. I think I have almost to come to terms with that now. So much more practical than selling a double bed or emptying one of the first floor rooms. With that decided, we can get on with living in our little nest on the first floor for the foreseeable future.

Prof R's appetite today was disrupted by his bowel. A petty concern to some but not to us. To Netty, it is a science. She spent her three hours helping him with it and she was happy, telling me the size and quality on her poo numbering scale, which is a mystery to me. If it's the right colour, not too hard, not too soft and doesn't hurt when he passes it, I'm happy.

He wasn't hungry when he woke from his exhausted afternoon sleep at 6.30 pm. Pooing takes it out of you (pun intended). Two mouthfuls of fish and mash were enough for him. But I did manage to entice him, before our final bedtime, when his hunger returned. Yoghurt and honey, tapioca (our first taste for years) a coconut chocolate pot and some fruit smoothie.

Totally irrelevant to his physical wellbeing is the increasing noise from our neighbours on both sides as their children grow, along with the size of their feet, and their ability to slam their front door. On our right, the five-year-old seems to be rhythmically hitting the wall. Every time the noise is unusual or loud, I go upstairs to check Prof R. Netty also jumps out of her skin, but I'm more battle-hardened. And because our left-side neighbours are also our saviours in an emergency, there will be no requests to "pipe down".

March 2 — Prof R is having a twilight morning. When this happens, he can respond enough to take pills and sometimes can suck up some of his coffee through a straw. I ask him what he sees but he can't tell me.

Mid-morning he's back to trying to poo. And saying he is hungry but wanting his bed after two bites and some mucus removal. On his way across the two-foot span from his chair to the bed he managed to lose his legs. I caught his weight, but it took a huge effort and loud instructions to propel us both forward to fall in an untidy heap onto the bed and save us both from the floor.

Once settled, and me saying, "What happened? Were you just upset?" he agreed that there may be some element of emotion attached to such sudden collapses. Because Prof R has his boundaries. Which is why we had said "no thank you" to the physiotherapist, and the occupational therapist, nor – a year ago – accept invitations to join the Parkinson's choir. Or the dotty brigade who met in the local hall. I supported him in his right to determine this part of his life. So much else was determined for him.

This time, I had been trying to persuade him to eat a little more and he wasn't in the mood to be told to do anything. Sometimes, persuasion works. This time it didn't. Fair enough, but it put us both in a temporary tight spot, which I need to remember.

Ten minutes later he was on the move again, deciding he was hungry after all. So the chair was set up, the food retrieved, and he ate about a third of the bowl. Better than nothing.

—

I weighed him this morning. He was 51.5 kg. I am going to weigh him again, because that is not good. Perhaps on a different surface. Although that never works in reverse for me.

Five minutes after lying down again following breakfast, he summoned me back to his bedside. He needed the toilet. Some days are like this, some are not. I try not to feel every muscle of my body aching. And if I need to leave the room for a few minutes while he is seated on the toilet, sometimes, he will remain seated as asked, and sometimes he will frighten me by getting up and being halfway back to bed when I return, without using his zimmer frame.

Because he was awake so much, we did a lot of grooming. Another hair wash, feet bathed, fingernails cut, and torso washed with bed bath wipes. And he allowed me to spray his armpits – which now seem to disappear up into his shoulder blades – with his crystal deodorant. It didn't settle him, but it is companionable and made me feel that we are coping, at least with his physical care.

Prof R pleased me very much tonight by eating my meat sauce and mash, even though it had been processed to look like a mud pie. And followed that with ice cream. Altogether, he has eaten much better today, although he was still up and down all evening until I went to bed in self-defence at 9 pm.

March 3 — Sunday. I have decided to go back to bed on a Sunday instead of dressing after we do the early morning toilet run for Prof R. Today that was 6.30 am. I always have a cup of tea, and a digestive biscuit, before dressing, but today I went back to bed until almost 9 am. I'm not sure whether it makes me feel more rested, but it certainly passes the time.

And because breakfast was late, I ate an enormous one. Spelt flakes, goats' milk, kefir and grapes, followed by two slices of toast – one with honey and one, lime marmalade. It's as if I am eating for Prof R, given he isn't eating enough.

When Prof R finally woke properly, he sat with his eyes closed as he ate his muesli. But he did eat it all. And then he lay down again.

Yesterday had worn us both out, but I was full of energy from my quiet morning, so I left him sleeping under two rugs and took the duvet away to change the cover. This is always like wrestling snakes, and at some point I lose sight of what I am doing and operate on instinct, mind disengaged, relying on the memory of where things probably are. It works for me.

Whoever said duvets are easier to manage than sheets and blankets must have had a maid, or at least a cleaner at £5 an hour. Although I do appreciate being able to throw it over Prof R's bare legs in the middle of the night without leaving my side of the bed.

—

I have been paying the ungodly sum of £2.50 per 25 minute episode to watch *Catastrophe,* which is brilliant. But when I asked my daughter if she had seen it, she said yes, it's free on All4.

It's been an erratic eating day. What I would class as "failed nutrition target". He's had very little appetite and none for hot food. His eyes want to close, he is so tired. Breakfast, yes, lunch, only yogurt and half a breakfast drink, no real evening meal. Ice cream.

March 4 — Monday. A wobbly start – some of these early morning trips to the toilet are marginal in terms of his leg strength. We test before we head off from the bed. But he had a cup of tea at 8 am and that hasn't appealed to him for a long time.

His fat eye is better. His scalp also looks a lot better. Or at least the 'flat caps' are under cover.

This is Netty's first Monday. I can still sometimes feel a bit directionless with this time off, but today I bought a new picture frame from the Factory Shop for a Rita Angus print that was crying out for one. I also went to the library and think I have found a gem – *Confidence*, a comedy of psychology.

Prof R finally ate seriously for Netty at 3 pm. His bowel motions continue to impress her with their size and healthy appearance. Given his food intake, where do they come from? Discuss.

March 5 — As if to answer my question, Prof R polished off cottage pie and mango yoghurt last night, but he had been Jack-in-the-Box since Netty left, so I wasn't feeling so chipper by 9 pm when he finally settled down.

I now manage the stress of this much more effectively, by keeping my voice in a low and calm tone, even when I am telling him that I am very unhappy because he is up and down and my meal has already been reheated twice and could he please, please, stay in bed for a while so I can finish it. I no longer feel the need to go into a darkened room and scream. That may or may not be a good thing.

This morning, we managed an 8 am trip to the loo, after a cup of tea and his assurance to me that his legs could hold him. But it was only my usual loud refrain "strong straight legs" that got us safely there and back.

Because this different bed is higher, landing his bottom far enough on to prevent a slide to the ground is a cliff-edge event. But it is so much better for his state of mind to have peed in the right place.

Overnight he had woken three times, the last at 5 am, to clear an impressive amount of mucus from his throat. So he has more levodopa in his system this morning than when he sleeps through. When I peeked around the door at 9 am his eyes were wide open. He was watching the mysterious flying creatures or objects he sees but cannot usually describe. This time he could. They were just white objects, like dots, he said. Although he seemed to try to say that at other times it is different. I said the levodopa can do that sometimes. He's not at all distressed by it.

—

Washing Prof R as usual this morning, while I change him from night pull-ups to underpants, it crossed my mind that his parents did us a favour when they had him circumcised. I shared this joke with Prof R, and he smiled.

As they tell you in the aeroplane, "Put your own mask on first", so one should remember priorities when considering who should get the first coffee in the morning. Today I made the mistake of giving Prof R the first one, so halfway through making mine, his bed alarm goes off and he needs the toilet. My coffee sits, waiting patiently, to be warmed up.

I have bought the dog a new dog food, which is 50 percent duck. And she loves it. But I notice it says in small print "for working dogs", so the mystery of why she is skipping around the kitchen has been solved.

Lunch will be in the folding chair in my office. In our small world, a whole floor full of rooms is like going global.

March 6 — Wednesday. Netty has been working with Prof R on his memory book. To me, it seemed like a naff idea when she first suggested it, but I suspect it just seemed too much like a *memento mori*. A portent of death. I was worried Prof R might find it so as well. But he doesn't. Now, I am impressed and find myself researching photos for her. She has already found his school, universities and other illustrations relating to his memories, but not yet the home he grew up in.

I've been battling my ignorance of how to take screen shots from Google Earth, and today succeeded in printing off a reasonable view of his Peckham childhood home, number 38. The triumph I feel greatly outweighs the value of the achievement. But Netty will be pleased.

—

For just a fleeting moment, during Pilates this afternoon, I felt as I did when a child. Or perhaps a young adult. Unencumbered by burdens and still full of possibility. It must have been the endorphins. Certainly, it is not based on reality. Pilates is hard for me at the moment. And I no longer feel like skipping down the road afterwards.

March 7 — Thursday. "Dreamy Daniel," as my parents used to say of me. Prof R has been in the twilight zone this morning but had coffee and pills. When he relaxes about being unable to get up, he uses his pull-ups for the purpose they are intended.

Overnight was unsettled, but any night when I don't have to leave the bed after about midnight is a good night.

I've been working with Prof R on his memories by showing him photographs from his university days that I'm curious about, but have no captions for. He rang his handbell last night to tell me excitedly that he remembered the name of the German boy he stayed with one summer – probably 1951, when he was about 14. It was Jurgan. I'm in sympathy with him in this process of files opening and closing. Quite a breakthrough when one opens.

Tina, our private carer, comes back today for two hours. She is kind and very nice but more of a baby-sitter than anything more challenging. Sometimes though, I wonder if Netty feels obliged to work a lot with Prof R, even if he is tired. That can have a knock-on effect for the next day – today being a good example.

—

It's not like me to enjoy a brisk walk into a cold headwind, but today I surprised myself. It was good to be out. Even better, when I turned for home, the wind behind me, I could feel smug that I no longer needed to worry about the regrowth in my hair. My hairdresser has skilfully blended it. Such small things continue to amuse me.

Prof R was happy tonight. He ate a lot and we talked of normal things, worrying about Tina, whose house sale in Yorkshire has fallen through, and whether our dog might be depressed. She has taken to sleeping a lot in the downstairs toilet. The dog, that is, not Tina. Every time I have to get up to go to Prof R, she leaves the couch and retreats. Tonight I have invited her to come upstairs with me. She is lying at my feet. It might be a solution.

When Prof R has a happy day, everyone is happy. Life feels worthwhile, in spite of everything. It's a welcome respite.

March 8 — My last dream before waking, I dreamt I was going to be hung, along with several others. For some sort of political or dissident reason. I was debating how much it would hurt when I woke up.

By 5.30 pm last night I was looking for an excuse to cook my dinner. I have this Russian roulette thing with Prof R – who will eat first? If he has had a later lunch, I gamble that I will get through mine without two trips to the microwave – if I start early enough. It's never an issue whether I am hungry or not. Unless I have had a giant chocolate cake at 4 pm I will always be ready for dinner.

Last night it was 3 am when Prof R needed the mucus cleared from his mouth and throat. We're pretty good at it, but how much nicer not to have to do this. I dread cutting out dairy products altogether, although we use coconut where possible. Perhaps that too is mucus-making.

While Netty was here, I went to see how the Abbey Physic Garden is getting on. It is still bare ground with new planting and signs that say, "Don't walk on the asparagus". But two apple trees are in full blossom already. At least I think they are apple trees. I'm not very good at identifying these things. Dozens of volunteers building structures and wheeling barrows. A busy and promising sight.

From late afternoon Prof R was on the move again, after a lovely mealtime and lots of chat and being settled comfortably back in his bed, presumably happy and contented and ready to rest. When he is like this, Jack-in-the-Box, I patiently count the unproductive trips to the loo until we get to five. Then I try the "bad cop" approach. Why are you getting up? Do you really need to go to the toilet – is your bladder uncomfortable – or are you just restless? Are you hungry? And so on. If food is not the issue, I say "I would like to be able to get on with making my dinner without being summoned constantly". He assures me he will try, and then 10 minutes later he is rattling his cages. And better than that, he is in whippet mode and has made it out of the bed and triumphantly on his feet without the zimmer.

When he sees I am angry or upset he can often realise that his behaviour is disruptive and will eventually apologise. And I tell him I love him but find it just too hard when he is like that. It's so much nicer not to have to be "bad cop" in the first place. But his restlessness continued later in the evening and on until 10.30 pm so it felt like a rather failed attempt at harmony and peace and love.

—

In between, perhaps unwisely, I was watching a two-part documentary on a major Parkinson's research project which had begun so hopefully and ended with funds being withdrawn by the drug company. The volunteers for that project were such stoic and brave people, with appalling symptoms, or so young that it was frightening. None of them seemed to have the type of Parkinson's Prof R or I would recognise.

They all, 42 of them, had brain surgery to install stents into their brains to overcome the blood/brain barrier. A growth hormone or a placebo, was injected directly into their brains. In several of them the improvements appeared miraculous, and all but two benefited, but they failed to meet the high criteria of 20% better than placebo, the benchmark of success. Even though, for obvious ethical reasons, in the second phase of treatment all 42 were given the growth hormone.

But when the funds were withdrawn, the improvements faded. All of them returned to their previous levels of disability, or worse. Like a horror movie. Where were the ethics in that scenario? It wasn't quite the best thing for me to be watching but it made me realise that Prof R had, in fact been "lucky" in the timing and scope of the Parkinson's side of his illness.

In spite of the poor outcome, I told him about it, leaving out the unhappy results. Something to talk about during toilet trips. How interesting it was, how amazing the trial. I think he was interested.

March 9 — Saturday. This morning I woke up at 6 am not knowing what day it is. Not just momentarily, but long enough to think it was Wednesday, Pilates day again, and feeling less than enthusiastic.

I must learn to sleep when Prof R sleeps, even if just a micro-nap. This morning, while he slept, I tried to watch a documentary film about Jane Jacobs, who campaigned to stop New York being overrun by modernism and motorways. It was a brilliant piece, but my head kept falling forward, or sideways, and I should have slept. Because this afternoon has proved to be a restless time.

—

In my list of achievements, I must not forget the rubber glove and the first digit – although more than one finger may be needed. I believe I have become fairly competent at helping Prof R safely when things go awry, and the 'goods train' stops halfway between platforms.

To keep Jack in his Box a little less stressfully, I spent an hour or more lying beside him on the bed, reading my biography of Penelope Fitzgerald. It's rather dense, so again, my head began to loll. But he stayed in the bed, so it was worthwhile.

—

We might boil in this room in summer. If I open the sash from the top, even just a few inches, the outside comes in. I like the bustle of inner urban living, but not when resting.

For afternoon tea Prof R had a melted brownie and another cup of tea. It seems to have become a much more successful drink to give him, although because of the milk, it might be more likely to cause mucus. Today has been a little less fraught with that.

March 10 — Sunday. Very stormy today, but with sunshine. The rest of the country has worse – wind and snow. Half the trellis on the brick wall has come down. About time too. It needs replacing.

Prof R is deceptive in his abilities, so much so, that I am surprised at times to remember that quite simple things are gone from his memory, never to be recovered apparently. He still cannot recall the name of the PM, nor can he retain his memory of how long we have been married – or even, at times, if we are married, but that is usually when he is tired.

The photos from his university days that I had hoped would shine a light on the past, for him are still a mystery. The Dutch girl with the windblown hair is only a vague memory. No name comes to him. Although he is very pleased to point himself out in any photo he appears in. What does remain clear is the detail of places, rather than faces.

More memory games this afternoon, while Prof R ate his way in series through breakfast, lunch and ice cream. Trying to isolate the areas of memory that are affected, we decide he has face blindness, especially in relation to grandchildren. He cannot recognise any of them. More jokes about his colander. But he does remember that Brexit is happening, so I brought him up to date with that.

Because we were eating in my office, which has more space and more light, we carried on talking while I trimmed his beard and his eyebrows, washed his hair, gave his upper body a once-over with a bed bath wipe, and changed his top. Afterwards he said, "That was about two days' work." But we are both pleased with the result.

The dietitian, Suzanne, comes tomorrow. I have my list of Prof R's foods ready for her. I hope she doesn't disappoint.

March 11th — Monday. Waiting for the dietitian, who has given us a 4-hour window.

I'm debating whether to use some of Netty's care time this afternoon to wash my hair. But have decided, that an hour at £13 tomorrow with Tina is better spent than an hour today, at £29 an hour. Although Netty is very good value.

Keeping on top of the management of the house is becoming an issue. I want to be more efficient with cleaning in particular. Currently, I wait for the sunlight to direct me to the next urgent job. Although I'm quite good at floors, anything above eye level requiring a stepladder becomes an embarrassment whenever a tradesperson is needed.

I have a friend, Kit, who has invented her own system, but given that the area she has to cover is far more contained than mine – a flat essentially – it might not work for me. I have got as far as writing in the diary once a week, "Start the motor on the car" (I may already have mentioned that) but no other tasks are formally scheduled except the rubbish and recycling. Would I simply be setting myself up for failure?

(In 2020, locked down due to Covid-19, I am again writing "Start the motor on the car" in my diary once a week)

Prof R has been far more mobile lately, when alert. The whippet is back, and I encourage it when he gets up just to have a look around. It's nice to see him behaving in a 'normal' way. Showing an interest in his surroundings. Asking me what is in the drawers of the chest by the bed. Gazing at the contents of my office shelves. Admiring the photographs, even if they are not familiar.

Suzanne the dietitian arrived with her Scottish sense of humour intact at 11.15 am and exceeded my wildest expectations. She had several tips I can use and ticked all the boxes I was already doing. While she was here, Prof R stirred, so I took her upstairs to meet him. He was nowhere in sight. The ensuite door was shut. I knocked and he had finished, almost dressed, having done a poo all by himself and a fair effort at wiping his own bottom. Ten marks to Prof R and nil to the bed alarm.

Because I enjoyed Suzanne's visit so much, I forgot to give Prof R his medication at 12 pm. By 1.20 pm, when Netty arrived, his eyes were a little glazed. And it wasn't just fatigue. But an hour later, he and Netty were happily doing their 'homework 'while I went to the shops.

Any day when two very nice and very positive people visit is a good day.

—

I spent some money. Not in the new shoe shop, where I had hoped to spend it, but in M & Co, as usual. A sensible shirt, £10 slippers and a sensibly priced yellow raincoat. Much nicer than that description indicates. Yellow is a big move for me. I am branching out. Let's hope no one laughs.

March 12 — Tuesday. It's possible that Prof R has more control over some of his symptoms than either he or I appreciate. Last night, as we settled down, and the handshakes began again in earnest, I (again) asked him to see if he could do something to ground them – place them under his body or between his legs. Last night he turned on his side and did the latter I think, because it worked.

It's easy to forget that, like me, Prof R knew quite a lot about natural health remedies when we met. Because his wife had been a physio, and studied Chinese medicine and homeopathy, he knew all the tricks for 'tiring' a muscle pain, and he had her electro-acupuncture machine.

I had always liked to think of myself as reasonably knowledgeable about natural health, and I had used acupuncture, but I had never known acupuncture could be given without needles. This was a revelation. We still have the machine and I have used it many times. We tried to treat Prof R's Parkinson's with it in the early stages. But Prof R is better at giving advice than receiving it, so he was reluctant to use it.

Now I have to make a special effort to remember how things were before Prof R became ill. What a good cook he was, and how sad his girls were when he stopped cooking for them and left it all to me. How knowledgeable he was about plants. How much he loved all the technical aspects of photography and film.

It all slipped away quietly when I wasn't looking.

—

Big Brexit vote at 7 pm tonight. I've been waiting all day for it, watching the debate when I could. And at just about 6.58 pm Prof R awakens for his dinner. So I took my mobile phone up with me and we listened to the vote together. It is something I will do again, when anything interesting is happening, because the blessed digital radio wouldn't tune to Parliament.

Since then, Jack-in-the-Box has been back in residence. It is the only thing, at this time of night, which tries my patience mightily, but if he manages a poo, as he did tonight, all is forgiven. The alarm wasn't warning me, just the scraping of zimmer frame on wood. So I've changed the batteries again in the pager.

March 13 — It is a sign of my own procrastination, when products need returning, that I have only now succeeded in contacting the toilet seat riser company about the broken fixing. This has taken me a month to do.

With Netty gently encouraging me occasionally to just ring up rather than try to manage with only one side secure.

And thanks to her, my new improved efficiency has been rewarded. Emma at the care supply company is sending us a whole new toilet seat. I am feeling overwhelmed with gratitude and stupid at the same time. Netty will be proud of me. Sadly, that also matters.

While Netty was here, I took the dog for a walk to the vet for a weigh-in. She has been on a reduced diet since she hit 13.6 kg in December. Today she weighed 12.4 kg. So she is doing better than I am. If only I had someone to control my food supply.

And she didn't disgrace either of us while walking on the footpath, despite not having had a proper walk since my sister left after Christmas. And even Stella was only walking her occasionally. The dog is maturing.

—

Something very funny happened about half an hour after Netty left. Prof R wanted to get up, but he didn't know why, which can happen when he is overtired. I tried to tell him this – that he really needed to rest – and he had a wee paddy, sat up suddenly and tried to bend the plastic lever that folds the zimmer frame.

My first reaction was to laugh, because I like seeing him energised, even if angry. But then I thought it might be an idea to intervene before he broke it off, or we would be unable to fold the frame. Both of us ended up laughing and he felt better.

March 15 — Friday. We're in calmer waters at the moment. The days are happier – more settled – and the nights less disrupted. Although he still wakes twice – around 1 am and then at 4 or 5. Sometimes I find myself waiting for the next trip. It seems easier not to be too deeply asleep.

—

Doris and Brian came again yesterday. His sister is the only person who can reconnect Prof R to his childhood. Who their neighbours were, going to the Speedway every Wednesday (Prof R had never told me that), the post-war Italian ice cream parlours. So many Italians came to Britain and so many of them knew what was missing from the British menu. Decent ice cream.

I love listening to them reminiscing. They have very funny stories. Especially Brian, whose mother was the queen of eccentricity and malapropisms. Her escalators became perambulators, and she once took him and some cousins twice around the circle line on the Underground before finding the right exit for the Royal Albert Hall. They had tickets for a show and finally arrived just as everyone was leaving.

Brian has another grimmer story from his childhood in the war. He once found a hat in a bombsite and when he picked it up, there was a man's head inside it.

—

But back in the world of the mundane, the new toilet seat is on. No more slipping and sliding and wondering if Prof R would shoot off the front of it during a more vigorous visit.

This morning I feel a bit weepy. Almost 50 people killed in mosques in Christchurch by gunmen. A soft target but yet another nail in the coffin of safe places to be. And poor Christchurch. The earthquake survivor. Where I grew up. The city I love most in the world. Although London comes a close second.

March 16 — Saturday. Prof R was comatose at 7.30 am so I took a risk and had a shower to wash my hair. Before I could dress, his handbell went. But he was able to understand that I wanted to dress first before giving him his pills.

I'm still glued to the news when I can be, feeling very connected to the events in Christchurch. Some will no doubt gloat that now NZ will know how it feels to experience terrorism. But Christchurch didn't need any more reminders of the fact that the world we know can change irrevocably without warning.

I have emailed family and friends. My sister and I exchanged emails without mentioning Prof R. It will take a while for this particular black cloud to blow over. And given I didn't summon it to begin with, that's a mystery. But presumably it would depart if I told them I have booked a care home for Prof R. They'll have a long wait.

March 17 — Sunday. I woke at 6 am. Prof R not stirring until after 7 am. I gave him his pills because he seemed awake enough to follow my instructions. And now I prop him up with my arm across his back. His mucus seems less. Symptoms come and go. It will be good if this one goes.

After his brunch I weighed him. It's always nerve-wracking but he was still 51.5 kg, the same as he was on 2nd March. At least there is no further loss. He's been very sleepy today. I had to wake him to get him to eat by lunchtime. But otherwise, he is feeling as good as he could in the circumstances. And he still enjoys his food.

In order to disturb Prof R as little as possible, I am using two duvets for the bed which I am rotating. I still hate them but can't think of anything better. He enjoys sitting in his chair watching me crawling and sweating across the bed, doing everything from one side, because there is a wall on my side. It's strangely satisfying. We both get enormous pleasure from clean sheets. I've been known to buy new ones just to experience the luxury of crisp folds.

March 18 — Monday. Prof R slept from 10 pm until 6.30 am. I can't recall if this has ever happened, although I suppose, when he was well, it must have. He wasn't able to get up, but he was able to take his pills and be happy to lie down again.

I, of course, have been waiting for him to wake since about 3 am, but I did sleep between time checks. Prof R was able to walk to the toilet and drink tea by 8.30 am. This is a big deal.

It's possible our busy evening made him so settled. We talked, he ate, and I used Netty's prompt sheets to run a mini quiz about the 1950s. Personal and political topics. When did they got their first TV (Answer: for the Coronation in 1953), how did his parents buy it? (From Gamages, bringing it home in the sidecar of their motorbike). And so on...

And does he remember Mary Whitehouse? Says the prompt sheet. And if he doesn't, it goes on to remind him. The morals campaigner, who gave film and theatre directors nervous breakdowns and took one of them, Michael Bogdanov, to court for his 1980 production of *The Romans in Britain*. She lost the case, and he was saved from prison, but she claimed victory for getting him to court in the first place. Ah, those were the days.

The prompt sheets are one of the reasons Netty is worth £29 an hour. Although Prof R and I often talk about our childhoods, the sheets tap into areas we might not yet have explored. Or haven't wanted to. Her background as a teaching assistant has made her the perfect companion for Prof R. And she is an 'ideas person' for me too. Tina, our Yorkshire 'nanny', makes no effort to work with Prof R other than to chat. And feed him. But that's enough some days.

—

Today was another Netty day.

After the brilliant start, Prof R was comatose at 10 am when I wanted to give him a pill and coffee. But I managed to wake him enough to do both. Even Netty has had trouble keeping Prof R awake today. Like me, she makes the most of every waking moment to encourage him to eat.

I have won £10 in the Age Concern UK lottery! Rather defeats the purpose of donating, but never mind.

March 19 — Another sleep right through the night. For Prof R anyway. I was worried how he would be in the morning, so woke him at 7.30 am for his pills. An hour later he was up, and in the toilet – almost before I could get to him. And he has eaten his breakfast at 10.30 am.

He did eat well in the end yesterday – but from lunchtime onwards. Dinner was after 7 pm and we kept going until 8.30.

I have taken some ideas from Netty, stealing a leaf out of her book. Stealing her thunder in fact. Googling things we are interested in for us to chat about. Last night it was the prisoner of war camps on Peckham Rye, which he remembers well. One of the huts remains and is being used as a children's play centre.

Then he was up and down, but only three or four times. Enough to be tiring but not as bad as it has been. And settled by the time I needed to go to sleep. Once in the night he began to have rigours, but it didn't last, and he didn't wake. They give me a fright though.

—

One of our best days today. Eating well. Walking a bit wobbly but not as bad as it has been. Sense of humour not far beneath the surface. Still nervous when I cut his fingernails but being brave.

And then at 5.30 pm he was still up and about so I asked him if he would like to come downstairs for his dinner. He said yes. It was a special evening because he hasn't eaten downstairs for many weeks. He sat at the table and fed himself with cottage pie and ice cream. And had a glass of wine, which he hasn't felt like for months. I knew this was going to be a rare glimpse for both of us of the man he was. So I took a photograph.

This happens. A day or a moment of clarity.

It's been a long time since the last one.

I kept waiting for him to tire. We watched the news. He was interested. And it wasn't until after 8 pm that he agreed bed was a good idea. When we got upstairs, and into the bedroom, he said, "Amazing, this looks just like home". His mind had dislocated the upstairs from the downstairs. He marvelled at what an odd feeling it was. What an odd illness he has. How his perceptions are altered. He could see almost everything. And understood that this wasn't always so. And perhaps it was debatable whether having the 'window' open on this knowledge was actually an advantage.

But he isn't sad about it. That is a blessing. I think we will have an up and down night. He hasn't moved his bowels for a few days, and it is pending.

March 20 — Wednesday. Netty drew the short straw in the bowel department. So, a successful afternoon for Prof R.

But he's been tired today, with one wake in the night and a pill at 1.30 am, and now we are playing catchup with food. It's 5.30 pm and I have given him his lunch and ice cream plus a fruit smoothie. Later I will try to get him to eat some salmon and mashed veg. He's happy. But he's seeing things he cannot describe. Perhaps because his afternoon pills were late. But a shortage of levodopa should not cause hallucinations. Rather the reverse.

I was supposed to go out and play at Whitstable with Ophelia and her parents, but they had to cancel. I walked instead.

March 21 — A very restless night for both of us. Prof R struggled during the evening to eat very much. And coughed a lot for the first half of the night, so that we tried to remove the phlegm that was plaguing him.

While I was downstairs with a cup of tea at 2 am I saw a live feed to New Zealand where PM Jacinda Ardern was announcing changes to the gun laws. The farmer lobby is a strong one and I suspect most New Zealanders would be shocked to know what types of weapons have been legal to obtain.

Prof R had a levodopa at 5.30 am and was still too dopey to move at the next pill time – 9 am. I tell him to just relax and stay where he is. Thank goodness for pull-ups.

Tina comes today. I will wash my hair. My body aches but I blame the Nike shoes I am trying to wear in. The ones that claim to be designed for people who are on their feet all day. The soles are so deep I keep tripping. It feels like I'm lifting a dead weight – the sort of shoes worn by the 60s TV family *The Munsters*. (Google that if you need to) And of course, they are not particularly flexible, so a whole new set of leg muscles are being forced into action. Because they cost £80 the legs will have to adapt.

—

People are coming out of the woodwork lately. It's amazing the lengths they will go to in order to track me down. They are not really interested in reconnecting, just sentimental or simply nosey. Who hasn't googled a few cobwebs from the past? But I don't feel a need to do anything about it. And I've managed to hide from a lot of them since I left Facebook two years ago. The best thing I ever did.

So we exchange a few perfunctory hail-old-fellow-well-met emails, and they go back into whatever woodwork they came out of. Some I don't reply to at all. Though if I really want to get rid of them, I write a long boring email and they never write back.

—

When I went to give Prof R his coffee this morning, I found his breakfast bowl close to the bed, half eaten. Two more pieces of evidence – muesli spills – were lying on the front of his top. It was a joy to see he had taken the initiative to eat without waiting for me or ringing his hand bell. But I also felt guilty.

He was so sleepy it was hard to see how he had managed it. I had to work hard to persuade him to sit in his chair for lunch and a catchup about Brexit, then he returned to bed. So I cancelled Tina. She would be struggling with him today. And he needs the peace and quiet.

With Prof R's slumbers seemingly stable, I had a bath and washed my hair. Halfway through blow drying the alarm went off. Almost succeeded – missed by a whisper. And after a big meal, Prof R was restless, so I persuaded him to come downstairs again. We watched the Brexit events in Brussels and then he tottered off to bed.

March 22 — Friday. Just for fun, I signed the petition to revoke Article 50. Of course, that would be totally anti-democratic and will not happen, but it felt like it was time to make a gesture. Plus I was bored.

We've had a 'normal' night, which means Prof R has woken about four times, (although I lost count) and went to the toilet and took meds. It is so much better when he is not comatose, although so much worse for me in terms of real rest.

I'm not in top form today. So tired, I have dragged myself around town while Netty is here, getting food for the little London family who are visiting tomorrow and buying brother-in-law Brian a present for his 80th birthday. When I showed the present to Prof R, he admired it but said he'd only met Brian once. I try to help him work out that this is not possible.

It would be easy to miss the things that are better, because they are more often absent. Prof R seldom has difficulty comprehending what I am saying now. Often, a few months ago, he would look at me puzzled as I tried to tell him something, and no matter how I reworded it or changed the volume, it would reach him in garbled form. We assumed it was his hearing. Well, if it was, it has improved. And the falls may have caused an inner ear imbalance that has now corrected itself.

March 23 — Saturday. As always, whether overnight medication makes a difference or not is still unclear. On Thursday night he was wakeful, had regular meds and seemed more alert in the morning yesterday.

Last night he was active until his bladder worked, so he had a pill before midnight, but he slept through until I gave him one, regardless, at 6 am. He couldn't suck on a straw to drink his tea at 9.30 am but I managed to get his two pills down him using the child cup which dispenses the water with more control.

Alex and Ophelia and the girls are due at 11.30 for lunch. I have decided not to wake Prof R unless he is ready to be woken.

—

What a difference a day makes. Or even a few hours.

He woke for his breakfast just as they arrived, and didn't want to come downstairs. So my son talked to me upstairs while Prof R ate. But later, when it was time for lunch, I asked Prof R again if he would like to come downstairs. And he did. Much to the delight of the children, who watched him descend the stairs on his stairlift. He ate at the table without my help while I took care of the others. And he showed no sign of tiring.

When he finally did tire, he went back to rest. But an hour or so later, when we were playing in the garden with the dog, Prof R suddenly appeared at the back door. The alarm had not warned me he was up, and he had made his way downstairs to look for us. And he had remained on his feet. It seemed like more than a minor miracle, and he stayed up, enjoying our chat, until late in the afternoon.

This day was the most special we have had in months. If it is a single event, so be it. But it is the third time in a little over a week that Prof R has decided he has a reason to go downstairs. He begins now to link the different parts of the house. He understands and enjoys the conversation.

He ate his evening meal in his room after the family had left and did not seem at all tired. What is this mysterious disease called Parkinson's? Someone on the radio today said it should not be called a disease, because it is not contagious, it should be called a syndrome. After today,

I'm inclined to agree. There are no rules, no stages, no common threads. To each their own.

March 24 — Sunday. Fatigue has only now set in mid-morning after a night of 4-hourly waking and peeing and pills. So the jury has returned a verdict. Regular overnight meds make no difference to the morning alertness.

And it is worrying when I have to cajole pills into a man whose eyes are open, but nobody is home. His head is raised and turned sideways for safety, and I see little squashed pills lodging in his gum, so that I say "swill and swallow" like a drill sergeant and feel like a bully.

—

When things change, it can be dramatic.

Prof R came downstairs after breakfast. We'd eaten, groomed, toileted, and chatted before he was ready to be resettled upstairs. I'd just had time to leave the room to go to the toilet when the alarm kicked off. But I hadn't had time to finish what I was doing. He was on the move. And when I reached him and asked why, he had one of his kicking displays on the bed. When that happens now, instead of feeling cross I am more proactive in thinking of things he can do to relieve his tension. Because it is a healthy sign that he doesn't want to sleep.

It's been a beautiful day. We went outside for the first time in months and he sat in the sun. All was well, until I left him sitting in the living room while I was busy in the kitchen. I always ask him to stay seated and he has been quite good of late.

But not today. He was wearing his size 9 shoes in feet that have shrunk to possibly a size 7. A trip, a thump, and he was on the floor. In pain from the fall but not apparently injured. The dog was licking his mouth when I reached him, which was causing him more discomfort than his battered hip.

I find I barely blink an eye now, apart from a hollow feeling of failure and resignation. Into the recovery position, checking what is hurting, comforting him and then going next door to get the neighbours. "Thank god it's Sunday", said the atheist.

This time Stacey's husband did the lift. It seemed that since Stacey had been on the specialist handling course, she now wasn't prepared to handle Prof R at all. And would only let her husband move him with my verbal permission. He couldn't do it alone. The livid colour of his face had me a little concerned, because Stacey kept saying that Prof R was as light as a feather, but I know a dead weight when I see it. Especially when I have handled it.

I must be at least 15 years older than Stacey, but I have been taught how to bend my knees and keep my back straight to take a weight, and I'm not afraid to give it a go. Public Liability wasn't an issue for me. So between the two of us, Stan and I got Prof R off the floor and safely to the couch. I reassured Stacey I was not seeking her help in a professional capacity, and was just very grateful. (I didn't mention Plan B, the men in the hardware shop, because it was Sunday, and they wouldn't be there.)

—

Prof R's been on the couch napping for two hours with just one ibuprofen and seems to be free of pain. So we both took a precarious journey to the first floor, then the toilet and hopefully safety. His legs are suffering from nervous exhaustion. Just like the rest of us. Safety is again dependent on the bed alarm working. It had better, because I'm cooking a meal. He says he's exhausted.

March 25 — He's hallucinating a little this morning. Mostly pleasant I think, but once or twice something he didn't like very much. I have given him one ibuprofen again to help when he begins to move. He went to the toilet twice in the night successfully, but his hip is quite sore when he tries to sit up and it will be bruised.

While Netty was here, I shopped for Prof R. New shoes – narrower for his newly narrowed feet – and a zip-up fleece top for sitting outside in the cool spring winds.

He is gradually finding his feet again and wanted to come downstairs, but I asked him to wait until tomorrow. He really isn't steady enough.

Tonight will be another Brexit crunch night in parliament. I watch when I can.

March 26 — Tuesday. This morning Prof R managed a pill at 6 am but was too comatose at 9.30 to take the next dose. This may become a serious issue and the solution is to take the capsules apart and put their contents into a 'carrier' that would not choke him. In the end, we used a toddler smoothie mix on a spoon, and I raised him as much as possible. It took a while, and perhaps can be done more efficiently, but it is only every so often that I'm unable to wake him enough for the capsules.

Hallucinating rather a lot. Too little levodopa? I brought him a coffee and he had trouble ignoring his invisible 'friends' long enough to suck on the straw. Although he did manage half a cup eventually.

Last night we ate together upstairs – fish pie again, because he can eat it – and when I offered him wine this time, he found it too bitter. It's such a mystery. Wine tasted good to him when he was in his magic moments eating downstairs.

March 27 — Prof R is still suffering the after-effects of his fall. Very unsteady on his feet so that every trip to the bathroom is fraught with stress. But technique is everything with the zimmer, so gradually we hope to do better.

My big son sent me a pair of new shoes called AllBirds. Wool and recycled materials. I feel very lucky. I even dreamt about them last night. Naturally, he thinks that is sad. But he doesn't know how much I love shoes. Anyone with feet they can seldom forget are hurting, is always searching for the perfect pair. For me, it used to be the perfect handbag.

I am managing the pills today without resorting to smoothie mix. If he can hear me, when I turn his head on its side, I can get him to take water and pill without choking. Although his swallowing is a great deal slower than it was, at least slow means careful.

Last night's dinner in our room seemed to take forever, but he is eating everything. Energy is a mystery. I can be fully enjoying his company and our mealtime, but by 8 pm suddenly my body is begging to be allowed to go downstairs and crash on the couch.

The physicality of helping him move can sometimes be considerable. He has to use his muscles as well, or I cannot lift or move him. This is when I need to bring him on board mentally. I need his help. Last night I said, "This is a job for two nurses, but you only have me, so we have to be very careful." If Kent Social Services saw us they would go pale, but they would also be relieved we don't need them.

—

At 10.45 am he must take two pills or things will slide. I manage to get one stuck to the roof of his mouth. So in went the smoothie to dislodge it. He's responding but only just. I use the torch, his favourite thing, to investigate his mouth after each effort to get everything down. I cannot sit him up semi-comatose, but his head is raised on the bolster. I may go back to putting the contents of each pill into smoothie. As the GP would probably suggest, if we ever saw one. But it's not an emergency. There is never a guarantee he won't choke, either way.

Netty had a busy session with him. And he is resettled. I went back to Pilates and enjoyed it. I have worn my new shoes out and feel sure that is why I hardly noticed the time passing.

I still find Netty unwilling to provide much in the way of advice regarding techniques for handling Prof R in bed. I'm assuming because she is not allowed to. But I did manage to get her to tell me the tricks of easily changing him while he is in his twilight zone and lying in bed. Apparently, they tear the side of the pull-ups to get them off, although she didn't then explain how to dress him again when he is not able to help.

For now, my focus can be on the indicative votes in Parliament, and wondering why John Bercow, the Speaker, has so much power.

March 28 — Thursday. Success getting Prof R awake at 8.30 am and to the toilet. Yesterday he had been so unable to move he didn't get to the toilet until lunchtime. The pull-up was full up. The wool bed fleece went in the washing machine. He had been prone too long.

Perhaps he is simply slowly recovering from the fall. But no complaint of hip pain so far today. He could be woken at 11.30 am for a pee, pill, pants change, mouth swab and tea. No appetite for breakfast yet, but a clean pull-up. He's lying on his side seeing something I cannot see. It absorbs him.

When Prof R holds his own cup to drink, sometimes he only catches every 'eighth wave'. Watching him – if he is using his 'bad' hand, the right one – is like watching your clothes thrashing around through the glass window of the washing machine. Except less relaxing.

He was very tired all day, so that I worried I would not get three meals and snacks into him. He had lunch at 3 pm, after I had given the lawn its first cut of the season. The afternoon was beautiful, the dog happy to be groomed, and me with the bed alarm pager on the outdoor table. Praying it would work, and it did.

At 7 pm I had to wake him from a deep sleep for his evening pills and food. It was a relief when he eventually woke enough to eat salmon (with everything but the kitchen sink) and chocolate ice cream.

His legs are a little steadier. We talked about going out one day. Taking a trip in the car. He is more interested in this now than he has been for months. My main question is, can I remember how to assemble the wheelchair?

March 29 — Friday. This should have been Brexit Day – our exit from the EU. But it flounders on, and Theresa May cannot make headway.

But here, it was a red-letter day. Prof R could be woken and medicated and even breakfast eaten by 11 am. His pull-ups were not put to use.

And after Netty arrived, I was picked up and whisked away to Whitstable by Ophelia, her parents, and two-year-old Violet. It felt like a birthday. They took me to a café by the sea for my first taste of fish and chips in months. And this fish was fresh, so fresh it fell off my fork. Hand cut chips with tomato ketchup. And seagulls the size of small aircraft just waiting for us to leave our outside table.

The weather was perfect, my only regret that I would not be at home to take Prof R outside into the sunshine. Netty can't do it yet. She is not familiar with the stairlift and needs to be shown its little 'weaknesses'. In other words, how it can trap you on the stair on the wrong side of the rider when he wants to alight. And she felt it would be too rushed today for me to give her a tutorial.

Netty brought some extra *Daily Sparkle* newsletter sheets with her, as requested. Terrible title. You'd need to have dementia not to be insulted by it. But a useful source of topic prompts for talking about the past.

March 30 — Saturday. Another beautiful day. Prof R sleepy, very sleepy, but eating everything. While he slept, I cleaned.

His pull-ups are definitely too large. He missed them altogether today, so we had a change of clothes and duvet. Happily, he seemed not to notice. I lie to explain the wet clothes and say, "Gosh you must have been hot". Because he often does detox that way overnight.

After lunch I took him outside. We used the walking stick as his 'extra leg', but he hasn't had enough practice to be very good at it. So it was, if not knife edge, not exactly relaxing either getting him down into the living room, new shoes on, and then onwards outside. Once out, we settled and stayed. And I cut his hair.

When he felt tired, and was ready to go inside he said, "I want to go home". He still often separates the levels of the house in a way that confounds even him. There is a spatial element to it that no doubt a neurologist could explain. But we no longer see the neurologist. He doesn't want to see us. And we're both glad of that.

—

The speech therapist rang me when I was out on Friday and said she would ring back. I'm not sure why we have been referred back to her, unless it is in relation to the mucus. Prof R's voice is generally strong enough most of the time. Or he can turn the volume up when encouraged to 'play to the back of the theatre'.

Tonight, he didn't manage all his food. Too tired. But not too tired for a glass of wine. I tell him that that by cutting his hair I have weakened his manhood, so I had better not cut his fingernails as well today. He smiles.

Unsurprisingly, he didn't feel like a session with the *Daily Sparkle*. Netty has received a photo from me of Prof R outside. Proof of success. Perhaps she will gain the confidence to do it too.

At 7 pm, I have tidied the kitchen and just flopped onto the couch when his alarm goes off again. This time, he feels like a tour of the first floor. He says he remembers the rooms but thinks he has only walked around them twice.

Resettled, wine in hand (my hand this time) I return to watching the animated film *Loving Vincent* about the death of Vincent van Gogh. Without iPlayer, Prime and Netflix I would be a very frustrated viewer. Vincent was interrupted twice more before I managed to finish dispatching him. And once, Prof R's alarm failed to work, and I found him on the landing upstairs. No amount of reasoning around safety enables him to stop doing this.

Sunday March 31 (Clocks change to summertime) — Overnight my body clock changed with my smart watch. I woke at 7 am, which gave me an extra hour to shower and wash my hair. Prof R is given his pill at 7.30, and goes back into deep sleep. I'm still pondering the wisdom of letting him sleep right through the night. It's good for both of us of course, in one sense. But I suspect his mornings are less responsive if he goes more than six hours or so without levodopa.

Today he is awake but very much still in his own world at 10 am and not awake enough to be taken to the toilet. Should I change his pull-ups? Often, he can go for several hours without needing to pee, so he should be comfortable and dry even if he has used them. I hate the thought of disturbing him to change them. Some physical needs – like essential pill swallowing – can seem like a cruelty.

—

The day that began with promise has become a battle to wake him and keep him awake to eat lunch. For the first time, he had a loss of bladder control in daytime, before I could rouse him. Not major, and I don't think he noticed the damp clothing, but still a first. And not in a good way. We have the fleece on the bed and for small spills it is quick and easy to sponge and rub dry. But now I begin to see the time rapidly approaching when pull-ups will be for days as well as night.

Eating called for repetition from me to keep him focused. "Darling, are you ready for another mouthful?" Or, "Open your mouth please". And so the day continued until bedtime.

April 1 — When Prof R woke in the small hours and was able to go to the toilet, I said to him "a pinch and a punch" and he knew what I meant. I thought "April Fool" might be a step too far.

He woke again at 6.30 am, and could walk to the toilet again, although he needs the zimmer still. This is a big improvement on yesterday.

Other than his sister, I notice his family seem even more reluctant to visit. Busyness is always the reason but it's not an excuse. Two of his girls have not seen him since the beginning of December. On his birthday.

It's ironic that my niece interfered too much and with too little knowledge, and yet his own daughters don't seem to feel the need to show an interest in his care at all. Of course, they have different agendas.

Ophelia and Violet turned up with an April Fool Day surprise – beautiful spring flowers, miniature azaleas, and a card that took my breath away with her heartfelt words of love and support. How often I thank Alex for choosing such a wonderful wife. The mystery is....... but only his mother is allowed to tease this way.

Ophelia took the dog and Violet for a walk while I fed Prof R, and pronounced her well behaved in the park. Violet behaved as well. Prof R was also well behaved. Then they had to go home to collect Hester from school.

Netty came and I met Tina for coffee at 2 pm. It was my first venture into socialising, and I enjoyed her company, in spite of her confession to homesickness for Yorkshire family, and some rather serious depression. I'm never afraid to talk about such things, having 'form', so we exchanged our favourite blues-chaser tricks. I hope it helped.

It occurred to me afterwards that it should have been me seeking comfort. And yet I have adapted to this life. It isn't normal, but treating it as such makes me accept it and I get satisfaction from the challenge of keeping Prof R afloat.

April 2 — Tuesday. He was afloat all night unfortunately. Four times, after days and even weeks of sleeping almost too well. The bed alarm wasn't working properly, so I had two frights before bed and one at 3 am when I was downstairs making a cup of tea and checking on the Brexit indicative vote results. The ominous scraping of the zimmer on wood is unmistakable. Without it he would probably wobble silently to the loo without my knowing it.

I decided all this activity is a positive, as I could give him levodopa four-hourly, but this morning we came close to the edge of coping on his first daylight trip to the toilet. His legs vary in strength almost from moment to moment.

—

Sometimes it seems pointless to keep this diary. (*No doubt, dear reader, you are inclined to agree.*) While each day is different to its neighbour, it is the same as many which have gone before. But how else to value each day? To feel these months and years have not been wasted? I'm afraid of forgetting.

One thing that is better – he is eating all meals and as many as two desserts. So his weight has edged up just a little – from 51.5 – 51.9 kg. As Hope would say, "Perhaps you should weigh him before his trip to the loo!"

Before bed, I managed to interest him in some more history research – this time the motorbike with sidecar his parents owned. He remembered it was a BSA, so I found a picture online and printed it out. It is now white-tacked to the wall where he can see it. Something for Netty to follow up on tomorrow.

April 3 — Today I will chase up the superfood prescription from the dietitian which should have been delivered by now.

Prof R has become comatose again. Only awake enough to take pills without opening his eyes. At 11.30 am I washed his face and gave him his next levodopa but could not fully wake him. If he has a full pull-up, Netty will not approve if I do not change him in the bed. But I've checked, and he is not wet.

Teresa May is now reduced to inviting Jeremy Corbyn to joint Brexit talks. All caused by her own party hardliners, who consider her move a betrayal.

—

After Pilates I took my spotted wheelie bag down to the chemist, and took delivery of 56 compact bottles of superfood for Prof R. I had not heard from the GP that the prescription was ready. I was told they would be delivered. But they weren't. Given they only have 300 cals each, I thought they were a bit lightweight, but protein is probably their main function.

While I am trying to write this, Prof R's alarm keeps going off. He probably has a pee on the line which has not yet arrived. Each run is dry. I am much better at hanging around upstairs when this happens, so that my nerves remain unfrayed.

His meal tonight was a little masterpiece. A mixture of onions, red peppers, wheatberry and other grains, and chicken. I should have photographed my own portion so he would know what he was eating. By the time I had put his through the food processor it could have been anything. But his has cream and honey as well. And tasted delicious.

As I was leaving the bedroom with the empty dishes, he said "How long is it till supper?". You would think this was an indication of hunger, but no. He was simply asking. I hoped he wasn't bored. We had done some online research in my office after the meal, looking for the theatres he went to as a child. But there were none he recognised.

Given his short energy span, it is difficult to get far beyond eating and drinking between lie-downs. Although I talk to him a great deal about the day. It doesn't seem inspiring to try to read to him. The news is as far as I get. He shows little interest now in books.

April 4 — At 1 am I suddenly remembered I hadn't put a parking voucher on the windscreen of the car. Yesterday, I had glanced through the front window downstairs to see a traffic warden photographing the car. Never a good sign. So I went out to ask him what the infringement was. My annual parking permit had expired last month. And I hadn't noticed.

There's always one thing that slips through the net. And this one cost me a £25 fine. Although, when I renewed the permit yesterday, the clerk told me I should have received a reminder. That didn't stop her taking the £25.

So, at 1.30 am I went outside and put a voucher in the car so that I would not have to appear early in my pyjamas to do it in the morning. It will be about seven days before the new permit arrives.

Prof R has had a good portion of a strawberry super-shake at 9.30 am. He is seldom hungry for breakfast until much later, so they are going to fill a calorie gap. I am on a mission to put weight on this man. He's sleeping a lot today, but eating well.

—

I have realised there is a rather obvious solution to finding activities he can enjoy. That we both can enjoy, in fact. I was researching WW2 rationing after a conversation we had, and found film archive of a propaganda film made in New Zealand, explaining rationing there. I left him happily watching it while I fetched his food. So much better than searching for books or magazines to spark his interest.

April 5 — Friday. The levodopa jury has been called back in.

Overnight Prof R woke twice, at the right time for a pill each time. This morning he was definitely more alert, although still sleepy and not wanting breakfast. He had tea and one of his super-shakes mid-morning instead, before spending considerable, and eventually productive, time on the loo. In this instance, I increased my medical qualifications somewhat by successfully assisting in the 'birth'. He is now resting from our labours. There is no one I would willingly share this level of information with.

I was telling Netty this afternoon about a TV drama series I'm enjoying about the Coptic Jewish community. She said, "I don't have time to watch anything like that." It would be easy to be offended by that comment. Or even to say, "I don't suppose you are getting up in the night to take anyone to the toilet though."

Nor is she spending the best part of her evening feeding her husband upstairs in a chair. But our evenings are friendly and fun. It's when he keeps getting up until 9.30 pm or so that my face begins to freeze over.

April 6 (Grand National Day) — Prof R's morning aperitif, courtesy of the NHS, goes down his throat, semi-prone, through a straw at 8.30 am, along with a cup of tea. Bliss for him on his face. He has gone back to sleep with the straw still in his mouth.

I've seen no signs of him watching his invisible friends lately. The level of levodopa seems to be immaterial. We're both very tired. It was an unsettled night. But I managed to get him to wake for muesli before 11 am.

But I should have put fresh pull-ups on him after breakfast. At 2 pm I couldn't wake him enough to do more than give him his pills. And when I checked, he had damp clothes. This is the first time I have had to put clean underpants or pull-ups on him in bed during the day. Because he can't get up. It's a new skill, and I stopped after managing new underpants, rather than trying to put on his pyjama trousers as well.

Downstairs, I had been cleaning, cooking and, in between, watching *Fleabag* and my Jewish TV series, *Shitsel*. It is my ultra-Orthodox Jewish homework. There had been no indication Prof R would still be in his morning semi-daze in the middle of the afternoon. But he eventually woke enough to wolf lunch and fruit jelly. We are definitely on track in the food department.

By 5 pm I was trying to interest him in watching the Grand National on my iPad. I've been a fan since my black and white TV childhood. Prof R does remember these events, but doesn't really engage when presented with them. Just as well, as I couldn't get it to work without the app. So I asked him if he could wait while I watched it downstairs.

At the 23rd fence his bed alarm went off. I almost wondered if I had called it down from the gods by tempting fate. But suddenly, desperately, I really wanted to see the end of this race, so I ran upstairs and didn't even attempt to try to explain. He didn't need the toilet, but was just on the move. I issued an instruction "Please lie down and stay where you are until I come back." He did.

—

We've spent a lot of time today trying to think of games or activities we could do together. Pick-up-sticks is definitely out we decided. Although the images it evoked kept us amused for quite some time. More source material for black humour. It isn't easy to find things Prof R can do.

April 7 — Sunday. It's been one of those days when I wonder how much longer Prof R can survive. He goes so far away. Even though I know he will be back, it's difficult to imagine when his eyes are open but not comprehending.

He is eating less today because of this. At 5 pm I am hoping to get his lunch into him. He didn't eat all his muesli earlier. This time I'm experimenting with how ravioli behaves in the food processor. The answer is, badly, but with fruit puree and cream it becomes both edible and delicious.

I'm slipping the smoothie drinks into him every hour or so. Just a few mouthfuls. When he is too sleepy, they slide out of the side of his mouth and down onto his shoulder. The dietitian would not be pleased. She says he should always sit up at 90 deg. And no, 45deg is not sufficient. And of course, neither of those is possible when he is unable to wake fully. He is raised by his tri-pillow and bolster and I always turn his head sideways. I don't believe prone people in hospital are not given food by mouth. Though if I rethink that, I suspect they don't get fed at all.

—

I've just washed my hair with one of his shampoo caps to avoid the risk of interruption. Three minutes into the process his bed alarm went off. And I laugh, because it only takes three minutes to use the cap. He is surprised when I enter the bedroom with hair awry and no glasses. "Remember I told you I was just going to use the shampoo cap?" Some lack of comprehension tells me he has forgotten.

But it hasn't been a busy day for me because he has been so sleepy. I've been able to do two more coats of paint on the water stain on the dining room ceiling where the bathroom leaked. It may never be truly covered, but who looks up, except to check the spot lighting? Or the cobwebs.

There must be a lot of chemicals in the shampoo cap because I can smell them when I use the straighteners. It smells like burning cloth. No matter, I am clean enough for a few more days.

Prof R's day ended as poorly as it began. The 5 pm lunch was a success, but later weak legs, bad tremor and an appetite only for NHS shakes, banana smoothie and jelly. But he will have eaten more than is obvious with all those little boosters. Dinner, another experiment with risotto, can wait until tomorrow.

April 8 — My mother's birthday. She would have been 100. It is also, Tina's birthday. Two more different people would be a challenge to find. Although that doesn't stop me reading my own horoscope.

I met Tina later for coffee and cake. We walked across the swing bridge and out onto the meadows. Tina has not explored the countryside here yet and has been missing her Yorkshire landscapes. I coughed madly through the rape field.

Prof R is a lot better today. Eating better, more awake. But Netty thinks he may be slightly liverish. His skin is tinged yellow around his eyes. I shall keep watch for that.

I've had no chance to buy a bowl suitable for soaking his feet, rather than just washing them. Netty offered to lend us a foot spa she has. But I don't like borrowing things.

My first husband bought me a foot spa once for a birthday present. I think it was after we had separated, although I don't place any significance on that. It rather took me by surprise. Such a 'domestic' present for someone in their mid-40s. Like being given a vacuum cleaner. And yet very nice too. I didn't use it of course – too much of a drag – and later gave it to charity. Right now, it would be useful.

In spite of myself, I am again counting how long it is since each of his daughters have visited. Four months for two of them – two months for one. The most recent visitor, Julie, will be back at Easter to pick up her great grandmother's sewing machine. It's lovely someone wants it.

April 9 — Tuesday. Prof R managed to get through the night dry. Although he was agitated in the early hours until he was awake enough to use his legs.

His last meal yesterday was the rest of his evening meal at 9.30 pm. I don't mind when he eats, as long as he does.

His sister rang me this morning to say she has been diagnosed with Parkinson's. She has no confidence in the neurologist fortunately, so will await further clinical evidence before being pushed into taking levodopa. I think she is very wise. So far, she only has a tremor and there is no reason why she should have the same experience as Prof R. He definitely drew a short straw.

I've written to the manager at the agency to ask how they arrange bookings for 'block care' requirements. I want to organise several full days of care when Hope has the baby. And it's not going to be easy to schedule. The manager says Netty can do it and her other clients can be covered by someone else. That's a relief. But it will be hit and miss timewise.

Prof R is not eating quite so well today. He's had tasters of milkshake, banana smoothie and two thirds of his muesli. But he's not firing on many cylinders.

Meanwhile, Teresa May is meeting Angela Merkel and Macron, angling (no pun) for a Brexit extension. After months of holding up well she looks so tired.

—

A meat sauce and more veggie mash have been made this morning. I'm looking for things I know need doing. If I sit down, I will only stiffen up. It may be time to return to gluten free eating. What a bore.

No sooner had those words left the keyboard when I spied, through our bedroom door, a little head rising above the parapet that is the bedside rail. He was hungry again. Which is good. It took a few minutes to determine this, as he had lost his voice. So I told him to shout. It always works. He is his own best speech therapist.

So now he has eaten lunch and fruit jelly and is back in bed under a clean duvet.

3.15 pm is much better than 5 pm for lunch. We may end up on track today.

Prof R is always tired when he has had success on the toilet. I tell him "No wonder you are tired. They don't call it a jobbies for nothing!" And all evening he was up and down doing dry runs until eventually he peed properly around midnight. By which time I had pieced together a film called *Paris can Wait*. It had to.

April 10 — It's unfortunate I have to keep relearning lessons from my university of life. Today, facing another day of stiffness and limping, I had an epiphany regarding food preservatives. Not all of them, but definitely some of them, like nitrates, have done this to me before. Either that or I can expect to need hip replacements anytime soon. Note to self: keep reading the labels and discard all but freshly made with no preservatives. Wine is an exception. I can handle sulphites thank goodness.

Pilates today. How tempting not to go. But I did. And our teacher told us she could see a huge variation between us and her younger classes when it came to balance. And before we got excited and misunderstood, she added "and not in a good way". Balance apparently is a marker for longevity. She had us walking one foot directly in front of the other. Like a cop testing a class of drunks. I failed. It's shit getting old.

When I got home, I scoffed several rice crackers topped with Stilton and onion chutney. It didn't make me feel any younger.

Prof R has eaten all his lunch and two desserts for Netty. There's no room for another booster shake.

After dinner, Prof R said, "My mouth is half empty". This happens when he notices his partial plates are missing. "So that means your mouth is half full." He hardly ever fails to see the joke.

April 11 — Thursday. Prof R was on deck earlier today. Very unusual. And all without levodopa overnight. So he'd had a cup of tea and one of his NHS booster shakes by 9 am.

I'm stiff from Pilates, and whatever else makes me stiff. And bored. There is only so much cleaning you either want to do or need to do. Brexit is in a deadlock and painful to watch. I've crushed a few cardboard boxes for the recycling and done some more exercises.

Prof R is simply sleeping between feeds, like a newborn. Except, when prompted, he can respond to my reports from the outside world.

—

I have received this month's account from the agency but the password, supposedly to protect Prof R's data, doesn't work, so I can't open it. I have double-checked the password. It still doesn't work. If they want me to pay them, perhaps they could act less like the secret service and more like a care agency.

It turned out the passwords had been changed. The bill was £1,145.50 for the month. We can't sustain much more than that. Although I know we will need to.

—

Later Prof R woke up for his early evening lunch/dinner and dessert before 6 pm. If a late breakfast is brunch, what is a late lunch and dinner? Pass. And at around 4 pm he'd had one of his NHS freebie shakes and some smoothie, so he was on track with his calories.

When he resettled, I had just downed my own dinner, before his alarm went off again soon after 7 pm. I always ask him if he is hungry, and this time he said yes. So I raced off to do a dinner for him. It doesn't take long. Chicken from the bird I had just twice-cooked, vegetables, pea humous, apple puree cream and honey all whizzed up and heated.

But while it's a triumph he is eating so much, I am otherwise bordering on tearful and a bit tired. My back is beginning to complain. I know it doesn't help that I am lifting him more than I should. And two meals in the evening is hard work when he doesn't talk.

The truth is I feel sad that I can't get a carer on a weekend so I can go out with my family. Or even spend an hour at one of the summer festivals. My daughter wants to come down in two weeks and Netty is not available. She suggests I apply for someone else to stand in. And even though I hate the thought, I know this is how things must proceed. Netty cannot always be our only choice.

Theresa May has been given a Brexit delay until 31st October. It's not a triumph, but a triumph is no longer considered an option.

April 12 — Friday. A good night. And by that, I mean I may actually have got about 8 hours of sleep. Prof R needed to get up twice, but I had been too tired after each trip to spend even half an hour reading my book.

And once again he has had a cup of tea and one of his super shakes by 9 am. It doesn't seem to wake him up though. The mornings are snooze time. Thank goodness for pull-ups when he cannot get out of bed.

A better day and certainly, Prof R is now eating better. In spite of seemingly becoming progressively more tired. So it is confusing, that in some ways he is better while in others he is obviously losing the battle.

And it's sad, especially if I show him photos of us in our early days. The days he has forgotten. And I look at the man in the photo and realise I have lost him, all but a small part of him anyway.

I have asked the agency if they can give me a replacement carer for a Saturday afternoon in April, the 27th, so my daughter can come down. I want to take her out for lunch. The manager made it clear this would not be easy, they would have to introduce a new PA blah blah blah.

How do these people run a business? What would happen in an emergency? I fear the thought. And I fear for the time the baby arrives, now that one afternoon on a weekend is clearly a big challenge for them.

—

Keeping calm and carrying on. I have the sense to know that I only hurt myself if I get sad or angry or depressed. No one else knows. Except Prof R perhaps, if I am sad and tired around him. And it's not his fault that care is so expensive and so hard to come by. As if they were giving us a gift instead of charging £29 an hour (social hours that is) and £32 if I am being unsociable. That is, wanting someone on a weekend or evening.

I have bought some more shoes – this time for summer and with memory foam for my punished feet and legs. They felt like fairy slippers. Let's hope they act like them.

April 13 (Hope's birthday) — The new morning pattern continues. Prof R is alert enough to go to the toilet at 9.30 and has both a banana smoothie and his super shake. The banana smoothie rather than muesli, because he collapsed back into bed exhausted and faint-headed after moving his bowels. Exhausted or not, he was hungry, and the banana smoothie can be fed to him in bed.

He is eating much more – especially in the morning – and yet not apparently gaining weight or noticeably improving his quality of life. Although perhaps enjoying food can be counted as QOL.

Netty said she loves our house. It's kind of her. Some are of the opinion we should have bought something with separate living rooms downstairs which could also be bedrooms.

I've talked to Prof R about what might happen later – about trying to get a medical bed which will fit in our room rather than contemplating a move downstairs. I'm never sure how much he comprehends about this future planning. But I always want to include him in my thinking. As long as it doesn't distress him. It could mean we pay for our own bed if the 'Powers that Be' refuse to bring a bed upstairs.

—

The mystery of how Prof R can move like lightening can never be fathomed. He's just done it again. Ten minutes after a previous dry run on teetering legs. He was closing the bathroom door by the time I got to the room. No zimmer, no handholds. Look mummy, no hands. And then wobbly again on the return journey. Strangely unnerving. You know where you are with a legless man. But he isn't. Never relax.

Ten minutes later I popped my head around the door, and he was on the move again. I'm sure it was another dry run, although he thinks not. It is an aspect of his care that I find truly exhausting.

April 14 — Sunday. A stressful night for both of us. At midnight Prof R was off to the toilet for the second time since I came to bed, and became cross when I tried to get him to be more careful with handholds and the zimmer. He attacked the toilet, not me, but it was very distressing. Trying to throw the zimmer frame and break the seat.

Getting him back to bed in one piece after that was one of life's low points. But I managed. And he realised he had put us both at risk. It was tears before bedtime for me and not to be repeated if possible.

The irony of my seat-of-the-pants skill level compared to the stringent operational rules Netty operates under, does not escape me. But would she really be able to deal with these situations differently? I could ask to shadow her, but it would unnerve her. She is always shooing me out the door. And I know she is not tasked with training me. She hesitates even to advise on handling. And because he is usually at the best part of his day when she is here, my concerns are not ones she is confronted with. I'm over-thinking again.

This morning he is positively jovial by the time he has finished his early cup of tea and a strawberry shake. While not up and about, he is more or less awake. And that is with an 8-hour overnight gap between doses of levodopa. His bowels are also active now mid-morning. He's doing remarkably well.

This afternoon I moved the bookcase away from in front of the Juliette door at the foot of my side of the bed. The door is ugly, despite the tongue-in-groove panelling, but at least now I don't have to climb over the end of the bed and down the step stool to get out in the night. Or fly across the bed after Prof R when he's on the move. The bookcase is now next to the chest of drawers on his side of the bed. It fits perfectly and takes Prof R's medical supplies. The books meanwhile are stacked up in my office. I have kicked the can down the road, but the accident black spot has gone with it. Safety first.

Tonight Prof R weighed in at 52.5 kg. A steady improvement. I'm thrilled.

April 15 — I'm moving the deckchairs on the Titanic again. This time, Prof R's books, mostly gardening and landscape, up to an alcove in the loft behind our former bed. I want to make room for the books I've had to remove from our bedroom bookcase. It's frightening to think that one day I will have to deal with them; I just have to decide "not now". Who would want them?

But looking at all these titles, I remember how Prof R loved and treasured his books. How interested he was in absolutely everything to do with history and landscape. And London. And gardening. His girls almost always gave him a book for Christmas and birthdays.

And now he lies half asleep in our bed while I move around him cleaning and shifting things. I cannot remember when he last picked up a book.

April 16 — Notre-Dame was on fire last night. There are few sights more distressing than an irreplaceable architectural masterpiece burning. I told Prof R and this morning he remembered again when I gave him an update. The good news is that the stone structure has survived. It's nice when we can talk in the old way about these things.

Every morning now I wake him with tea and a super shake by 9 am to keep his appetite alive. It seems to be working. Although he shows no desire to get up at that time, even to go to the toilet.

The manager at the agency has found a PA to fill in for Netty on 27th April. He, Darren, will come next Monday to shadow Netty and get to know Prof R. It's a relief. I can now take Hope out for lunch and there will be another person on board for backup.

I have painted the Juliette door and hung my best robe on a hook to make it look like a design feature rather than an eyesore.

—

Prof R has eaten breakfast, lunch and dessert in one hit at 1pm. Just in time to be nicely tucked up when Tina arrived for her two-hour stint. She brought leftover chicken stew already puréed for Prof R. A very nice surprise.

But I haven't solved my joints problem yet. I walked like a cripple downtown today.

April 17 — Wednesday. The latest scan confirms Hope's baby is a girl! Only one set of names to trawl through. Lots of clothes from two older cousins. Very good.

Sleep is very restless for both of us at the moment. Prof R and I that is. I wake almost every hour. Waiting, I think, for him to try to get up. He makes several half-hearted attempts at various times and then draws the covers back over himself. I need to relax.

A did relax this afternoon, with Tina. Meeting her outside 'office hours'. Eating and taking her on a walk along parts of the Creek she hadn't discovered yet.

But here the neighbours are driving me mad. Perhaps it's just Easter holidays, but I hear sounds that could be Prof R rearranging his zimmer frame, but are just as likely to be a head-banger next door. I've just checked, and it is definitely a head-banger.

Prof R is sleeping soundly after his evening meal, delicious leftovers from Tina again, and a chat about my mother's watercolour paintings. We both decided to hang one on top of the now faded Rita Angus print in our bedroom. It's been a long time since I revisited these 'daubs', as my mother would have called them. She underestimated them. Even in their raw state, they are so evocative of New Zealand and Canterbury that we can feel ourselves there.

—

Netty helped Prof R make a novelty face-towel rabbit for Easter. It's sitting above the bed with something where its stomach should be that may be chocolate. I haven't investigated. She said Prof R was frustrated, which doesn't surprise me. A towel rabbit isn't going to float his boat, light his fire or give him the will to live. Although miraculously one thing he has never lost is the will to live. But he is too frail to really want to do a great deal.

I asked him at dinner if he was fed up and he nodded. But what to do about it? Almost every day I ask if he would like to come downstairs, or venture out, or have me read to him. But he is really too tired, frustrated or not. Lying down is his favourite thing, possibly because then he has both oxygen and blood in his head, rather than in his stomach or his feet.

April 18 — A change this morning. He is not so keen on his tea or his super shake. And when he had his mid-morning pill at 11 am he was not hungry for breakfast or the shake.

I've been baking a cake. Chocolate for Prof R's youngest daughter Julie, her hubby and the children who are coming tomorrow. Not 'sans dairy', which young Harold requires, but she will bring dairy free hot cross buns for him. It is her birthday on 22nd and her husband's on 23rd, so it seemed appropriate. The bed alarm went off when the cake was due out of the oven. Law of Sod. But Prof R was awake enough to say he could wait a few minutes.

I sent my sister a scan photo of the new baby to tell her it is a girl. She has not been in touch at all for three weeks. She replied "that's sorta good news". I guess she thinks it's time there was a boy. She had nothing else to say. I'm not sure why I persevere. Except I know she is probably just feeling low.

I feel ancient today. Trying to ignore the fact that everything hurts again. Deciding not to take ibuprofen. Hayfever may also be the culprit. Prof R says he feels rubbish, but he has much more excuse than me. To make him feel better, I have given him a foot soak in Dead Sea salt. An appropriate name. He sheds skin like a snake and the water was full of it.

Halfway through my salmon fillet tonight the bed alarm went off, but it no longer irritates me. I'm so pleased with the way Prof R is eating. And I'm waking him more to check if he is hungry. Usually, his appetite doesn't appear until lunchtime. Tonight he had mains, jelly and an entire super shake, which alone has 300 calories.

It's been a beautiful day. My push mower had another outing. The dog poo has been collected. We're ready for our visitors tomorrow. Sadly, the treadle sewing machine has developed some rust while it's been in the shed. I hope that won't put his granddaughter off.

—

Prof R showed his muscle this evening. So much food made him restless. While I was tied up in technology and password changes, he was on the move. I hear him rather than the alarm telling me he is up. So I race up telling him to please stay put while I finish what I am doing, as I am online; and he is getting frustrated at being stopped.

He fancied a wander, and began trying to wreck his bedrail (which he hates) and the zimmer. As usual, I find it bizarrely refreshing, to see the energy, the power he still has in his muscles when the adrenalin is running. I tell him so, and he can see it too when I point it out. When he was calm again, we talked about life and its random chaotic nature. Comparing the disasters in our lives to those of our parents. I feel I have graduated in several health issues, having now had considerable experience, past and present; but I have no desire to go on and do my Masters.

Good Friday — Though what is 'good' about it I can't imagine. Celebrating a crucifixion is not. Although I'm very partial to hot cross buns.

Prof R is restless. This is good from a nutrition point of view. He had his breakfast mid-morning and his lunch at noon. But he is not resting as much as he needs to if he's to be on deck for the family arriving mid-afternoon.

My eyes are red. Hayfever and a few unshed tears I think. Prof R said today he would like to go home, home this time being London. We talked about our favourite houses, the ones we have owned together. Brookside in New Zealand wins, and the London house.

Then I came in here to write the diary, and he-who-is-supposed-to-be-resting was on the move again. After agreeing to rest. When I entered the room and asked him why he was sitting up he said "I'm not" because by that time he had lain back down again. "Ha ha" said I.

The truth is he probably needs a pee. His last trip 20 minutes ago was a dry run.

—

6 pm: The little family visit was good medicine for both of us. Visitations are rare and therefore more significant. We haven't seen these grandchildren of Prof R's for over a year. After that sort of time lapse, growth and maturity hits you between the eyes. It's wonderful to talk to the new 'them'.

I managed to ruin the dairy-free hot cross buns they brought with them by absent-mindedly putting butter on them, but young Harold forgave me when he had sweets and coconut chocolate ice cream as compensation. He couldn't have the chocolate cake I had made, but I was ready for that.

Step-granddaughter, lovely grounded girl, is as tall as I am at 11. She has an interest in all things vintage, so she went home with my train set and a wind-up steam engine, along with the sewing machine. The machine caused so much trouble to her parents, I hope she loves it. An absolute swine to get out of the shed and into the car, with her poor father nursing bruised or broken ribs from a bike fall, just to add to his advancing MS.

Middle boy, aged nine, also has an interest in all things old, but his main interest lies in people. After he had almost demolished the sewing machine examining its inner and outer workings, (and breaking the fragile treadle belt) he insisted on knowing my birth year, in order to compare my age with grandpa's. He pronounced that when I turn 70 later this year I will be "officially old". I thanked him for that observation. And put him in charge of wrapping up a large section of the chocolate cake to take home for everyone to have later.

Harold-the-dairy-free, aged four, had changed least of all. Except he can now write "the" and draw a flower. He complained that I had given his sister lots of stuff and he got nothing. I pointed to the bag of sweets in his hand and he was silenced.

They all took the dog for a walk in the park and pronounced her behaviour "very good". Even though middle boy had to run back home for an extra bag when she decided to do a substantial poo.

Before they left, they admired my mother's watercolour on our bedroom wall, saying it reminded them of Quentin Blake. They asked who the artist was, and when I told them, raised eyebrows and open mouths. And perhaps questioning their own judgement. One of life's special little moments. I salute you, Mamma.

Prof R has suffered no ill effects from all the stimulation. I wish they would come down more often.

April 20 — Saturday. Another beautiful pre-summer, summer day. Prof R is bright and early onto the toilet before 9 am. Clearly yesterday was medicine that has lasted.

Having abandoned wheat a week ago, I now find myself scoffing two hot cross buns left behind by the little family. Two of the four I had burnt in the toaster before choosing to grill the survivors. An early lunch I tell myself. But I will be curious to see what happens to the aches and pains. They have already improved avoiding gluten.

—

A friend has sent me a news item about 'recomposing' – the disposal of a body by accelerated natural decay. Legislation is being passed in the States to allow it. I wonder if burying people in a shroud in approved places is just as green. Quicker for one thing. Cheaper too. Although the thought of any sort of underground option makes me shudder. Was it the Victorians who had a coffin option with a glass window and a breathing tube ... just in case?

—

With Prof R's blessing and cooperation, I managed a bath and a hair wash before dinner.

April 21 — Last night I nearly lost him on the floor. He seemed to lose his legs on our way back from the toilet. We had almost made it. But I held him up and did my loud voice "straight legs darling" until we could collapse safely onto the bed.

My heart rate takes flight, but he never seems particularly fazed by these episodes. I guess if you don't have to ring for the ambulance you don't fret about it too much.

It was a restless night again, with his legs getting active for a while in the small hours. Before I went to bed, I had managed to put him in his pull-ups where he lay. He was too sleepy to get up. It's a technique I need to master. But we managed. When he can't help by lifting his hips it will get interesting. I must ask Netty for a tutorial.

My sister is still sending me snappy cross replies to any emails. I really must leave her alone for a while. But I had really wanted to tell her that Mamma's painting was a hit. It's hard to resist all normal communication.

—

Men are unfortunate in old age when it comes to grooming. Hair sprouts everywhere, just when and where they don't need it. This morning I used a tiny pair of Swiss Army knife scissors to trim inside Prof R's nostrils. My chimpanzee cousins would be proud of me. I believe I may have been born to groom.

Prof R's eaten enough today to make me suspect worms. If he doesn't gain weight, it will be a metabolic issue rather than nutritional. He had three desserts at lunch, and was hungry again an hour and a half later. Dinner was fish pie and ice cream (again).

I'm wondering if eating well later in the day contributes to restlessness. Again, I am resorting to delivering him the safety lecture. He tries to get out of the rail, forgetting that it is there for his own safety. He wants to walk around, forgetting that sometimes his legs fail him and at other times they are unreliable at best. We talk and talk, and I feel like a rat on a wheel, saying the same things over and over.

It isn't just the dementia, it's a lapse in awareness of the reality of his physical limitations. But the dementia does stop him remembering that he alone is ultimately responsible for his own safety. We can have rails and alarms and hand bells, but if he is feeling determined to do his own thing, he will be at risk.

That fact that all this occurs in the evening doesn't help with fatigue or patience for either of us. Often, after a pep talk, he will vow to stay put until I come to bed and then discover that suddenly he needs the loo. And I will hear him move again just as I have resettled myself on the couch with the dog. He wonders how I can do that – know he is moving when the alarm has not gone off. Wooden floors and a zimmer being kicked is the simple answer.

April 22 — Darren comes today to shadow Netty.

Another early morning for me, woken by dreams and a headache. At

5 am. The sort of headache that goes once you get up and move around. But I helped it along with two ibuprofen and two cups of tea.

Every morning now the first pill ritual is the same; some time after 7 am. Prof R doesn't fully wake, but he can hear me and follows my instructions more or less. Well enough for me to be fairly sure the pills have been swallowed. Then I tell him to relax, stay where he is and go back to sleep.

My dream was, for once, about my true age. And attempts to get a job. Being rejected at interview due to my age. Usually, age does not come into my dreams. I am always of some indeterminate, yet mature, era. Probably late 40s. Clearly advancing age is beginning to worry me. And lack of purpose.

—

My niece has been in touch asking for some of my mother's paintings. It's an excellent idea and I have begun photographing and emailing them to her. So she can choose which ones she would like me to send.

There seems to be a time and place for reawakening interest in things from the past. I have carried those paintings for a very long time – at least 30 years. I've hung the framed ones on my walls but never really thought too much about the others, other than to treasure their existence. Now, I see afresh the immense charm and value in them. I reappraise them with new eyes. And they remind me of childhood I suspect. I begin to long for home just a little.

—

Netty and I are officially geniuses when it comes to problem solving. Two birds killed two birds with one stone today when we managed to nut out a solution to making space for the zimmer to park. The bookcase on his side of the bed had to go – again.

We went into Prof R's office with a tape measure and decided his desk, although enormous, could be turned sideways in the narrow room. Other

paraphernalia could go under the desk and the bookcase would fit in the
available wall space, while still allowing the drawers on the desk to open.

The second 'bird' we killed was where to put the collection of medical
kit Prof R needs, which I had put on the bookcase. The answer was to
move the small bookcase on top of Prof R's office desk to the top of the
chest of drawers by our bed.

Netty left at 4.30 pm, but added instructions that I was not to move
the furniture by myself. By 5.30 pm I had moved his desk and by 6.30 pm,
after Prof R had been fed, the little bookcase was on top of the chest of
drawers and fully loaded.

There I had to stop, because Prof R had gone to sleep. But not before
he had hobbled to look at his half-reconstructed office. Very pleased.
Moving the large bookcase can wait till tomorrow. I'm on fire with this
stuff. It's so satisfying.

Darren, meanwhile, came mid-afternoon and impressed me as much
as he needed to. Mature, intelligent, a business background, clearly
needing a new career in his 50s and very suited to this one. I'm looking
forward to good reports from Prof R.

April 23 — Across the road to the hardware store at 7.30 am to get batteries
for the bed alarm pager. I never tire of appreciating how marvellous it is to
have such a resource so close. And it is as safe as it will ever be to leave
Prof R for the 10 minutes I am away.

By mid-morning I had finished the room redesign and we are both
pleased with the result in the bedroom. If it were not for Netty's
input of ideas, I wouldn't have attempted the ambitious move of
Prof R's desk. The result is an entirely new room – more spacious,
less cluttered, altogether finally finished after looking like a 'work in
progress' for two years.

But there is no whippet in the house today, so Prof R has not been able to visit his completed office. I'm seriously worried about his mobility, namely the gradual loss of it, and have ordered a narrower zimmer which should be much more manoeuvrable outside the bedroom as well as in. Today, I have done a training session with him, trying to change his preferred technique of pushing the zimmer out in front rather than letting it take his weight. This has been an ongoing issue with the zimmer ever since it arrived. I'm hopeful the new one will be less cumbersome for him to use.

It's not easy for him to fully understand or retain what I am telling him. Spatial recognition issues seem to be affected very much by his type of dementia. And we are only guessing which type that is. So he will acknowledge what I am saying and then carry on moving his own way. It's hugely frustrating to feel unable to help him. And what will happen when his legs no longer hold him at all? Some days that moment seems a lot closer.

Eventually, late in the afternoon before dinner, his legs were good enough to make the journey. He was thrilled. But as Netty says, he has started "plaiting his feet". It's a recipe for disaster.

April 24 — Wednesday. A disrupted evening and night. More fruitless trips from downstairs because he seems simply restless. He's not sure why. More pep talks about the rail and its importance. Like so many things in life, it just has to be accepted.

At about 8.30pm I asked if he was still hungry and he pronounced he wasn't, but he hadn't had his dinner yet. (Note to self: perhaps CCTV isn't such a bad idea).

In the night, the problem was mucus, which has been reasonably dormant lately. And then his legs out and pressing against the rail. The blessed rail. Without which we could not function. He may not love it, but I do.

I have bought Dickens *The Uncommercial Traveller* in the hope it is one book he may like to be read from. (*Six months later I found an old edition hiding on his over-stocked bookshelf*)

Meantime, in the realms of the unimportant but interesting, I'm getting fatter. Another kilo added in the last month. My relationship with food continues to puzzle me. I'm aware of wanting to eat. I assume it's hunger, but perhaps it's not. Fatigue? Grabbing healthy food on the go, but clearly too much of it. I've gone off eggs for lunch. And our dinners are also healthy with only vegetable carbs or rice noodles. Blitzed for Prof R. And he gets the cream and honey, not me. I'm eating gluten free bread now too, to help with the aches and pains. So it's not about the 'what' it's about the amount.

—

Prof R has been very sleepy this afternoon. He was more alert this morning before Netty came. She texted me when she couldn't wake him to give him his pills, but I was in Pilates class and my phone was muted, so she soldiered on, as I would have done, and she finally managed it.

The incident reminded me of one of Prof R's favourite anecdotes. He had his camera stolen once when he was in Rome. Young and naïve, he approached a traffic policeman on point duty and reported the theft. "What you want I should do about it?" was the reply. It still makes me laugh.

He's very sleepy at 6pm. I managed to get him to take another super shake because he has only had breakfast. And after that, he practically choked on a gallon of mucus which I caught for him as it left his mouth. It really is no surprise he feels he is not hungry when he is carrying that in his throat.

Later he was able to eat chicken and veggies, mulched to a pulp of course, and later still, cake and ice cream. So the day ended with me being pretty satisfied with his intake. That observation makes him sound like a much loved vintage machine. Or a prize steer.

But I feel overall he is much less steady on his feet now.

April 25 (ANZAC Day) — Mr Parky caught me out this morning, sleeping deeply until late, except for tea and pills and a super shake. His pull-ups couldn't cope. So a bed change, including electric blanket, was the surprise result. His fleece, which I thought would contain leakage, did not. Shorn fleece on a synthetic backing, good enough and cheap enough for hospitals, but not good enough.

While he was sleeping and leaking, I had reorganised my office, moving my desk to the wall near the door. It isn't really an improvement, nowhere near the thrill of Prof R's office transformation, but it did force me to organise and clear out. And like Prof R's office, the room looks more spacious. Fiddling while Rome is burning.

When Prof R did wake, he caught up on muesli, lunch and two desserts. As long as he does that, I don't worry. Especially when he has hoovered up a super shake. He loves them. They come in three flavours – vanilla, strawberry and banana. It takes all my willpower not to sample them myself. The 300 calorie count, which suddenly looks enormous, helps.

I took him on a tour of the first floor again, to show him my redesigned office. Then he walked to his own office. But his legs are very weak. He used the walking stick, but not very well. I shadow him but try not to grab. I can be guilty of helping too much.

After all that, he didn't interrupt my meal tonight. I had to wake him at 7 pm for his pills. But it was my fault for giving him cake and ice cream at 4.30 pm. Once awake, he ate his chicken and veggies and more ice cream. No one can accuse him of not eating.

April 26 — Friday. Not such a great day for the patient. He has been sleepy. I managed to wake him for toileting and super shake by mid-morning, but he didn't wake for Netty for 'breakfast' until 2 pm. And by then his bladder was on the edge of disaster.

I came home from my walk at 3.15 pm to wash my hair and was

confronted by more wet bedding and clothing. Poor Prof R. This time, as it was Netty, he was more aware of the implications and had said to her "What is going to become of me with this illness?" She cheered him with humour, and he has recovered his. But this moment of clarity voices the fears we all have for him.

On the positive side, I managed almost 9000 steps along the Creek track. It knackered me, and my feet and legs are complaining, but given they were complaining before I left, I take no notice of them. I met a woman with her dog who told me she'd had breast cancer for four years and last year it was bladder cancer. I didn't tell her how grateful, in comparison, she made me feel.

Prof R slept all afternoon and missed his lunch altogether. At 6 pm he began with pills and was persuaded to eat. Once begun, all was well. We ate and talked for two hours. About the loss of native birds in Britain over the last 50 years. The RSBP say there has been a decline of 40 million. How they count is anyone's guess, but we will take the figures at face value, mainly because the more we thought of different British birds the more we realised how many we had not seen. Or in Prof R's case, perhaps he hasn't seen for years.

It had made us feel New Zealand birds are so much more interesting, which isn't the case. They are more colourful and more present, and often larger and louder, but that is all.

April 27 — Saturday. My little expectant mother and her baby's father come down for lunch today. Darren will have his first session with Prof R.

He's slept right through the night, which makes me fear for his pull-ups, even while being grateful for the sleep. Much more awake this morning. By 10.30 am he had eaten breakfast and had a banana super shake. I had woken him before 10 am because I wanted to pre-empt disaster in the bed department. And as it happened, I noticed the first small tell-tale damp patches on the back of his pyjama bottoms as he walked to the toilet.

This time, I have put pull-ups on him again so that he can relax while Darren is here. Yesterday, the wet bed with Netty was a trauma for him that I don't want to repeat.

April 28 (Market Town Doggy Day) — Prof R is not at his best today and neither am I. He was very happy with Darren, but it seemed to over-stimulate him. Late afternoon and evening he was restless and awake.

After a lovely rare afternoon with Hope and Simon, I found myself hovering on the edge of tears on our return. Almost immediately after Darren left, I became imprisoned upstairs. Prof R had just woken and was on the toilet. He thought it was about 7.30 pm and wanted his dinner. If Darren did offer him food, Prof R had apparently refused it. I settled him with ice cream and smoothie and managed another precious hour with the kids before they got the train.

I cannot say in words how it felt to feel my daughter's baby move in her womb. I had been thrilled by the earlier pregnancies and felt very close to and concerned about my dearest daughter-in-law during her births. But nothing prepared me for this new emotion. Except perhaps now I have more reason to feel everything more acutely.

—

Until after midnight, Prof R was wakeful, with lots of problems with mucus that together we eventually succeeded in dealing with. Then again at 3 am he was up for the toilet. Which is a good sign of course.

We are going to be introduced to a third PA tomorrow. Helen is needed because they cannot fill one of the days Netty will be on leave. I'm pleased. The bigger the team supporting us the better. The more likelihood I can get away when the baby is born. It's my major focus at the moment and a nice distraction from our sadder moments here.

—

Later: The helpful Helen has now been asked not to come tomorrow. She had written to tell me she will not be a regular on our team, merely filling a gap. She is largely administrative and only does PA work when there is a shortfall. We don't need yet another short-term person. Darren is enough. It's too exhausting for Prof R.

We're thinking, thinking, thinking, about a solution to this care situation. Talking it out, we eventually returned to Hope's idea of a type of au pair. An idea I had never really taken up. Then I began thinking of a trained companion. And then I thought of Tina.

What would it take for her to leave her care home job? If she needed 21+ hours a week we could take her on for the long haul. If she was happy with £13 an hour. Much more than the £10 she gets in the care home. We couldn't afford those hours with the agency. They are never going to be an affordable long-term solution for us.

I am meeting Tina for coffee on Wednesday. No hint to her yet of what I am plotting. Even if she is not ready to make a move from the care home yet, we may be able to plan for the future. I'm allowing myself a small buzz of possibility.

April 29 — When he is good, he is very, very, good. But when he is bad, he is horrid. And he was horrid all last evening. No doubt overtired. And able to listen to reason but not to follow it. I was afraid he would be reckless, and I wouldn't be able to manage him physically. More and more it reinforces our need for more support.

I woke at 6 am today so it was safe to take a shower. A rare event.

More thinking about a private carer has made me decide to offer the job to Netty first, as a courtesy, and because her approach to care is more educative. That doesn't mean she would be better than Tina, just different, with a different energy (no doubt there are rules around not poaching agency staff) but as it turned out, Netty didn't actually know as much about personal care as I thought she did. Mid-morning, when Prof R was comatose, I decided to change his pull-ups. They had been on long enough. Ripping the sides merrily as she had instructed, I removed them without difficulty. But when it came to putting on the clean ones, I came unstuck. Prof R could not roll onto to his sides for me or raise his hips. After struggling for some time, I covered the critical parts of his 'underlings' with the new pull-ups as best I could, left his trousers off, and let him return to sleep.

When I saw Netty, and asked for a tutorial, she said "Actually, I've never had to do that". So not hands-on end of life care experience as I had been led to believe. And not encouraging. Any thoughts of hiring her full time were dampened, although I did ask if she would be interested, and fortunately she admitted she liked the freedom of her current contract.

Helen, who I had cancelled, came with Netty anyway. She had not read my email about not bothering. But that was of course, no bad thing, as at least she has seen the environment and been shown how Prof R operates.

—

The new zimmer frame arrived and is indeed ultra-slim. But the box wasn't, and the poor delivery man had to wait while I cleared the hallway of shoes and bags before it would fit through the gap.

Today I have managed to walk over 9,000 steps and it will be well over 10,000 by the time I have finished. If I can do this twice a week and Pilates once, I will feel I am doing enough for my aerobic fitness not to be classed as 'sedentary'. Such a negative word.

For the second time today, just before 5 pm, I changed his pull-ups again. Not because he was obviously wet, although his clothes were damp with sweat, but because he is comatose again. This time, he managed to roll onto one side for me so I could pull up the back of his pull-ups. Result!!

April 30 — The last day of April. No real sign of summer yet, but definitely the desire to get out and do more, with and without Prof R. Who, by the way, had a quiet night and slept well. Unlike me, who had insomnia, possibly brought on by stuffing two chocolate brownies into my mouth at about 9 pm.

Much more 'normal' this morning, with a super shake and a cup of tea at 8.30 am, although his eyes began to roll up into his head before he has had the last drops. Not awake enough for a trip to the toilet. But by 10.30 am he was just awake enough for me to persuade him that a pee was a good idea, if his legs would work. And they did. So he was dry, clean, medicated and back in bed by 11 am. No appetite for breakfast yet or another super shake.

When we have a morning that works, as this morning has, it seems unnecessary to have another person in the house many more hours than we currently do. But Prof R's wellness is so unpredictable. I can lose sight of my desire to get away when the baby is born, or have a block of care when Sydney son Douglas visits in August. That is when the costs will be prohibitive.

—

I have filled in my postal vote application for the EU elections, although I may spoil my ballot paper in protest. When I talked to Prof R about it, he said he would quite like to vote. Guilty, guilty am I of assuming he would not be engaged with it. So, I will see if I can get a form online for him. He has to sign it, which is his biggest challenge.

This 'normal' day continued through dinner and into the evening. I am able to watch a film – *A Serious Man* – without intermissions. It is so unnerving; I am up checking him while my cup of tea brews. He is sound asleep.

I don't know why I still plan to take him out. He is so frail it will be a miracle if he is awake long enough or has the strength to get into a car or a wheelchair. But I remain hopeful nevertheless. Netty never mentions wanting to attempt it. Another assumption that never eventuated.

May 1 — Wednesday. Another 'normal' day. Tea, super shake, poo etc. In fact, breakfast as well, at about 11 am and teeth cleaned in time for Netty. We do like to impress Netty with our efficiency.

She likes my concoctions for Prof R and says I should do a recipe book for soft foods. No one else seems to have done so yet. Or not that we can find online.

After Pilates I met Tina for lunch, and like a panther, I crept up on her verbally to sound her out for a private job. How was work? Did she prefer the care home to private care? What would her ideal job be? Number of hours? And then she said she had received an offer of work from another couple – not many hours to begin with – so I pounced and said, "But we want you to come and work for us!" And she was thrilled.

So I had read the runes correctly. She will be perfect. So much more knowledge than any agency people, for most of whom it is a second career. She just waits for permission before offering help. In 30 seconds, she had told me how to encourage Prof R to roll on his side when he is comatose. If I put his arm straight down his body on the side I want him to roll to, and then put the other arm across him in the direction of the roll, it will be much easier. Simples! Netty doesn't know that.

Pilates was tough enough to make me feel a bit sick today. That is a good sign. I am working hard and not slacking. But I was glad when we finished.

May 2 — Prof R weighed in at 53.4 kg today. Although you wouldn't notice it, I'm very pleased nevertheless. But he's sleeping a lot. I'm hoping Tina won't be bored.

A huge box arrived today with one month's rations for me. It's called JanePlan and I have ordered it because it means I only have to worry about Prof R's food and will be less tempted to just grab anything for my own. Or worse, I begin to eat the same food I am blending for him, most of which is designed to build him up.

———

Caught a falling poo this morning for the NHS – mine that is. Two more to go. Cancer check. I am so grateful for these poo tests every two years.

———

We had a terrible night of phlegm and coughing and disrupted sleep. It's a mystery why this occurs sometimes and not others.

The other 'unfathomable' is his whippet moments of muscle switch-on. There was another just after 5 pm today when I was elbow-deep cooking chicken for our meal. As soon as the wok was at full heat, the bed alarm sounded. When I reached Prof R, he was just sitting up, so I asked him if he could stay in bed for a few minutes while I dealt with the chicken. Did he need the toilet? No. Could he wait? And he said yes.

But downstairs, I could still hear the bed alarm, so I switched off the gas and went back up. He was sitting on the toilet. No zimmer, no drama, no obvious difficulty in arriving at his destination. But when he returned to bed, it was all wobbles and handholds and weak knees. The autonomic nervous system works best undisturbed.

May 3 — A perfect night. No coughing. No mucus. No reason why this should be. But during the night he does have periods of violent tremors. They don't seem to wake him up, even when his hand is beating on his chest.

But a peaceful night can mean a very wet man. And by 9 am he was. Fortunately, he was also awake, so I could change both him and the bottom bed sheet and under-blanket. The pull-ups can't cope and become a wick to the rest of his clothing.

The bed change has been managed by tackling each side separately, without removing the duvet. This is probably a skill I could have learned during a holiday job at a hotel, or at Girl Guides, but it felt like an achievement.

When Netty is here today I will be shopping for more effective continence products. I suspect I'm a bit behind in my research.

—

I have ordered Prof R another apron, the black one being far too indiscrete when ice cream is spilt on it. I have gone for stripes. The ice cream will show, whatever we do, but one more apron means we can change it daily. We refuse to resort to hospital paper disposables. The real problem lies with the spoon. No spoon can cope with melted ice cream efficiently, and it must be slightly melted, or it is too cold for his mouth.

By 4 pm Prof R was over-tired. And over-stimulated. I don't know how to broach the subject with Netty, because she takes such pride in being proactive with him. By 6 pm, even after a sleep, he said he couldn't remember she had been. His legs are very weak. Where is the man who got to the toilet on his own yesterday when I wasn't watching him?

I asked Netty which day she would like to work when we go down to one agency day. It is hard for her not to feel offended that I have chosen more support hours without using the agency. A little defensively, she pointed out that a care home is much more expensive. And so it is, for 24/7 care. But that level of care is not what we are getting. And if we were, we would have to mortgage the house. And of course, it is not as good as home care.

I'm hoping it won't spoil our relationship with her.

Prof R is too tired for our usual evening chat and is back in bed at 6.30 pm. Perhaps he will be restless instead. I am supposed to go and warm up one of my diet plan meals and I feel unusually without appetite. I know that will pass the minute I smell it.

—

I was putting chickweed cream on a rash on the back of Prof R's head when he said, "That is where I was shot". So I asked when that could have happened and he said, "When I was at the BBC". It was a shotgun, he said, and a spray of bullets. I talked gently to him about the logic of it and where perhaps the memory had come from. Perhaps when he had been strafed in the street on his way home from school by the lone German aircraft. The bullets sprayed the fences. I suggested that might be what he was remembering. And he agreed.

I know that dementia patients often feel they have had a head injury. It is an explanation for how they have lost their memory. I remind Prof R of his fall last summer, when he split his head and it had to be glued. But that wound wasn't on the back of his head where his rash is.

May 4 — Prof R's hands look as though he is wearing them inside out. The veins are generous tributaries on an arid ground. He is so thin. But his hands are beautiful because his fingers are so long.

It's been a very strange day. Prof R has been out of sorts at times – forgetting where we are and why. "Is this a hospital?" etc. and when I said he would remember later and hopefully he would forget that he had forgotten, he laughed. So his head is in two worlds, one of which is very much the present.

And to top things off, I accidentally lopped a slither off the top of his little finger on the left hand. Clipping his fingernails is always fraught with mutual nervousness and for good reason. He has bled enough to make anyone feel guilty. And I am abject, apologising and promising I will never let it happen again. Because the clippers will be retired. At least we know his circulation is excellent.

Sometime later, when I had thought him sleeping, (no alarm again), I found Prof R askew in the bed leaking from a livid bloody plaster. Horrors. But more unfathomable, the bathroom and toilet looked as though someone had been haemorrhaging, and I was puzzled by the bloody finger-mark on Prof R's lower abdomen.

A guess: He must have been leaking from the plaster when he last went to the toilet. And if I was with him on what I thought was his last trip, which I was, why hadn't I seen the blood? And cleaned up the bathroom at the time? And re-bandaged him? The only possible answer is that Prof R had got up and gone to the toilet a second time, without setting off the alarm, and returned to bed without my knowing. This is a mystery that will never be solved. But good ammunition for more guilt.

He's eaten well regardless of his unhappy day. I do my best to comfort him. But it can be hard to make light of the distress, and I don't attempt it. But I did give him a foot bath in Dead Sea salt which may have helped.

His eldest daughter Hannah rang, crying down the phone because she hasn't seen her dad for five months. She wants to come on Monday. I tell her that's fine, but Netty will be here, so I will be out. My heart is not moved. Or only a little. I tell her to relax and breathe. Come when she can.

May 5 — Sunday. At 6 am Prof R and I tried to get him on his feet for the toilet and failed. His legs are just too frail at that hour.

But he was able to get up by 9 am so the bed was saved. He is so tired after our sessions of food and chat I can't imagine that we will succeed in taking him out while he has so little energy. Perhaps the energy of a month or so ago will return. Phases are not all downhill.

I cut his hair again to make it more manageable. Now he looks like an escaped convict. Only thinner. But short hair does suit him.

May 6 (Bank Holiday) — Prof R's bowel drove him from the bed at 9 am this morning. This is good – both for him and the capacity of the pull-up. I am sure it is the magnesium citrate that is making his digestion so much more efficient. But the effort makes him so tired, he crawls back into bed and drinks his tea and super shake through a straw, eyes closed.

Our nights are messy, in that he is restless, and I wake every hour or so. Another cup of tea at 3 am this morning, but it doesn't worry me.

Netty came this afternoon. I have finished proofreading her sister's children's book. It was a nice, if boring, diversion. Fantasy talking animals and magic are not my thing.

Prof R is subdued today. Either depressed or withdrawn into his own world. It's not easy to tell. It means he has eaten less. Only two super shakes, muesli and ice cream so far by 6 pm. It's so much sadder when he is like this.

I watched a documentary with Louis Theroux on Dementia. He was in Phoenix Arizona, an Alzheimer's hot spot. Usually, I find Louis less than sincere, but he did an excellent job of this. It made me realise that Prof R and I are fortunate he was almost 80 before things got really bad. And the type of dementia he has does not cause a ruckus in the neighbourhood.

Prof R did eat his fish pie and dessert in the evening, so all was not lost.

May 7 — Tuesday. The new routine early morning trip to the toilet at around 9 am continues and is so good for Prof R's self-esteem. I'm not sure he notices if the pull-ups are wet or not, and they always are, but he does know the bed is not and neither are his clothes.

But he's still more tired than usual. Breakfast is only half eaten and it's 1 pm. Ice cream has been eaten however. And half a cup of tea afterwards while he almost slept.

Instead of using a shampoo cap on him I gave him a barber shop hot flannel treatment. His hair is so short it is absolutely adequate for washing it. And so much less stressful than the cap. And on the subject of caps, his cradle cap has gone, which is a blessing. Two treatments with the recommended 'anti-everything' livid red shampoo was enough.

—

I'm all domestic as usual. A new top drawer for the fridge freezer has been ordered. (to replace the one I kicked) I totally object to the cost, £50 and £8 delivery charge, but the alternative is not intelligent either.

My 'new' iPhone XR arrived, and it was gratifying to set it up without losing my cool or my sanity. The best test for dementia you could hope for.

Setting up face recognition was like watching myself in a coffin. How unkind can a self-image be? Then I outdid myself by successfully using Google to find out how to clear my old phone for reuse. Hope has decided she would like it.

I'm hungry still after my JanePlan lunch. Their dinners are much more successful.

Prof R finally played catch-up at 4 pm with lunch and dessert, followed by dinner at 6.30 pm. He took me by surprise at 6 pm because I thought he might not be hungry so soon. And I was, as usual, halfway through my own meal. But it's always a relief.

May 8 — Prof R thinks he wants to get up at 8.30 am but he is not with me. Cannot answer questions. So I tuck him back in. I'm still so stiff in the mornings I can hardly move. What am I doing wrong?

Well, the answer to that question is this. Several things. None of them related to stiffness. One of them: I threw away my old sim card instead of putting it in my new phone, and spent half an hour searching through the rubbish sack to find it. I'm good at searching rubbish sacks. So I did find it. Lesson learned (again), as they say, so annoyingly.

But we both had a good afternoon – me with kiwi friends and Prof R with Helen this time. I have relented. But I have cancelled Darren on Friday. Three different carers in one week are probably two too many. And he was exhausted when I got back today.

Later, with him restored, we had a lovely evening chatting and eating, so all is well.

The 'mucus nights' have not recurred lately. It's easy not to notice the good things. They deserve a mention.

May 9 — My sister is back in touch. Normal transmission has resumed, except I wonder if she is losing the plot a little. When I mentioned there is short-mat bowls here, she said "Prof R could be left alone for that length of time". When I said he couldn't, she said "Is he ready for the care home?" I could have said, "But Stella, we never left him alone when you were here last year". But I decided not to. The less I tell her the better.

Another little flurry of anger from Prof R this morning. But they are now rare. I was trying to get him to walk inside the zimmer frame rather than pushing it ahead of him. And he lost his temper and tried to throw it. I had to grab him and propel him unceremoniously onto the bed to prevent a fall. As always, he was apologetic. And no wonder he loses it sometimes.

—

Tina came to discuss our new arrangement, and was nervous, as was I a little. We're not quite sure how this is all going to work. But it will, I'm sure. She wants Monday to Thursday, 10.30 till 4.30 pm, so it's already a compromise for me. I preferred 11 am to 5 pm. And Netty may decide she can't do Friday.

Prof R was interesting. He woke while Tina was here and she fed him while I made us both a coffee, but later, when he rang his bell and was hungry again, she answered his call. And he took one look at her at decided to lie down instead.

Once she had gone, the bell went, and I gave him his lunch. He and I will both have some adjusting to do. Later he took a tour of the first floor with the much more user-friendly zimmer. He sat at his desk and opened every drawer. It was lovely.

But in the night, we were back on mucus alert. It was very bad this time, but eventually we cleared it.

May 10 — Friday. The good thing about GPs being overworked is that they don't have time to interfere. Tina told me about a resident in the care home whose GP tried to stop her Rivastigmine, claiming she couldn't be getting much benefit after being on it for 10 years. Her family intervened, insisting on its continued benefits. And they won.

I have been in the mood today to discuss topics that Prof R appeared to be interested in, even while I thought he would not. The evolution of the female body and pelvis which has led to inefficient childbirth; the philosophical questions of autonomy – Simone de Beauvoir believed this to be the goal of child rearing. Sometimes I just feel I want to talk to someone about all these things and Prof R is the last man standing around here, so he gets it.

I did ask him if he touched on autonomy in his studies of educational psychology, but he thought not. Because it occurs to me it could solve the problem of loneliness and lack of purpose in old age. If we could rediscover it, if we ever had it, or simply discover it if we hadn't. And so many women lose it along the way to the needs of others.

—

Prof R has slept a good part of the day, starting his breakfast at 11 am, following the earlier tea and super shake. Lunch was at 4 pm, then dessert of ice cream, followed by the rest of his breakfast. At 6.15 pm he was ready for dinner. It doesn't matter a jot when he eats as long as he eats.

The pharmacy delivered another two months' supply of the super shakes. We look like a milk factory.

May 11 — Saturday. The day begins as it typically does just now.
7.30ish first pills.

He settles back to sleep.

8.45ish I take him tea and a super shake.

9.30ish we test his legs for the toilet. Today, all was well.

He settles back to sleep.

Breakfast is at 11.30. I am trying repetition of "are you hungry?" until he says "yes". He needs time to connect with his stomach sometimes. And his bladder. Often says "no" to a toilet question until I say, "worth a try". Then he often pees.

But by the time he lies down again I am all talked out. It's tiring when there is comprehension but little response. At least, I know there is often comprehension. Perhaps not always. Or perhaps he is just bored.

Quality of life seems remote today. There is no energy left in him for going downstairs or anywhere else once he has eaten and peed. It's very disheartening. We are supposed to weigh him tomorrow and he says what I fear – that he'd be surprised if he's gained any weight.

May 13 — Going, going…that's how the last two days have felt. Circling the drain. Prof R is leaving me in his mind more noticeably now. It's going to be so much harder when he eventually does.

Eldest daughter Hannah finally came yesterday, and I asked if she noticed much change. She said, "He's very thin" but didn't mention noticing a decline in his mind. Perhaps when they have visited previously, he has had bad days. His birthday last year certainly was. Or perhaps he managed to be a lot more responsive to her when they were alone. She enjoyed her visit she said.

I made the mistake of weighing him again last night, even though I knew it was a risk. He has lost almost a kilogram again. I realise I should be weighing him at the same time and only once a fortnight. I must also ask myself why it matters that he gains weight. The main thing is that he does not lose it.

My niece has asked for half of my mother's painting collection to share with Stella and I'm pleased.

I have bought another mini cactus to replace the latest one to die in our bedroom. And a big cactus for Netty because it will be her birthday on Wednesday.

Prof R ate well for her, so perhaps I should not be too downhearted. He's a sprinter. Although he never used to be.

Rather like the dog, who managed to sprint out of the front door yesterday with Hannah when she left for the train station. Instead of using her new ability to return when called, she followed her nose and disappeared. I simply kept calling until eventually she returned at breakneck speed; missing the front door on her first pass before realising her mistake. At which point, instead of telling her off, I rewarded her in the hope she would think it worthwhile to return next time.

May 14 — Our ballot papers for the EU elections have arrived. It will be interesting to see how Prof R chooses to vote. And whether his hand will allow him to sign the paper.

At 10 am today I tried to wake him by washing his face with a hot flannel. He snoozed on. And as his medication wasn't due until 11 am, I left him to sleep. But it will be touch and go whether his pull-ups can out-perform the delay.

It's been a generally sleepy day for him. So much so that he concertinaed breakfast, lunch and dessert into the hour between 3 and 4 pm.

I've been spring cleaning and filling charity bags. When Tina begins work in June, I will begin seriously tackling the garden sheds.

And then, without warning, at 4.30 pm Prof R told me he would like to get up – not to eat, just to get up and do something. So, I took him downstairs and out into the garden.

These adrenalin moments have to be seized as there are very few of them. It was sunny and he didn't fall. At each step my heart was in my mouth, but we made it out, and we made it back. A very good effort. Smiling is harder for him now so the photo I took is a bit grim.

The trip out seemed to make him restless for the rest of the day and into the evening, never my favourite time for responding to his hand bell. He cannot help it when he looks at our bed and says to me "Is there room here for you?" He has lost track of where he is in the universe. "Which house are we in?" It passes.

May 16 — Thursday. Yesterday was an 'away afternoon' for me. My feet have finally been done by the podiatrist. They still hurt, because they have been eviscerated, but they will feel better.

Later, Prof R and I tried to watch a YouTube tour of Norwood Cemetery – where his grandparents are buried and which he knows well. But he cannot concentrate for long. The iPad screen is perhaps too small. Netty had also tried but found her screen too difficult for him to view as well.

—

I tried a medication experiment yesterday. Not waking him at 11 am for levodopa and waiting till he woke up nearer 1 pm. It made no difference at all to his cognitive and other functions while Netty was here. So by the end of yesterday, he had taken two fewer levodopa than usual. I noticed that overnight he shook less. The previous night it was tom-toms till dawn.

Netty was very pleased with the amount of food he ate on her watch. He also had a good dinner. So why does none of it stick?

I semi-woke him as usual this morning at about 7.15 am because I still want the day to begin with the opportunity to have the necessary functioning processes in place. But less is definitely more, as everyone tells you, when the illness becomes advanced. There is no guidebook.

In the end, at 11 am I chickened out and woke him for levodopa and a cup of tea. But he had drifted back to sleep before I could give him one of his shakes.

Mysteriously, he had no tremor at all later when I gave him his breakfast and lunch at 1.30 pm. At 2 pm, after only having breakfast, he wanted to get back into bed, so I bribed him with the promise of a coffee. It worked, and he had coffee followed by lunch without even noticing.

But when it came to filling out his ballot paper for the election, he accidentally spoilt it by beginning to write his birth date into the signature box. I had thought we had two copies of the paper, so I raced to get his second one, but there was no second one. It was instead a letter correcting the instructions that had been sent out with the first one. So Prof R has not cast his vote. I mind more than he does.

Dinner was at 6 pm and by 7 pm he was telling me he hadn't eaten. But he did remember I had changed the bed linen at 5 pm. Very odd. I brought him a second helping, and he began it and then faded. Conceding perhaps that he had had his dinner after all. I joke as usual that I will leave the dirty dishes by the bed each night so I can prove to him that I have fed him.

It's been another evening of bell ringing. Quasimodo himself could not compete. And at 10 pm his top was soaked with sweat and needed to be changed. Mysterious the cause of these sweats. But he slept well.

May 17 — Friday. Acorn Stairlift's Ethan rang me today to discuss our maintenance account. Which I have chosen not to buy. I explained we only used the lifts infrequently. Clearly totally bemused by his client's needs, he asked, in his 'good news' voice, if Prof R was no longer reliant on the lift? I began to laugh inappropriately. He remained perplexed even after I explained why I was laughing, because he had no sense of humour and a boring job. I told him to put the details of whatever scheme he was trying to sell me in the post.

One interesting thing he did ask, was would we want the lifts removed? I had no idea they offered that service, and no doubt there would be minimal remuneration, but I suggested gently that the offer was premature, given by then he had been told Prof R was largely bedridden, not dead.

—

Netty couldn't get him to eat any more successfully than I could today. By evening, he had only had muesli and drinks. The longer it went on it seemed the less aware he was of any feelings of hunger. It called for desperate measures, so I began a serious charm offensive on the food front. Two spoonful's of something chocolate first, and then the suggestion of something savoury. Yes, perhaps he would. And I heated up both lunch and dinner so he could choose.

He ate the chicken and avocado lunch but very little dessert and that was as far as he could go.

The irony does not escape me. Me, exhausted from lack of food thanks to the cruelty of JanePlan, and he, also exhausted, partly from lack of food. But not realising it.

Today may well qualify as one of his worst eating days ever. And his responses become fewer. Very little is initiated by him except a refusal to eat. Or a race to the toilet. He's doing well in that department during the day. And the pull-ups cope overnight.

May 18 — Saturday. We began little better than yesterday, as he woke for the toilet and a body wash mid-morning. But he only ate half of his muesli, if that, at lunchtime.

Later he managed lunch and at 7 pm dinner. And then he decided to wake up. I am not a fan of the active evening, even though it's great he wants to do a tour of the first floor at any time. I have to work hard to hide my lack of enthusiasm. And just hope he doesn't notice.

And after the walk, he asked about when he could expect food. This is the second time he has forgotten that he's already had dinner. Although I had joked I would leave the dirty dishes by the bed, of course I hadn't. No evidence, so I asked him if he was hungry and he wasn't. Enough evidence??

10.30 pm, a try for a pee and 11 pm another try, this time successful.

May 19 — A new day and a good start. Tea, super shake and off to the toilet by 9.30 am. This time his bowels were so efficient I reminded him of his years of constipation and how much better it is now. It's unscientific to give all credit to the citrate magnesium but it is tempting.

My eldest son Alex just asked if I would like a Facetime. It's his birthday, but I'm mid-way to taking a nappy-laden bag downstairs so I've delayed the pleasure till I have a coffee in my hand.

—

Prof R has barely been here. His life is peeing, pooing and eating and the rest is all sleep. Sometimes he is responsive when amused or engaged by my conversation. As he was this morning when Douglas called from Sydney to talk about coming over in August. I was giving Prof R his breakfast as we spoke, and I invited my son to say hello. All Prof R could say, when asked by Douglas how he was, was "exhausted". It says it all.

I cannot believe how awful it has become for him. The only blessing is he is losing his awareness of this. There is no curiosity. No ability to initiate a topic. When asked what he feels like having – drink, ice cream etc – he resorts to 'What is on offer?'. "All the usual suspects" is the tempting reply, but I go through the list.

We've had no excess energy tonight – no request for a second dinner. Just a toilet trip at 9 pm when I offered him a super shake. He cannot lie down soon enough.

May 20 — Prof R's face begins to look like the chiselled bow of a ship. Very sharp and narrow. Today he managed to stay awake and eat breakfast, lunch and ice cream for Netty. Perhaps I will weigh him after all. The dietitian is due again tomorrow.

He did do something rather interesting in the morning. While getting up to go to the toilet. I helped him sit up in bed with his legs over the side and then his upper body swung like a pendulum from the vertical across to the side, where he buried his face in the bedclothes. It wasn't meant to be a joke, but it did look like his intention. Presumably just the lack of energy to sit upright and a head too heavy for his muscles.

—

There is always a little surprise in store each day. Tonight, after a really good meal and dessert, Prof R felt like one of his super shakes. I had chosen a different straw, but there was no warning of a problem as Prof R soldiered on. That was until the shake began to come out instead of going in. Suddenly, explosively, his mouth fountained forth. His tightly closed lips finally failed to contain a mouthful that he couldn't swallow. And of course, he was unable to tell me. We concluded the straw was too big and it delivered too much.

Well, that was our initial conclusion. But after he had cleaned his teeth and was spitting into his basin a quagmire of mucus began to erupt from his mouth. Like ectoplasm in a horror movie. I was rolling it out onto tissues as fast as I could. No wonder his swallowing had been hindered. Mystery solved.

On a higher note, we weighed him and he is 53 kg, which is not high by anyone's standards but is relatively high compared to lowest point. "Holding his own" will be the verdict of the dietitian, I hope.

May 21 — Tuesday. The dietitian arrived between two poos. And Prof R was awake. We both enjoy these visits because never has there been a health visitor we didn't like or feel supported by. She was no exception.

We learnt a lot. Such as that the prescription for Prof R's super food should have contained three daily booster 'shots' as well, and never has. But given they are pure fat, and can slow bowel motions, I think we have literally dodged a bullet. Wei Wei will request an extra super shake a day instead.

We also learnt that the Speech Therapy people should have talked to us about swallowing. The last dietitian had referred us, without mentioning swallowing, and when the therapist called, she talked only about speech and language, not swallowing, so we had sent her packing, in a very nice way of course. And she took Prof R off her list.

So now I have to ask for a re-referral to talk about swallowing. The dietitian was concerned about the mucus, in that it indicates he isn't able to swallow it, and therefore food could go "the wrong way". A euphemism for it could go into his lungs and give him an infection. Which we are aware of already with the food, and are doing our best to avoid. But the mucus – thick enough to lay bricks with, could also be a danger. It had never gone that far. He coughs before that can happen.

Annoyingly, she insisted on weighing Prof R again herself, so of course her scales showed him weighing a kg less than he did last night. Which translates to an overall weight increase in the last two months of only around half a kg. Why do we feel like we've failed our A Levels?

When she left, after visiting the toilet, I discovered she had left both seats up. Fear of infection? Or just interesting?

—

Doris and Brian came bearing chocolate cake. Prof R scarcely knew they were there, he was so tired from his morning. He didn't eat and returned to bed. They helped me repot a tree instead. At first, they couldn't be bothered, and said they would do it "another time", so I had to dig my toes in. It was too heavy for one person and "another time" seldom comes.

May 22nd — Wednesday. Prof R was exhausted after the two visitations and let me know this by ringing his handbell every 20 minutes all evening. Fortunately, he didn't have the energy for a tour.

A very disrupted night followed, with Prof R's right-hand tremor reaching such a velocity that it became a blur. I reached over and covered it with mine and said "stop". And it did. Who knows how much control his subconscious mind may have? But these disturbances usually send me downstairs for a cup of tea. I find it hard to return to sleep.

Netty found him tired too but otherwise as usual. He only ate breakfast and ice cream with her. When I returned, he slept and didn't eat his lunch until after 6 pm. And more ice cream. He was struggling with taste and texture and generally feeling fussy. Wanted to lie down, and then said he was hungry once settled. I'm wondering if his sense of appetite is becoming harder for him to detect. Once back up again and seated and gowned, he was presented with his last course of the day, posh sausage and mash (which means cream and honey). He 'sent it back to the kitchen'.

In the kitchen, the chef added this and that in her laboratory and re-re-presented it. It tasted brilliant. I had to restrain my tasting role. But he fiddled. So I played my last card – a surprise for him – raspberries, He was keen to try those, but after apparently successfully eating two of them, suggested he save the rest for the morning.

The evidence for his reticence became clear (yet again) when he expectorated a mutilated raspberry from his throat while visiting the toilet later. Back to the laboratory with the raspberries. And I need to chase up the swallowing therapy.

Eating time at Prof R's zoo didn't end until after 9 pm, and later, for light relief and relaxation, I watched a new documentary on Margaret Thatcher.

May 23 — Oh the irony, that the conversationalist, me, cannot get a response.

Today has been an exhausting round of questions from me and minimal responses from Prof R. But he can speak when pressed, and seems sometimes unaware that he is not responding. So, would he like the cup of tea or a super shake? Answer: "yes". When will I learn? For him, perhaps it's like living inside a glass box. If only we knew.

But he has eaten breakfast, or most of it, and most of lunch and some chocolate dessert – all at near normal times. It's going to be a challenge though to get three of the super shakes into him each day.

In the end, Prof R did eat his salmon and mash but no desert. His appetite is declining. Everything is in decline. Conversation, energy, engagement. It gets sadder every day. The bell goes more often now. He mainly just wants to know where I am. When Tina comes, he will have more company.

She and I have worked out our business agreement and she has decided to set herself up properly as self-employed. It's a much better idea than cash under or over the table. She needs to keep herself in the National Insurance loop or her pension will suffer.

May 24 — Friday. Both Prof R and I find it harder to be aware of what day it is. I have commitments to keep track of, but he doesn't. It sparked a discussion – would we even need to know what day it was if we were totally self-sufficient with no interaction with organised society? Perhaps the supply boat visit could be measured in sunsets rather than dates. It would be important not to run out of favourite foods before the next boat.

He's very tired today; but taking his pills on time and managing the toilet and a super shake.

I trimmed his beard yesterday while he was lying down. So much easier, and a good result. I can hear his ring hand tapping on the bed rail as I write. Not long now before the bell sounds.

At lunchtime – before Netty came – the muesli was eaten. And with Netty he ate lunch and dessert. So, we may be back on track. But later, I made the mistake of giving him a super shake at 5 pm and it spoilt his appetite for dinner.

May 25 — Prof R is perplexed by his illness. He says, "I don't know what's going on" when I say, "Is there is anything you would like to ask me"? He gazes at the ceiling with eyes that appear to see something, but may not.

—

The dog finally looks like a proper Scottie dog. All those 'skinned rabbit' grooms had made me forget what she was supposed to look like. The new look suits her. But she bit the hand that groomed her – a mobile grooming van and a tough opponent – so she is an unwelcome return client, and we will need to return to our old groomer.

She came upstairs to show off her new cut. Prof R's responses are muted but I think he enjoyed seeing her. She cannot be placed on his lap now because he cannot bear the weight.

When I tried to tell him that I have finally succumbed to having a Smart Meter installed, I'm not sure he remembered what they are, or really understood what I was talking about. They have had such bad press I have been avoiding this moment. I explained that it was a requirement for the new best tariff. But it's not clear now what hits and what misses. His words are failing him. He told me that much.

He did understand when I talked about RHS Chelsea but is not really interested in the detail. Or in watching it on the iPlayer. Awake times with him are all about trying to stimulate his interest in something – anything. Even the most delicious food is eaten now without any obvious enjoyment. And most amazing – he will sometimes say no to chocolate. And yet he can understand often when I joke about something, and will smile. Or perhaps he simply understands my intention.

In the realm of boring but important, we have test-driven every pull-up on the market and the last one I bought – reluctantly – from Boots turns out to be by far the best fit. Ironical, because Boots must be almost my least favourite brand. I try to boycott chains which force you to buy their products by under-stocking those of their competitors.

—

We've now got a new problem. Prof R summons me with the bell and doesn't sit up to activate the bed alarm. I explain it's harder for me to hear the handbell, and then later ask him if he knows how the bed alarm works and he says "no". That's when I say, "never mind".

It means I cannot go outside at all if he cannot sit up to set off the alarm. These little failures can be more than frustrating, they make life almost impossible.

May 27 — Monday. A lovely day that nearly ended in disaster.

My little family came for lunch outdoors, and later Netty came for her usual three hours while we went to the playground and had tea and cake. Before we went, I put the downstairs pager on vibrate so it wouldn't ring while Netty had Prof R out of bed upstairs.

Later, after she had gone, and I had answered his hand bell several times to tell him we were here and just nearby, my daughter-in-law Ophelia noticed the pager – still on vibrate and flashing. I ran upstairs, expecting to see him already in the ensuite toilet. Instead, I met him in the main bathroom at the top of the stairs, just pulling up his pants after using the toilet. There was no zimmer, no toilet frame, no riser seat, nothing for him to hold onto, but he was standing. He had needed to pass a motion. He had cleaned himself.

I said "Oh hello, so there you are! That's rather clever." And then quietly and slowly returned him to the bedroom with my hand as a crutch and my heart in my mouth. He was plaiting his feet and sliding on the wooden floor. When he was safely back in bed, I apologised for not hearing the alarm and asked him if that had been a good experience, to independently go to the toilet successfully. He said, "Not really, that floor was very slippery".

I'm still practising breathing out. There is never a time when it is safe to be off duty, unless someone else is *on* duty. We escaped this time. But I need to remember that when we have visitors, and I am distracted, it is a dangerous time.

May 28 — Awoke this morning to deafening silence. Our door-slamming neighbours are away for half term. Shortly thereafter, men arrived to dig up the pavement beneath our bedroom window. I suspect it might be a leaky water pipe because we lost our water for a short time last night. They have been drilling, banging, wheeling squeaky wheelbarrows and generally keeping Prof R half awake, when he'd prefer to be asleep.

Douglas, for whom plane tickets had been bought for late July and early August, will now need his tickets changed. Neither I nor his father had realised his London siblings will be away for precisely those dates – in Thailand. I'm sad it has to be postponed. Who knows how Prof R will be by then?

—

Alex is full of enthusiasm for my forthcoming 70th birthday. He wants to make plans NOW and while I am touched by his caring thought, there is nothing I want to do. The suggested lunch at *Bibendum* would be hollow. I've only been there with Prof R. It's where me met. It would be too sad.

After the workmen had left, we had a companionable dinner and another trip down memory lane. Memories that he can still access with my help. Travels we have done. Funny disasters. I avoid the unfunny ones. His mind is clearer this week.

May 29 — Wednesday. Prof R is back to eating everything I can put in front of him. I am easily pleased.

Netty found him bright this afternoon and with more clarity than we've both seen in the last few weeks. She asked him for his assessment of how he is, and he said, "pretty normal". Miraculous. Being brighter and more awake has its downsides. I have to be more alert for the whippet. There was one escape bid today, but I was able to 'cross his bows' before disaster.

While Netty was here, I walked across the water meadows to the little inlet where all the small boats hide. It was the best walk I have had in months. No sore feet or legs. My Allbirds shoes causing me no problems. And I hit the magic figure of 10,000 steps.

—

My awful-but-necessary diet plan finishes on Friday, but I still have some pre-packaged meals to eat. They are almost indigestible at times, but by the time I get to them I hardly notice, I'm so hungry. The total weight loss will be disappointing, but it is a beginning.

Douglas and his father have managed to get his tickets changed to mid-August. Early enough to hopefully beat the baby's arrival so he can spend time with Hope. I'm thrilled it won't be October. What chance Prof R would be too ill to know he is here? And Prof R is very fond of my boy and will be keen to see him again. On his last visit, two years ago, we both stood in the kitchen and cried after his departure.

May 30 — Yesterday was yesterday. Today is a different story. Prof R has been tired. Too tired to eat more than a milkshake and two or three spoonful's of muesli until 2 pm, when he said he'd prefer his savoury lunch. Even then, he couldn't eat his chocolate dessert.

While he has slept, I've been sorting through another box of mine. Treasures, all of them, and very enjoyable to revisit. Even a diary from

1963 that I managed to keep until the school year kicked in, when I petered out. "Lacks discipline".

Dinner was redemption of sorts. He ate, but with little apparent enjoyment and equally small conversation. These are the times I become most discouraged and depleted. Neither of us appears to be making the day worthwhile.

The plumber did finally come to look at the tarpaulin he left on the shed roof in January. He will quote for a repair, but with him, any time he actually gets around to doing the job will be a miracle. The upside is, when he does finally show up, he is a good conversationalist. And they, like plumbers, are in short supply.

—

I watched the first part of a Panorama documentary on the crisis in social care. I'm hoping to learn something. And I did. Where the boundary likes for responsibility between the council and the NHS. Councils have to fight to cross that barrier.

May 31 — Friday. The contents of the rivastigmine pill I gave Prof R this morning were stuck to his forehead when I brought him a coffee at 9.30 am. The casing was on the pillow. If I have ever questioned the value of that drug I certainly don't today. He was unable to follow instructions to suck on the straw to get his coffee. A second attempt to give him his pill was successful.

Without these little surprises, Groundhog Day would be on a loop. With variations, but all on the same theme. What did we do to describe endless repetition before that film? The variation was that Prof R is content. That is where we are winning the battle for his wellbeing. Usually, I can meet his needs. His physical ones at least.

I have reached the halfway point in my weight loss. What a tedious month it has been, but I will soldier on. A 4 kg loss is not to be sniffed at.

But I will try to do without the help of JanePlan.

It's a Netty day today, so I have a list of things I must do. Prescriptions, pull-ups, double cream and supplements. And perhaps some more tempting desserts for the patient.

—

The pharmacy delivery service becomes more comical. Even though I am grateful. This morning, half of Prof R's medications arrived. And I know why only half. Because only half had been ordered – the first half – so they then put in an order for this, the second half. But have not delivered the first half. I hope you are keeping up. Fortunately, I plan to visit the pharmacy today in any case.

Something that intrigues me is the size of Prof R's pupils. They are almost always pinpricks. I have compared them to mine in the same light and mine are larger. If he was losing the ability to process light you would expect them to enlarge. Some research is required.

The evening was so quiet I could watch Russell Davies *Years and Years* – the third episode – without interruption. I think it may be excellent, but the jury is still out. Comparing it to *Endeavour* – which is just a crime series in essence – it doesn't seem as clever or as crisply produced.

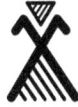

Summer 2019

JUNE 1 — Saturday. Prof R is very tired again today. But seems content. Every time he wakes, the poor man has food funnelled into him until he cries halt. But he cries halt before he's really done justice to it.

The weather is beautiful. The sash window is open, and the curtain is billowing gently in the breeze, but he is warm enough. And just has a light duvet cover on him or he will overheat.

—

I've been taking photographs of things in the shed that need to go – my bike, the battery mower and there will be others. No one in the family seems to want them. At this stage, I am only putting them on the neighbourhood website. eBay is too public and too much bother.

I'm hungry and trying not to think about it. Possibly I simply crave carbohydrates and fats, but the feeling is the same. And my so-called but undiagnosed arthritis is also attacking my hips. I have read that for every pound of weight I lose the joints will have four pounds less pressure on them. Incentive enough.

My heart health age, when I checked it at NHS online, is 70. I don't think I can argue with that. Although 69 would have been nice. This preoccupation is all Netty's doing. She has urged me to ask for the health check everyone between 55 and 74 should get. She's just had hers. The

NHS apparently send out letters every five years so they will probably hope I reach 74 before my name comes up.

Meanwhile, I have done a double take on discovering my blood pressure is only 113/65. This is now considered normal apparently, and clearly due to the low salt diet. I once, about 20 years ago, had my application for a gym membership refused because my systolic pressure was 110. They didn't want people passing out on the equipment. Now I would probably get a pat on the back. Though I may be passing out by the time I have lost the next 4 kg.

Now I must go and put almond oil on the dog's flaking tummy. Always this happens when she has been groomed and washed with the wrong shampoo.

A child outside is imitating the call of a collared dove. This is why I like living in an urban environment.

—

By about 5 pm some days I have run out of steam, mentally if not physically. It depends how many times the hand bell has been rung, or the bed alarm activated, when I am trying to achieve something.

Today it was mowing the lawn and clipping the edges, which I told Prof R I was going to do after he had half-eaten the latest meal. When I completed the task, returned to the kitchen and began making his next meal, the bell tolled again. And this time it jangled. That is when I know my rope has begun to stretch.

This is not fatigue as we might remember it from our corporate working days. This is the fatigue of the firefighter on duty in the Watch House. Waiting for the alarm. Unable to lower the alert level. I'm hoping my complaining body has settled down by tomorrow.

Later, I found myself talking to him about courage. Not exactly the "brave little soldier speech" but along those lines. I told him I knew he wanted us to do better. I need him to help me as much as he can, through the times when he feels desperate, or it will be too hard for us to manage. He agreed. He is used to being rescued and this time I can't.

June 2 — How I dread waking Prof R each morning to give him his pills. He is so blissfully asleep at that time, but by 7.45 am it has to be done or he will not be on deck later.

—

I'm feeling a bit down about my sister as time passes and I don't hear from her. It seems that now she and my niece have what they want – the parental paintings – they no longer need to be onside with me. Just then, instead of writing 'onside', I almost wrote that they no longer feel the need to 'groom' me. And that is the truth of how it feels.

It is easy to become insular and inward looking in the situation we are in here. Everyone else has more things to think about, other than the daily round of health issues facing us here. Being aware of that, and remembering that, will help give me perspective.

I have had *The Moon and I* from the Mikado in my ear as a worm. It drove me to get up in the night and find a recording of it on Google. Purely by chance, the recording was from 1967. I know where my worm has come from, but 1960s school productions are a long reach back, and a strange thing to invoke at this time. It is a beautiful song, but it made me sad, which is also an unnecessary thing.

—

Prof R has had another of his disrupted evenings. I tried making sure he ate as much as possible, because he becomes picky with his food at night. But it hasn't helped. He has just said he wants to go home. Quite often said, but not really explained. I think he means he wants to be where I am. So, I explain as usual.

June 4 — Tuesday. Someone else in the neighbourhood definitely has a hand bell. Someone other than Archie next door, because I just raced upstairs to answer it and Archie is at school.

Yesterday was Tina's first day on the job. We're both relaxed about the operating strategy, and she is professional and keeps brief notes.

I found the freedom rather heady, and immediately put half a dozen items from the shed for sale or free on our local neighbourhood website. I did this without first checking that the electrical garden tools actually work. And then someone on the site asked me. Task for today.

I also walked. 10,000 steps and in some new streets tucked away behind the Quay with little Kentish-style newbuilds in them. Very charming. Then, to celebrate the fact that I have completed a month of sugar denial, I had a Portuguese tart. But only after first checking how many calories it would cost me. Only 180. So maybe I'd eat the whole thing rather than half? It seemed like a price worth paying.

—

At last, an email from my sister today. Business as usual and no mention of our mother's paintings or whether she was pleased to get them. I refuse to 'hit the ball back' by asking her. What is it about no-go areas in families? Crazy and unnatural behaviour. An over-sentimentality about things we both treasure; making a great big production of it. Silence from my sister is a sign of a big production for her.

—

It's raining today and what a difference it makes to my schedule. Basically, it's too wet to do much in the shed. I have tried. I don't particularly want to go out. Hopefully it will stop. I don't like walking in the rain.

Tina is sitting in the little kids' sitting room with nothing to do. I feel I need to look busy even if I just want to watch *Politics Live*. This is going to take some getting used to. She offers to do anything I want her to do. Food prep etc. I don't want her to, partly because she needs to be on duty if Prof R's alarm or hand bell go – as has just occurred. Tina has gone in to him. That's all I want her for. If she gets bored, I may lose her. But I prefer to run my own house at the moment. As things progress with Prof R her tasks will intensify, but I will still be alone most of the time.

But what luxury to have her. And I know she would step in and take over if I was run over by the proverbial bus. She lives two blocks away and it is security to know she is at least willing to do this, even if, in the event of such a disaster, she is unable to for some reason.

She has asked me to brief her on food preparation in case of the above emergency or if I am called away to London for Hope's baby. And she has suggested I freeze several meals. I know she is right, but the truth is, there is no fixed food plan. Variety and flexibility is what I aim for. Creativity is needed when his palette is changing and challenging him every day. She is a person who takes pride in her skill as a cook. And while it's important she knows what foods he can eat, in an emergency she will also have to use her initiative. There is always easy-to-prepare food in the fridge — it overflows. The food processor is on the bench. The back-up toddler food and apple puree is in the cupboard. Open the fridge door and take your pick. As long as it has cream and honey added to it, with luck it will taste good.

After Tina had gone, we had our usual evening of eating and bell ringing. But he still ate less than normal. He says of Tina, "she's big". I tease him that he is 'fattist,' and he denies it. But he is a person who notices such things. Even though I remind him he was very big when I met him. And I worried about that. With Tina, I had only worried that she might have difficulty with stairs, or the tiny ensuite, but she is very fit. And can walk me into the ground probably.

Overnight I have put a pillow against his back in the hope he will stay lying on his side. He has pink patches on his bottom again.

June 5 (75th anniversary events for D-Day begin) — Prof R woke stiff from being confined by the pillow. But cheerful and ready for coffee and milk shake before 9 am. And afterwards, when I had washed his beard with the same spray I use on his bottom, he asked if there was any coffee left. So I will make him another later.

Tina is settling in, and by that I probably mean that I am settling in to having someone in the house. It isn't easy. After she has gone, I find myself being critical of the things she hasn't done – like tidying up Prof R's things on the shelves or leaving the sofa in the children's room dishevelled. I go around after her, straightening the throw rug as I would for the dog.

But of course, that is just me being protective of my space. It's not personal to Tina. And I am getting her advice about side support pillows in bed. She advised getting a V-shaped pillow to tuck around Prof R's bottom and keep him on his side. I have got one. Our local drapery shop was better equipped than John Lewis, having pillowcases for it as well.

—

A lot of D-Day event watching today in between chores and Pilates. Prof R is being told blow by blow what is happening, but it is hard to know if he cares. I continue to tell him everything that is going on, outside in the world, as well as here. He is isolated enough, and sometimes peers out of our bedroom door to remind himself what is out there. It makes me feel guilty, even though I cannot persuade him to leave his room most days.

Panorama's second episode of its documentary *Crisis in Care* really focussed on care in the home and was well worth watching. There is a trend towards what we are doing here – micro-providers of care working for themselves. I must tell Tina she is a micro-provider.

June 6 (D-Day proper) — Prof R had a relatively peaceful night apart from coughing, which makes me try again to persuade him to turn onto his side. He is hard to move unless he is co-operating.

All the people being cared for in the documentary seemed motivated enough to make their care less of a battle. Turning him in bed if he is not willing is going to be a major thing for me to overcome. I have to learn how to do it whether he is a dead weight or not.

—

A beautiful day today, so I made more headway in the shed. A large suitcase was wheeled to the Cancer Research charity shop and the nearly new zippo scooters have gone onto the neighbourhood website. It seems criminal. But there is no room for sentiment here. And no one in the family wants them.

Prof R said to Tina, when she answered his bell, "Be ready to help when needed." Maybe he had been listening to my D-Day commentary after all. But I think he is warming to her. She can be a source of some good ideas. And I am enjoying our lunchtime chats. We mostly talk about care issues, but conversation is easy.

My only worry today was that she did not attempt to wake Prof R for his late morning medications. Some instinct told me to check. She thought it a shame to wake him, which it is, but it cannot be left too long. It's a fine judgement at times. I have discovered that she is not used to being responsible for medications in the care home, so both of us are equally likely to forget them.

At lunch he requested "a proper meal". Muesli being no longer appealing. But the 'proper meal' on offer came back to the chef with a complaint about texture. I managed some alchemy, and he ate it.

The evening shift begins when Tina leaves. This is when he wakes up. Tonight, he has requested fish pie. In the end, the most we have achieved today is to get three milkshakes into him for the first time. I tell him we need to speed up consumption or we will end up with the sort of stockpile that would see us through a war. (*Or, as it might have turned out, a Covid-19 lockdown*).

The fish pie, doctored with spinach and cream, was given a cursory taste before being declined. He will see it again, albeit in a different disguise.

We did our homework for Netty – Q &A with the *Daily Sparkle*. What an idiot-sheet it can be. Dated today, the 6th June, with no mention of D-Day. Perhaps the dementia police decided it would be too upsetting for the readers. More likely, they hoped they didn't even know it was happening.

June 7 — Friday. A peaceful night. Prof R moves onto his back regardless of the new V-shaped pillow tucked around his bottom. But it's important for him to move and it's easier than having to turn him myself. I will need a special slip sheet if/when we come to that.

Friday is my weigh-in day. Another 1 kg gone. Strangely, I don't feel any triumph, probably because it's more of a tedious journey than an adventure. And I was nervous about weighing myself, in case this week has been a failure. It's my first week without JanePlan doing the cooking for me. But I have clearly broken all bad habits. 'Nibble nibble Nana' has gone. But I'm keeping 'mum' with the children about this project of mine. It's easier.

—

A new departure this morning, literally. Prof R had more than pee in his pull-ups. Hopefully he didn't fully realise, although I think he is past caring about such things.

I was lucky it wasn't the full 'Dam Buster'. Netty got that later. But in the right place.

Prof R is sleepy again. Netty had no time to use any of her props – her book of WW2 and photographs of D-Day celebrations. He had no energy to do more than eat and toilet and sleep.

Later, he ate a meal for me, but no dessert. Netty has given me a notebook to write my little alchemy recipes in. "A little prod" she says. Because I have done nothing about writing them down. She is sure I could fill a gap here for people preparing soft and pureed food. Certainly nothing from the NHS. Just a general list of obvious food groups. Like something from the 1950s.

Because I'm making up meals as I go along, note-taking is a good idea. But it is not something people would want to follow slavishly. It's all about what healthy normal foods are in the fridge or cupboard and how they can be balanced and adapted. Plus daily supplements. Then you just add cream and honey if you want them to gain weight or withhold it if you don't.

This evening has been eerily quiet. He has not stirred since about 6.30 pm. Ridiculous I should find I miss his hand bell that can drive me so mad. Or the bed alarm that makes me jump out of my skin. But I'm not happy he is leaving me.

June 8 — It's becoming harder to wake him for his morning pills. (Note to self: put this statement on a loop?) This morning it was 8 am. But eventually he does surface enough, eyes still shut, to swallow them. He knows it is critical that he does, but his mouth must be so dry. I'm not waking him in the night to hydrate him because he is drinking well during the day. So well, I wonder if it is replacing food. At lunchtime today, he drank almost two beakers of water, half asleep. He won't eat lunch until later, but it's still unusual.

Earlier, I brought *The Trooping of the Colours* to him on my iPad. He enjoyed it for as long as he had the energy. Enough to see the Queen in her Scottish carriage and quite a bit of the parade. But he had to lie down for half of it, while I held the iPad in front of him. I was pleased though, very pleased, that he enjoyed it and was engaged by it. That doesn't happen very often.

It's poignant, watching the Queen travel alone in her carriage. Without her consort. While it would be laughable to compare the royals to Prof R and I, there are parallels to the sadness of it all. Not that Elizabeth shows any signs of tiring. She was giving the horse flesh a thorough once over. How lucky she is to be so well at such an age. An absence of austerity may play a part in that.

—

Big late lunch and minimal dinner. He preferred ice cream. But he is eating less overall, and it's harder to get enough milkshakes onto the menu. I want him to eat his 'real' food first. It's not just about fat and calories.

June 9 — Sunday. Coughing overnight signals me to prop him up to try to remove the mucus. But it is not forming in the terrible amounts we were having. Perhaps the increase in his water drinking is helping. It seemed to be the only advice.

His legs are losing power, but he still manages to get to the bathroom with two hands on the zimmer and two of my hands beneath his bum, guiding him as well as supporting his weight.

We both laughed when I accidentally made rough contact with his testicles. "Oh, my goodness, I've hit you in the nuts!" Not too roughly clearly, thank goodness. And just as well no one is paying me to do this job. I might have got the sack.

A man is coming at 2 pm to take some vintage kitchen chairs and a curtain pole. Only because they are free of course. But it saves me a journey to recycling. The charity shops don't want them, and I don't want to deliver them. If I can't carry it, or bag it, it goes to the tip.

—

How contrary is the human mind. Now that I only have weekends totally alone with Prof R, it feels like freedom of a different kind. Just the two of us.

And speaking of contrary, it is definitely worthwhile to record my concerns about his eating. As soon as I have done so, it gives him an opportunity to prove me a liar. By 12.30 he had drunk two milkshakes and eaten his muesli as well. At which point I retired to have my own lunch.

Prof R's 'lunch' at 4 pm, turned into a war zone. Chocolate ice cream (melted) spraying down his front, the hit and miss of spooning wet food, a sneezing attack rendering him helpless, and motoring through tissues, while I contemplated shaving off his moustache. Instead, when we had retired from the fray, I trimmed it. Never let a medic swab it for bugs, Prof R, whatever you do. Both exhausted, we retired.

—

This afternoon I sold the two scooters for £30 and got rid of some chairs and a curtain pole. Now I have someone seriously interested in the electric mower. Things are looking up.

June 10 — Monday. Tina is back today. Prof R is sleepy, but I managed to give him coffee and a milkshake before she arrived. Now she is trying to get him to have some breakfast while she gives him his late morning pills. Good luck with that. I can hear the bed alarm tweeting as he returns to bed.

I am looking for a book for Tina that I fear I may have recently discarded. A good illustration of why I do not like getting rid of books.

Tuesday 11 — Prof R is almost too tired to talk today. He isn't eating much. I'm writing this in the hope that he will prove me a liar as the late afternoon wears on. Tina has gone and managed to feed him his breakfast. I had warmed it up this time. And it worked.

Yesterday I was talking to Prof R about how lucky we have been with our careers. A 'counting our blessings' session. And he said "Yes, being a TV producer". At which I said, "Oh, you didn't tell me about that. Are you thinking of the radio interviews with young people that you did for the BBC?" At that point he conceded that perhaps he might have been a bit confused. It's the first time this has happened. He could always remember his career, even if he sometimes wished for the path not followed.

I have been walking in Market Town's main cemetery today. It is beautiful and large, with lavish flowers and decorative work on the graves. And toy plastic windmills for the saddest graves – the children. They are larger versions of the miniature garden sand-saucers we made at primary school. Almost competitive it seems. So beautiful that I took photos. But when I posted them on my family photo-stream, equally deathly silence from them. Unspoken thought perhaps, "Why on earth is she taking photos of graves?"

Some days walking is harder than others and today it was easy and effortless. I begin to wonder again if Pilates is good for me. Tomorrow is my weekly class.

And so it came to pass, that at 5.30 pm Prof R did prove me a liar, and was on the move. He ate his lunch and ice cream. But it was a bit too late to hope he would eat dinner.

June 13 — Yesterday Prof R was asked by Tina – by way of conversation – what would be the one thing he would like that day. And he said, "my sister". When I reminded him later that he had said that, he looked perplexed. And even a little amused. And we both know why that is funny.

But I told Doris, and she will visit today if possible. Although she and I both know it would have been a random thought rather than intentional.

——

A restless evening and night yesterday until 2 am. Bell ringing before I came to bed and coughing afterwards, which I listened to before deciding whether I need to sit him up to try to remove the mucus. We did have to do that. At 2 am it was a trip to the toilet, which is good news as it means a drier Prof R in the morning.

Every day I look into his eyes and wonder about the pin-sized pupils. It seems in whatever light, that they are small. Again, I think, "More research required". Just out of curiosity, not with the hope of any worthwhile outcome. Perhaps that is why I keep forgetting to do it.

When people phone, as they sometimes do, I can feel I have nothing at all to say. Our days are only peppered by politics or horrible weather. Or what new thing I can think of to concoct for Prof R's meals.

I have discovered that my NZ drivers' licence is valid until I am 75. How civilised. It begins to concern me how many doors here, and in the EU, may be closed to me after my 70th birthday. Well, Brexit will probably trump old age in that department.

Doris and Brian visited late afternoon. I'm not sure how rewarding it was for her, but I hope she is not too discouraged. They visit less and now I do not blame them.

A better eating day, with Prof R managing three main meals and one dessert. Only one milkshake but I will trade nutrition for fat any day.

June 14 — Friday. A quiet night with no coughing, mainly because we 'cleared the drains' before he settled for the night. And I did not give him a later levodopa. I sometimes think he is more settled without it.

At 8 am and far too soon for his legs, Prof R tried to get up for the toilet. We sat on the side of the bed, waiting and talking and changing his top, but still his legs could not take his weight. He has lain down again, without fuss. While I can only reassure him that his pull-ups will cope.

When he did finally get to the toilet, I decided to wash him thoroughly – that meant the foam wash. I sprayed, and washed, and suddenly his entire 'front-piece' became immersed in suds. I had used a bed bath wipe to remove it, which is wet, and accidentally activated the foam. It's the first time that has happened, because I usually use it with dry paper towels on his underlings. Poor Prof R was clinging to the rail, running out of steam, while I frantically tried to remove the suds burying his nether regions. In the end, I decided it wasn't actually soap of course so would not irritate him. Let's hope I'm right.

Netty came this afternoon, and I took the car for an outing – the first in three months. It only went as far as the recycling centre, but it was a relief to find it is still in good operating order in spite of my neglect.

June 15 — Saturday. Another quiet night. No bedtime levodopa and a jolly good spit as a nightcap.

Alex now wants to take me to Berners Tavern for my birthday. I love his optimism.

—

Prof R is very sleepy today. Half his breakfast eaten at 11 am and lunch with dessert at 3 pm. Hardly a feast. After having his feet washed, he had no energy for his hair. It remains a job that doesn't get tackled except on a good day.

On days like today, when he is tired, his legs are almost unable to get him to the toilet. It worries me because I know that one day soon he will be totally unable to do so. And when he did get there, he neither peed nor pooed.

Tonight I will put two magnesium citrate tablets in his dinner to try to get something shifting. All his supplements are in his breakfast, so it matters if he doesn't eat it.

What I love about Prof R is his continuing ability to surprise me. By 4 pm he was ringing his bell, and he stayed up, interested in being entertained for a couple of hours. I had found a box of photos in my shed cleanout and brought some up for us to go through. It made me feel sadder than it did him. All those years and the people who have come and gone. And of course, his beloved second wife. Without her loss our lives would have been so different.

He's eaten his evening meal now which I have laced with the two magnesium citrates as planned, plus two capsules of slippery elm. I will be hoping for an 'outcome' tomorrow.

June 16 (Fathers' Day) — It is so discouraging trying to give Prof R something interesting to do and having it rejected. I have sorted out more photos for him, but this morning, after breakfast, he has had an attack of the sneezes and just wants to lie down. Maybe later.

I have noticed I am generally less my usual cheerful self. Usually, I can jolt myself out of a blue moment, but it gets harder as this illness progresses. Strangely, having Tina more makes me feel less useful. I've become accustomed to this job I am doing, and it has given me a purpose. Which is a distraction in itself. If someone else takes over, and I can go and do something recreational, just for me, it makes me feel rudderless.

Clearing the shed is less rewarding than I'd hoped. More time to think about what next? I prefer to live in the moment. Having no friends here only matters when I have time for them. I have employed the only friend I was meeting for coffee. I don't want to have coffee out anymore. It's boring. Especially as I choose not to eat cake.

I have reached that point on this restricted diet when I am in danger of thinking about nothing but food. It may take 28 days to change a bad habit but being hungry – or believing I am hungry – lasts forever. Food was one of my consolations clearly. Nature wants it so. Today I broke ranks and ate a piece of cheese.

———

Five minutes into spooning lunch into Prof R's mouth I was cured of all altruism. It was "too thick", "too sticky", and after watering it down, "too everything" it seemed. I felt like throwing it at the ceiling, but instead I went down to the kitchen, split it into two bowls, whipped up some peeled tinned tomatoes and added them to one of the bowls – plus some more cream and honey. And lo! He ate it.

My irritation barometer was further tested by his new custom of pointing at something rather than asking. He points at the water beaker, or the tissues, or something obscure that I can't interpret and then I say "speak" because I know he can. But I kiss him as I put him back to bed because his life is shit.

There has still been no bowel movement by this evening. He ate chicken and tomato, with raw peas and mustard and cream, followed by ice cream and creamed rice. So he is eating well today. Even if he did complain about the texture of his meal again. I persuaded him that it is preferable to keep eating 'real' food than some unrecognisable mush. He agreed, and managed to eat the lot.

There was little interest from him in the new batch of photos I have found. But I was very interested. At last, photos of the mysterious Pam. The woman he left his first wife for. New pieces of the puzzle continue to surface.

Back in the 'now', I have given him two tablespoons of Syrup of Fig. It would be tempting to give him more, but I will wait until tomorrow.

June 17 — When Prof R is too dopey to drink from a straw, he will always be able to drink from the baby cup, with its plastic 'teat'. It has the perfect delivery system and doesn't make him choke.

Last night was punctuated right through with his hands 'taking off' and not landing again for several minutes. If it went on too long, I landed them for him. It can work.

At 6 am, I managed a shower. It's usually safe to do so. He doesn't really surface now, even after pills, until much later.

June 18 — I draw a veil over yesterday. It began well, but became the first day of illness I have had in several years. Just a 24 hour stomach flu, and I managed to get by without serious incident or giving it to Prof R.

—

Still ferreting through the shed, I get excited by more photos that Prof R barely glances at. But at least I will know they are there, and his children can take over when necessary.

I've begun worrying about process. What will need to happen when? There are few clear guidelines. Tina says that when Prof R can no longer walk I will need to turn him every two hours. Day and night. To do that I will need a slip sheet or I won't be able to shift him. And what of bowel incontinence?

Also, and crucially, what paperwork will I need at each point, including the end point? I find it better not to think about that but it's unavoidable and perhaps I can forget it when I know I am prepared.

The weather is beautiful, but as usual, it is not forecast to last.

The leadership debate tonight and the 'clown' will be sent in. Can I bear to watch it?

—

I have now found so many private papers and letters belonging to everyone but me, that I can go no further on that front. It will be a legacy for others. But I have filled the car with the detritus for recycling.

Tina had a nice surprise this afternoon when Prof R wanted a tour of the first floor. She hasn't encountered one of these events before. It made a welcome change for her.

When he is like this, perambulating, it can continue into the evening. He wanted to come and help me cook the dinner. This is when I find it very hard to explain this is not possible and why. He has forgotten he is ill. And it makes me miss those ordinary everyday things even more.

I continue to talk to him about everything I am doing in the shed and what I am finding. He acknowledges much of what I am saying, telling him of house transfer documents I have found, or certificates for one thing or another. Also, the revelation that he seems to have been addressed by the moniker 'Dr' in one of his senior Psychology Dept roles. I'm presuming it is an honorary title, as he certainly doesn't have a PhD. Never a shrinking violet, if he had he would still have been calling himself Dr.

He told Tina again that he wanted to go home. This happens more often, and today I asked him if he can recall what home he is thinking of when he feels he is in the wrong place. He couldn't recapture the moment, but next time he says it to me, I will ask him to describe 'home'. He was as curious about it as I am. But he may be curious constantly about where he is. It would be hard to know.

June 20 — Thursday. I seem to be parting a few veils this week, mainly because of what I have been discovering. But also because Doris and Brian came again yesterday, and took Prof R down memory lane in a good way. The shops, the people, the streets, the theatres of Peckham and the Rye. And Prof R could recall much of what they were saying.

It was such a good visit that Prof R has been more energised. He surprised Tina today and increased her education at the same time. She was caught on the toilet when the bed alarm went off, and by the time she had finished, met him coming out of the bedroom door. There was no stopping him, although she tried valiantly to keep tabs on him as he side-stepped her and galloped to his office. She hasn't seen Mr Whippet before, so now she knows. She is a person who doesn't believe what she hasn't seen. Which can be a problem. She doesn't believe he is 'frozen' in the morning, because he has defrosted by the time she arrives.

He made another break for freedom tonight, because the bed alarm didn't work. But my ears are finely tuned to his noises. Like rats in the ceiling, he has a sound signature. I met him coming out the bedroom door and deflected his advance by saying, "Do you want the toilet? It's this way". With a determined steer in the rear. And it turned out he did want the toilet. Which is always a bonus. And while he sat, I changed the battery in the bed alarm.

Now he is tampering with the hand bell as I write, and I want to mention the most pointless part of my day. Which was ringing the GP practice to request a home visit, simply because Doris and Brian urged me once more to do so, as if my life would depend on it. Because they had reason to believe that if Pro B died without a GP having seen him within the previous three weeks, there would have to be an inquest.

I felt such a fool when I spoke to the duty doctor. My explanation for asking for a visit being only that Prof R needs to be monitored by the practice. And hasn't been seen for months. It seemed so trite. The GP, refreshingly honest, said they would be lucky to visit housebound patients as often as once a year. But he took time to ask questions and find out how things are, until concluding, as do I, that there is no need for a doctor to be involved unless the situation worsens.

I am surrounded by other professionals I can call on. Doris and Brian have idealised the stature of the doctor in home care in a way that has been consigned to history. One that neither our GP nor the medical practice recognise. Although I suspect they are right about the risk of an inquest.

June 21 — Friday. We are back to bell ringing in the evenings and a general confusion about why he is where he is and "What is that bloody rail doing there". It is so hard to communicate with him when he is like that. At least, in a way which he can understand. He gets furious with me and I lose patience too and feel like stomping out. Instead, I have been known to stamp my feet in situ, to distract him. And then it passes.

So tonight has been the same. But the day was productive. There is a lot to be said for the joy of rediscovery in a shed. Today it was the 8 mm films and projectors. I want to get mine transferred to DVD. For a huge price we can have them digitalized of course and 'enhanced', but I prefer mine raw.

—

Tina lacks confidence but not ability. When she knows her way around more, things will be easier. Lack of confidence is dangerous. She hates to ask questions, so will do things like throwing all the drink bottles into the rubbish bin because she doesn't want to ask me how I recycle them. What if she didn't know what to do about a missed pill dose? Or am I overthinking this?

I happened to be in my office yesterday when I overheard her ask Prof R, when he turned up his nose at the meal offering, if he would prefer scrambled eggs. My confidence in her drained along with the blood from my head. Scrambled eggs are too dry and would take his breath away. Literally. She knows his food is softer now than scrambled egg. I need her to get the alchemy skill, if I'm not there, when my offering is too thick, or too slimy, or similar. A spoonful of honey and a healthy dollop of cream or fruit puree. I keep stacks of little pots of puréed apple that end up in almost every meal.

Why did I expect her to know all this? She has clearly been simply delivering food rather than being in charge of its preparation. But even so, I thought, how would she know about which foods are safe for each patient.

—

Much more understandably, she lacks even my modest familiarity with technology, and the phone in particular, because her career in care has not called for it. She asked me again today about emergency procedures and numbers, because she hasn't transferred the written details I gave her onto her phone. And now I realise she doesn't know how to.

She is conscientious and worries about procedures in times of medical or other crisis. But the vital piece of paper with the critical numbers has been put tidily in the back of her work logbook. Fortunately, she has one advantage. Her husband is a techno whiz. He can put the numbers in her phone for her. I suggested she take advantage of this. Note to self: never be afraid to take advantage of this yourself. Such people are in short supply.

This entry reads like a critique of Tina. But it is also a critique of me. It makes me realise I must do a better job of briefing her about how things work. This is a household that runs on automatic with most of the knowledge in my head.

The whole time I have been writing, Prof R is fidgeting next door. The folding chair leaning against the bed has crashed to the ground. I'm trying to ignore it. I know he is neither under nor on top of it. I have told him I will wait until he is feeling more settled before I come to bed. That is supposed to be an incentive for him to settle down.

June 22 — Saturday. The age of reason is not working when Prof R becomes confused. I have no idea how to defuse it, but eventually I did manage last night. But not after failing miserably for several hours as he kept thinking he needed to get up to help with something or we had someone arriving at 9 pm or he saw a shadow behind the door so who else was here?

I am convinced it is my conversation that he picks up parts of and then runs with what he thinks I have said. I need to be careful how I tell him things; that I am slower and clearer in my speech. Even though his hearing seems fine, his mind is not keeping up.

Eventually, by a process of elimination, I persuaded him that I had confused him with the information I had given him, and that there was no event or person or thing he had to do. But it makes me so sad when we 'fall out' and cannot understand each other. We both get cross and tired and (me) desperate when communication breaks down.

—

A man is coming to pick up the carpenter's workbench today. That may be what sent Prof R into a spin; me telling him about it. And Lucas next door, for whom a normal life is slipping ever further away, is 20 today and will be having a BBQ in the garden. At least there will be lots of happy noise.

I found Prof R sleeping just now, apparently with his eyes open. I can tell he is still asleep because his eyes are looking at his upper lid. Not easy to do if you are really awake.

Today he has been calm and relatively happy and eating all his food. But he sleeps in between toilet trips and food. I have taken the risk of working in the shed with the bed alarm on the garden table. It has become addictive. Today I have found an old typewriter of Prof R's. Plus, two more pieces of garden kit to put on the neighbourhood website and the croquet set, which no one wants.

—

That was written at about 5 pm. It is now 7.20 pm and I have been managing a man who was on the edge of madness for two hours. It had begun well, with a walk together to my office, where he sat while I showed him photos of Marrakesh from Alex and Ophelia's holiday. He seemed happy, walking with the zimmer to his office and back again, before he began to lose the strength in his legs. I hastened him back to his room to sit and that is where his mood changed.

Suddenly agitated, trying to walk off in all directions, refusing to stay seated when I wanted to fetch his meal, so that I had to say there would be no meal until I could be sure he would be safe. When he agreed, and I returned, he ate only a small portion, before rejecting it, so that I had to race downstairs to produce another, which he also only ate a few spoonful's of, before rejecting that too.

I asked him how he felt. "Confused". I told him to ask me questions so I could help. He couldn't or wouldn't. It became an unpleasant encounter, with him showing his frustration like a two-year-old, but very much harder to manage. Not because he was violent but because I feared a fall. Certainly hard to reason with. But I kept trying. "Would you like me to wash your hair?" and when he didn't reply, and I asked why, he said "Waste of breath. I washed it myself."

I became a hostage to his misfortune, unable to leave the room or eat myself. When he was shaking the rails or trying to express his anger by getting up recklessly, I considered ringing Doris and Brian. If this continued, I would need help.

But just as suddenly as it began, it left him. I was sitting opposite him, our knees touching, and I felt his body suddenly calm. Whatever it was, I felt it too, leaving him. A departing demon. "It's gone hasn't it?" I asked him. And he said "yes". I said "Welcome back husband. Lovely to see you." And he replied, "Lovely to see you too." His tremor also stopped. He looked and was exhausted. I was relieved. Very relieved. He agreed to lie down, and I can finally get something to eat myself.

—

But I need to write about it first. How to prevent this happening again? I will look at how the rivastigmine may be interacting with his chemistry differently. It is possible to reduce the dose and stay at maximum safe dosage, because we are slightly over (with the neurologist's blessing). But perhaps over time it may need evaluating. These are decisions we have to make ourselves. Neurologists don't 'live in'.

Next week I will ring my dementia advisor to ask if this is something I have to expect. I hope she does not say yes. There is a dementia type called The Sundowner. Sufferers who become determined to be active and preferably leave the building as soon as evening comes. I do not want a Sundowner.

Now, food.

June 23 — Sunday. After a little light reading yesterday, I have concluded that Prof R is indeed a potential Sundowner. I did everything right, trying to keep him calm. But nothing will prevent it happening probably, so the medications may not be involved.

By the end of today we will know.

I'm trying a new system for remembering Prof R's pill times. The kitchen timer. When I am busy or dealing with people, I can forget to notice the time. I have an alarm I can set on my watch, but as the pill times can vary, this is a pain to set up every day. The timer is quick and easy and very loud.

The day became a peaceful harbour of good moods, hair washing and eating everything put in front of him. The storm has passed. But I see a noticeable decline in his ability to share thoughts with me. As conversation diminishes, our life becomes harder. Although what would I know of his feelings about that?

June 24 — A local school Reception class teacher called Sarah has just left with Prof R's German Adler portable typewriter. It weighs a ton, but she is delighted with it. She will use it to help the class with letter recognition. What better end to the life of an old typewriter once owned by a professor?

A big scandal here (again) about care homes and dental neglect. Once again an elderly woman had her dentures fused to her gums and had to have them surgically removed. Prof R fortunately saw the dentist last year while he was still mobile. I keep his dentures upstairs because they hurt him to insert, and eventually he stopped noticing he didn't have them. I have no idea whether a dentist would visit him at home.

June 25 — A little cry of "help" this morning at 6 am after much thrashing. He had managed to jam his legs down between the railing and the side of the bed. Because his muscles lock, when I move his legs he complained loudly. But once moved, he was much relieved and not in pain. That means I now need to put a bolster or similar between him and the railing at night.

———

Yesterday another calm day, with Tina finding him very active at about 3.30 pm and walking him twice around the landing. He was heading for the stairs when I arrived back. But Tina did not need help. He was by then too tired to take the stairlift down. And she will not be prepared to tackle that on her own. Netty doesn't.

She is still nervous about being in charge on Saturday. I am going out for the day to meet an old and dear friend at Batemans, Kipling's home. I reassure Tina that it is really no different whether I am out for one hour or six. An emergency can happen in an instant. She agrees.

But it concerns me that she is nervous at all. After so many years of experience, working alone with someone as ill as Prof R still seems to daunt her. I still believe she can do it, but I wish she did too, or it is not ideal for his safety.

When he is with her, he seems often to ask if he can go home. It may confuse him that she is with him rather than me, but he is used to carers by now. She says it is common with Sundowners. I have asked her outright if she will feel able to work here if he becomes hard to manage at such times. She assures me she will.

———

A quiet day with Tina today, with Prof R sleeping a lot and eating a little. Which is just as well for her because she has agreed to a 5-9 pm shift at the care home. Keeping her hand in. Moonlighting too. A sign she sees the writing on the wall.

I've been buying cooler clothes for Prof R so the weather will no doubt return to cold within a few days.

Tina had a solution for briefing her about the things I need to share that happen between her shifts. She suggested I keep a handover notebook. After today, when I kept thinking of other things I needed to tell her, and worried about the things I would forget, I have grabbed the idea with both hands.

Previously, I had thought of asking if I could put notes in her book, but I felt she might not like to work that way. But the more I think about it, the more I think it would be better if all the information was in one place. However, a separate notebook will do.

Prof R had a treat for dinner. Tina is evangelical about her slow cooker and brought him some leftovers. It smelt amazing. He scoffed it with pleasure at 6.30pm and then woke at 8.30pm saying he hadn't had any dinner. I persuaded him to have a milkshake. Better than the chocolate dessert he had left untouched in its dish.

June 26 — Wednesday. Yesterday Tina and I noticed he had put both his rings on one finger. Months ago, I had to take them from his third fingers and put them on the first. They were falling off. This morning, the rings were back on their separate fingers. They are important to him and he hates to lose them.

I washed his feet before Tina got here, because I don't want her to feel she has to do it. He sheds so much skin that it is a bit of a messy job. This morning, his feet were in 'lockdown', so when I lifted them he grimaced. I promised him I would do them later in the day in future. And by the time his socks went on he had no pain at all.

—

Tina has tried to get him up for the toilet and breakfast but all he could manage was his pills. The overnight pull-up is still in place and we may have to change him in the bed. I say "we", but I know it would be best not to interfere with Tina's care if I want to avoid confusing Prof R and undermining her.

It's all too easy to see the flaws in care home regimes when they are applied here, at home. Such as the regulation morning body wash on the toilet, when he is most tired and just needs a top and tail. I have told her not to worry about the torso until later.

I know she is bored. That is why she has returned to doing odd late shifts at the care home. The first time she did it, she didn't tell me. Just said she "had to go somewhere" and raced off. Worried, I suspect, that I would object. But the second time she let me know. I'm glad, as it keeps our relationship honest.

—

There's something going on today which appears to be strike action. He rang his bell. Tina went into the room, he said he was hungry but when she asked him to get out of bed, he said no. She has offered him a milkshake instead, which is safe to have in bed, and he accepted.

Tina told me she was worried when Prof R picked up his Swiss Army knife. I said, don't worry, he wouldn't be able to open it, and she said yes, he can. He opened the little scissors and practiced using them. Prof R never fails to amaze me.

—

Tonight, we had what can only be described a Nutella fountain. This was not as it sounds. Not diarrhoea. But a tsunami of a different kind, more of a lava flow, that never stopped coming. And it's sticky. When I had filled the toilet with paper, I knew I should have risked flushing halfway through. The limits had been reached for the plumbing. When we could finally retire from the toilet, I donned a glove and dug all the paper out of the bowl again. Safely bagged, I could relax. We don't want a second visit from a man with a mechanical drain cleaning machine to ream out all the pipes again.

Earlier, Prof R had done as Tina and I predicted, been awake or wanting to eat or just ringing his bell ever since she went home, after about four hours on a couch for her and two actually doing something with Prof R. No wonder she is bored. He only ate his breakfast for her, and has had lunch, dessert and an hour later, dinner with me. I managed to get him to allow me to eat my meal. As soon as I have cooked it and placed it on the table, invariably his bell will sound.

So, do we have a Sundowner? The jury is still out. But by 8 pm I was asking him to be a better man. He said he would, until the next time he rang the bell. "I just want to contact you" and I joke he was lucky I didn't want to contact him, after the dance he has led me. But no matter how often he cries wolf, I will answer him. There is always going to be the one time he really needs me.

June 27 — Prof R has been awake again tonight and this time I have surrendered to the experience and just sat with him. It is so much easier and less stressful than trying to snatch moments downstairs.

I'm surprised he has been so alert, as his day has been a good one. Early breakfast and lunch and dinner on time at 6.30 pm. But at 8.30 pm he offered to make me something to eat. How sweet of him, you might think. But I know a hint when I hear it. Is he hungry? Yes, because, he says, he hasn't had his dinner yet.

To jog his memory, I reminded him that his dinner had been a special treat, because he ate it in bed. That helped him to believe I was telling the truth. Why he had this 'treat' was because when I had helped him up to eat, he sat on the edge of the bed and gently toppled sideways. When he does this, it seems callous to continue to propel him towards the chair. So I propped him up with the tri-pillow instead. And fortunately, I had already eaten, so I could think about his stomach rather than my own. If he's hungry, I will feed him.

———

He is still awake, at 9.30 pm and we have sat companionably all evening, listening to Jazz FM. He tells me often that he loves me and looks as happy as a boy on a first date when I tell him I love him too and we hold hands. I know these are times for me to cherish. And I do. It could be easy, at the end of a long day, to forget that. What could be so important downstairs?

And today I made progress. After another trip to the recycling centre, I have now opened the door to the second shed. The excitement never ends.

June 28 — Friday. We were not wrong to medicate Prof R with levodopa overnight when he was more active. No matter what the neurologist might think he knows, he is wrong. Because last night I gave Prof R a pill at 10 pm, just because he was awake, and he woke for a toilet trip at 3 am. And was able to walk there. So it does make a huge difference. But his legs were not very good, we must admit that. So the trip was a bit fraught. Nevertheless, it means I don't have to rush him to get to the bathroom this morning.

It was lovely to see Netty again today, after her fortnight's holiday away. I realise how much I miss her. She has a different approach to care which includes Prof R's mental as well as physical wellbeing. But he showed her some of his frustration nevertheless – just with toilet paper. He was restless, asking where I was. And then, in a few moments of true clarity, he saw his situation for what it is and told her he was worried about what would become of him. He also told her he wanted to help me, when she said I was sorting out the folding picnic table to give away. I'm glad these moments are few and far between. They are distressing. And not just for him.

I have succumbed, and ordered another month of JanePlan food. This time, the ones I liked more and with less gluten. It is tedious counting calories on top of everything else. I just want to grab and eat and forget it.

We finally have another home appointment with a speech therapist for mucus control. Next Wednesday at 11.30 am. The timing is perfect. But whether Prof R will respond to any efforts to help strengthen his swallow remains to be seen.

This has been another evening of bell ringing in the middle of my meal, so I took it upstairs with me, and sat in a chair with a book and my teeny glass of wine while he slept. If I left the room to go to the toilet, he woke up. But now I am out of the room and reading and writing in my office and so far, no tinkle, tinkle. I might risk making a cup of tea.

June 29 (the day of the mini heatwave) — Saturday. How funny we are, raving on about one day over 30deg when Europe is seriously sweltering in temperatures of 44deg plus. It's always the lead item on the news. We must be the laughing stock.

The house is managing to be cool enough at 32 deg so far. Downstairs is lovely and our bedroom is balmy but very pleasant. Much cooler than the loft. Prof R is under a sheet.

I should not feel so relieved when it is a 'no Tina' day but I am. It's not easy having someone in the house for so many hours a week. Especially when they are mostly here in Prof R's quiet time. I should get out more, I hear you say. And you are right.

Prof R got out. A nice calm walk around the first floor at 3.30 pm, having said "no" to an offer to take him downstairs. Back in our room, he cleaned his teeth and then said he wanted to go back to bed but "not here" pointing at the bed. He had lost his sense of place. Perhaps because I had placed his chair in a different position. Or he was remembering the loft.

I showed him a photo of the blue folding picnic table I was giving away and he didn't recognise it. When I mistakenly pressed him to remember it, he then said he did. But I'm sure that was only because he felt that he should.

I also talked to him about his eldest daughter Hannah's 50th birthday today – several times – but he didn't respond.

I couldn't rouse him for his evening meal. Maybe later.

It reached 34 deg here today.

June 30 (Cooler, and much nicer for that) — Sunday. Prof R did finally have dinner last night by 9 pm, and a few minutes after I had resettled him, he began to ring his bell. But this time I asked him to only ring it when he needed me. Really needed me, because I would be coming to bed soon. Miraculously it worked.

His girls write to me or ring telling me how much they are thinking of us, but their life events – some serious, some just football – seem to take precedence. The longer they stay away the less they need to come down.

I have been reading a book by American journalist Michael Kingsley – ostensibly about the challenges of the ageing baby boomers and their legacy but really obsessing about his own Parkinson's diagnosis. He describes what is called "The Parkinson's personality" and it is unflattering. It also, unnervingly, fits the Prof R I first met almost to a tee.

But now that Prof R's responses are minimal. It is hard to imagine the man who, in company, could barely manage to put his own trumpet back in its case.

—

Sunday's have become my domestic day. Cleaning, which is harder to do when Tina is here, though perhaps it's just that I don't want to pay her so that I can clean. It feels as though the time should be spent more productively.

Prof R is eating well but not dessert. The melted chocolate ice cream piles up, sitting on a fridge shelf, neglected. But the milk shakes are making up for it. I am afraid to weigh him because the dietitian will use her own scales as usual and we will be doomed to disappointment.

I have sticky hands from using a no-water wash spray on Prof R's head. No doubt his hair will be sticky too when it dries, although if it is, that means his 'underlings' will be sticky too. He hasn't complained of that so far.

He seems to respond best to jokey conversation about everyday things. If I talk about Wimbledon, or politics, he knows what I am talking about but is totally disinterested. As he seemed to be about Hannah's 50th birthday. So I joke about sticky hair or the fact that the dog couldn't dislodge a hairy leaf from her fur.

Prof R is having one of those days where about half of what comes out of my mouth sounds, to him, like gobbledegook. Probably because often it is, but he is not deaf. We know that. He can hear a pin drop. But the meaning of what I say can escape him. Then he looks puzzled, and I get fed up and talk louder...and slower...all the things we are not supposed to do ...eventually he gets it.

His bowel has made a couple of pre-emptive strikes. Sending out scouts. It's been a few days since the last full-blown assault.

At 9 pm tinkle tinkle, and he is looking for food. I give him a super shake before he asks when dinner will be served. He has totally forgotten, as often happens, that he has had his meal. So, I give him his chocolate dessert and then, when he is still hungry, I go and get some creamed rice and give it to him with honey.

He is coughing tonight and plagued with phlegm, so we try to deal with that too. And I give him some syrup. Syrup, honey, butter and even olive oil, can stop throat tickles. Not cough syrup, which is suspect, but any pure syrup will do, and we have Syrup of Figs. Killing two birds as usual.

By 9.45 I can leave him to get ready for my own bed and put the house to sleep. And the dog.

July 2 — Tuesday. At 3.40 am this morning, while I drank tea on the couch and watched BBC World, a veggie box was delivered by Milk and More. They gave me a hell of a fright. Not least, once I realised what the sound was, because of the ridiculous size of the pack of white onions. And a sack of both new and old potatoes. When will I learn *not* to order these? Two people do not need veggie boxes. One-and-a-half people even less so. Tina will be offered the overflow.

I was on the couch in the small hours because Prof R had such a restless first half of the night it left me with insomnia. He had spent a very peaceful day with Tina, sleeping a lot, while I went out to play with my New Zealand friend Chris. And was still sleepy until I fed him dinner. But by 9.30 pm he was wide awake.

So was I. For different reasons. My day with Chris had been both delightful and overwhelming. We had so much to say to each other after several years since our last meeting. It had been a wonderful day and I was buzzing. And a bit upended.

—

Today was another 'Nutella' day. I caught the first rear-guard action in his overnight pants and Tina got the rest in series, throughout the day. It does not mean his stomach is upset, just that his bowel messages and muscles are changing. We both marvel at the stickiness. Shall we blame the honey or the cream? (*I'm glad I didn't realise then that it also meant he was dying*).

Every day is different, and this was no exception (joke). But we were not happy when Prof R was unresponsive verbally for much of the day and was not eating until late afternoon. He did eat eventually, and felt better for it. And then he was alert enough for me to amuse him with the tale of the vegie box. And rough wash his hair and cut his fingernails. Without injuring him.

July 3 — Surprise, surprise. How often I begin a diary entry with those words.

The bed alarm went off before 9 am and Prof R was alert and ready for the toilet. I am tempted to think it is the new pill regime I began today, but I doubt it. Changes have seldom resulted in useful change before. But today we began the pills at 7 am instead of 7.45 am just to see if I could improve on yesterday. Which was a dreadful day.

Later: Our wish was granted. But probably not for the reasons we might hope. He was just well for no reason at all. And eating normally. So, a temporary respite from worry, until 11.30 am when the speech therapist came. Megan tested his swallowing, pronounced it still reasonably strong, but emphasised again he should be vertical to have anything by mouth, not just food.

She has again raised the issue we had largely managed to avoid. How to give Prof R fluids and pills when he is too tired or too sleepy to sit bolt upright. I've been living in hope this man of many pillows could safely be given liquid and pills at 45deg with his head turned sideways to prevent it "going the wrong way", but there's no avoiding the fact that there is still a risk of them entering his lungs and causing an infection.

The hunt is on for some easily deployed sitting frame for raising him without stress when he is in bed.

Otherwise, this day was one of his best. Chatting, engaging with us, and no low mood.

July 4 — Thursday. Prof R has retreated again. A very withdrawn day, with the only difference being his mood, which seems calm and not sad.

Poor Tina didn't like to wake him for his pills, but now I have instructed her to do so. I'm not prepared to risk allowing him to drift. Or drift further than he needs to.

While he was sleeping, I was busy online buying a dual-mechanised bed. King size, oak and looking pretty normal, except they are 4 inches longer than a standard bed. It has to be custom-made to suit our individual heights and weights. I am measuring the space at the end of our current bed and there won't be much room. But I'm relieved to have a solution that is not a hospital bed. If he must be bolt upright for liquid and pills when he is comatose, it is proving increasingly difficult to do it manually.

—

It's my turn to be sad. I have continued with my clear-out of the small shed and found old files of Prof R's. Seeing the life of a man who was meticulous with his records, or at least appeared to be, brings home how much he has lost of himself. And how much I have lost of our lives together. So much easier to block it out and live in the present.

It's 5 pm and he is lying in bed with his eyes open but barely responding to me. No words, just a flicker of expression. If he follows past patterns, he will suddenly emerge and start eating. And I have to give him his pills at around 6.30 pm.

Finally, at 7.30 pm, he was awake enough to eat – dinner and two portions of ice cream.

July 5 — Friday. Waking him for pills is becoming impossible. He is as stiff as a board when I try to lift him into a sitting position. He simply can't do it. We manage 45 degrees or so and it just has to do. He cannot wake himself at these times. I have ordered a cheap temporary adjustable bed rest that I hope will help until the new bed arrives.

Breakfast at 11 am and coffee. A big improvement on yesterday. Then straight to sleep. And a tinkle from his bell half an hour later, looking for company. I wait till his eyes close and sneak out. When he is in bell mode, I daren't risk going outside.

Netty took over at 1 pm and found him responsive and eating – but not the ice cream. Netty has new 'props' – mostly war time memorabilia – and they are perfect for Prof R. And me. I'm very interested.

Netty and I talked about his dwindling mobility. So, it was no surprise when he woke at 5.30 pm as Whippet Man. We haven't seen Mr Whippet for a while. Long enough for me to think he might not return. So as usual, when I come to these conclusions, he proves me wrong.

This time the bed rail was proven to be extended one notch too short, and I found him halfway to the toilet only seconds after the bed alarm sounded. But fortunately, he didn't fall. Unfortunately, he didn't eat either.

Now it is after 7 pm, I want to give him his medication, and his food, but because he is so settled, I'm hesitant to wake him. There are no rules of engagement.

He woke himself eventually, for dinner and a pee at nearly 8 pm and none the worse for his pills being late. Now, just after 9 pm, he is waiting impatiently for me to come to bed. I'm exhausted today, even though it has been beautiful weather, so I won't be arguing. Two bad nights of sleep do that to me. Just insomnia and restlessness. Not Prof R's fault. Although I think I find it hard to relax if I am worrying about him needing help in the night.

A really very ordinary day. I prefer them.

July 6 — Saturday. My big day spent in London with my own darlings. At Kings Cross Coal Drops Yard. I was very amused when Hope gave Alex a pair of crystal whisky glasses for a late birthday present. I said, "If any of you like crystal, I've got a shed load." And didn't add I was about to sell it on eBay. Who knew a liking for crystal would skip a generation?

Prof R and Tina managed so well in my absence, I will no longer feel guilty. He has eaten and slept and she, for whom seeing is believing, can relax too.

With me, he did eat some dinner, but late and without enthusiasm.

And he was restless enough in the night to stop me sleeping well for a few hours.

July 7 — As it is Sunday, with no carers, I have decided to experiment (yet again) with Prof R's early morning pill regime. I have tried to wake him several times, but he opens one eye, and then the other, and promptly closes them again. I am going to wait and see what happens. He is too heavy to propel into a sitting position comatose.

At 8.45 am I lost my nerve, raised him as high as I could and put the tri-pillow behind him. The effect is only head and shoulders above the parapet, but it was the best I could do. He could hear my instructions and took his pills. It is another month at least before the mechanical bed comes.

Sunday is domesticity day in our house. All the things I don't want the carers to do are done on Sunday. Hair washing or cutting, feet bathed in Dead Sea salt, bed linen changed and washed, and food prepared.

But I also chill out and watch a movie. Or tennis.

The foot soaking is rewarding. The salt not only dislodges the dead skin which normal washing doesn't, it also softens his toenails so I can trim them if necessary. If it's a while since we have done this (because Prof R is often too tired; and today was such a day) there is an awful lot of 'product' from the feet. I can't work out if it is salt as well, or the creams I use daily after normal foot washing, but I am always astounded. Each foot therefore needs its own towel, and my clothing seems to wear the rest.

He has been very sleepy today, so no hair wash. I told him I had finally heard from his son Michael, thanking us for the birthday presents, but still, he barely registers. He did raise a smile once, when I told him his youngest daughter Julie had suggested I have the old camping stove packaged up and couriered to them. "In your dreams." We both got that joke.

Dinner was at 7.30 pm, the whole day delayed by the late start. But at

10 pm I got such a shock when he asked for his meal. I should have been delighted but so shocked was I, that it was ill-concealed. "You're hungry?? At 10 o'clock at night?" A rather uncontrolled rant in fact, overcome quickly when I saw how perplexed he was. If he was truly hungry? Yes, he was. And I ran downstairs and grabbed today's leftovers for tomorrow's lunch and whipped it up. He ate it, and followed it with a super shake. Impressive.

Now, at 10.30 pm I can finally go to bed myself.

July 8 — One of my favourite songs is Cat Stevens' *Bad Night*. 1967 but never deliberately forgotten by me. And when nights are rough, it becomes my mantra. Because it's upbeat, and I can cope.

And last night was rough. Rotator hands for several hours before a toilet trip to pee at 2 am. I know I did sleep at some point, but it wasn't exactly restful.

And this morning, bright and early he was ready for the 'off' again. By 7 am I decided to give him his pills, and later, about 9 am, all became clear when he managed a very decent bowel movement of several days' gestation. Not dry, not difficult, not Nutella, no cause for concern. Followed understandably by an earlier than usual breakfast before Tina arrived.

Tonight, after she left, he has been eating an early dinner and dessert and remained active enough to have his hair 'washed' with a shampoo cap. Tina had been interested in having a tutorial on how to do it. Tempting to say, "read the label", no tutorial required. She credits me with far more knowledge than I actually have.

I am constantly amazed that care homes clearly specialise their staff into very narrow roles. Or, less charitably, simply can't be arsed training them. I know she is good at body washes and toilet care, but she has experience of very little else. Including pills. Yet she's certainly capable enough.

The other missing ingredient – working with Prof R to stimulate him intellectually –isn't such a mystery. It's almost bound to be due to lack of time in a care home setting. Netty and I can fill that gap.

Today I wandered the vintage shops looking for childhood items that would trigger memories for him. Annuals, or books from the 40s and 50s. So far, I have drawn a blank. There are plenty of vintage toys and books for younger children, or about trains, but there are not enough well illustrated ones, regardless of topic. I thought I was getting warm when I found the Fleet Air Arm and merchant navy brochures, but even they are more words than visuals, and Prof R is not easily focused.

On my way home, I passed the open door of Market Town's 'cathedral' and could hear the organ playing. When Stella was here, she had discovered what time the organist practices – Monday afternoons – and sometimes went to listen. But I had either forgotten that or not really remembered. Now I did, and went in.

It was one of the most moving experiences I have had. She was playing a piece by a French composer – she did tell me his name afterwards, when I asked, but it took an online search to help me remember – *Méditation sur le Salve Regina* by *Léonce de St Martin*. It was very beautiful, and I videoed it for my sister, while I wept silent tears. I will want to listen to it again.

—

It's now 7 pm. Prof R interrupted my own meal earlier, ringing his bell, but when I asked him if I could finish eating first, he was perfectly happy. Time now to help myself to my espresso glass of wine. Not so fast, his eyes are open. Just when I hoped to watch Wimbledon.

And I didn't watch Wimbledon. Prof R decided he was hungry and wanted his dinner. As always, I remind him he has had it, but if he is still hungry, I will make more. Because any hunger is so welcome. So I have done, after ranting silently to myself a bit about wanting to watch the tennis. And when I brought his meal upstairs at 7.40 pm, he had gone back to sleep. This is a respite, but not for long.

July 9 — Dinner last night was eventually at 8.30 pm, and thereafter all was quiet.

This morning. Things remained quiet. So much so, I was unable to lift him sufficiently for his pills until after 9 am. He is again locked in a prone posture. I've had to decide that it simply doesn't matter. The new bed will make all things possible.

It will have to. Because the adjustable back rest I ordered arrived today and it's so large it shunts the user halfway down the bed. And will be impossible to leave in place overnight or deploy with one hand when I want to give Prof R his morning meds. It is quality, I will say that. I picture the perfect home for it being on a beach somewhere, the owner having planted their bottom in the sand rather than on a mattress.

—

When Tina had gone today, I dusted the 'playroom', which is her escape room, and found her discarded water bottle in the wire paper bin I have there. Why does it seem such a mean thing to do? I have removed the bin. Solved.

She is very kind and good to Prof R and he appreciates her efforts. She told me today that he had squeezed her hand. That is kind of him. Or he cannot tell any longer who is his wife and who isn't. But I don't think we have reached that low point yet.

I do enjoy Tina's company. It's good for me to have someone to talk to in the house. I feel her lack of motivation to do more than clean and feed Prof R. But maybe her smiling face is enough to brighten his day. I hope so. He's so much operating on one cylinder today he seems content with just being cared for and loved.

I have discovered more recordings of the French composer of the organ music – Leone de Saint Martin. He died in 1954, but his music sounds very contemporary. Online there are clips of him playing improvisations at Notre Dame, where he was the organist. I have now listened to the piece often enough to have an ear worm.

—

Dinner at 7.30 pm tonight. Later, when Prof R was standing up from the toilet, holding onto the rail with both hands, I told him he looked as though he were water skiing. But he didn't see the joke.

July 10 — Wednesday. There was a second dinner last night, but at 9 pm rather than 10 pm, and I was ready. So, no surprise. Four meals a day is a very good thing. We may get praise from the dietitian yet.

This morning, tired of manhandling and bullying him into a sitting position, I relied on the 'three pillows and a bolster ' method. (Not as romantic as the film I stole that pun from). They raised his head sufficiently for his pills. It will have to continue to be good enough until the new bed arrives.

(Confession. I discovered last night that I do mind him squeezing Tina's hand. Silly the things that still matter.)

The day that began well with coffee and a milkshake at about 9 am deteriorated into disinterest and not eating. It's 5.30 pm and he has eaten virtually nothing, in spite of Tina's efforts. I have just washed his face and hands and groomed his nails to help him rest. His agitation is not obvious, but he is not feeling good.

After several days of four meals a day, a let-down is to be expected. But we always hope he will not have these days. He gazes into my eyes apparently unseeing, although he responds to my questions. And no, he isn't hungry.

While I was at Pilates, he told Tina it was his birthday. She explained that it was an 'unbirthday', like Alice in Wonderland, which I thought very clever, and she sang him the unbirthday song. He then told her it was time she got on with her work. How he makes me laugh.

He interacts with her very differently to either Netty or me. Today he put his hand over her mouth when she was chatting while trying to give him food. He also spat out his breakfast, something he never does. But he wasn't cross. Just disrespectful, which is not how he would want to be judged.

After Pilates, because I often feel rather light and relaxed and energised, I browsed the record and vintage shops. It's good to remind myself of life outside.

July 11 — Prof R finally had two milkshakes before retiring last night. (As opposed to retiring for the entire day, although it can be difficult to tell the difference).

This morning, he is awake but again cannot use his muscles to help me lift him for his pills. Instead of having his pills, he had his skin nicked (again), this time while I was trimming his nose hair. Guilt-ridden (again), but still unable to get him to rise, even after such abuse from his wife. The nose shows no evidence of internal damage and has stopped bleeding with an application of Germolene and tissue pressure. Elder Abuse (with capitals).

By 9.30 I was still trying to lift him into a sitting position. It would have been easy to panic, but eventually I managed it and gave him his pills. That bed can't come soon enough. But a better day overall, if rather comatose. Breakfast eaten and lunch. Ice cream at 4.30 pm.

—

I almost made a friend today when I was walking by the Creek. Sitting in the shade (28 degrees today) eating cherries, and a woman of my own age came up and sat at the other end of the bench. We remarked how peaceful it was and then awkward silence. So we chatted. It was both nice and a bit annoying, but we exchanged names and she told me to call in if passing. She lives alone, likes to garden, and has a view of the Creek. I also learned she is estranged from her son and daughter-in-law. How grateful am I that I cannot say the same?

—

Although I sometimes feel Tina's hours here are too long, today I felt sorry when she left. She helped me lift Prof R for his pill before leaving. Having this new worrying phase dents my confidence. I have left him fairly propped up so that things are not too fraught later. But there is always the morning.

Dinner was unexpectedly on time, at 6.30 pm and he ate well. But the lights go out in his eyes after about 40 minutes or so. He returns to bed gratefully.

July 12 — Friday. A better sleep and a more alert man this morning, able to sit up enough for me to give him his pills. But he only has coffee and a milkshake before Netty comes at 1.pm.

I've begun taking things from Prof R's stash of technical kit in the shed down to the Cancer Society charity shop. He had two converters from video to DVD unopened. There's no point in offering this out-of-date stuff to any of his daughters. I'm already beginning to worry about the family video film I have converted to DVD. That it should now be digitised.

We have two new plants at the front door for the princely sum of £1.50 per plant. Garden centres cannot compete with the market. And given Market Town no longer has a garden centre, it's just as well.

I weighed in today at 60 kg. The boredom and hunger are paying off and I will reach 58 kg by the end of the month. It sounds good until I convert it to stones and pounds. I will still be 9 stone and it sounds enormous compared to my youthful 8 stone 7 lb. But I know it will be enough for my face.

July 13 — Friday. A 'normal' morning. I added one pillow to give him his pills at 8 am. It'll have to be enough. He wouldn't eat more than a few spoons of muesli around 11 am when I had washed and changed him while he sat on the toilet. But he had a coffee.

"I wish I could magic you well" I said this afternoon.

At least Simona Halep beat Serena Williams in the Wimbledon final. That was a plus.

Later. One of his awake evenings. How I loathe them. I sit with him to avoid the constant bell ringing. But there is so little to say. Instead, as displacement therapy, I wash his hands and put cream on them. Or ask him if he remembers that I also sleep in the bed with him. He never does. But he is witty, despite it all. When I say I wish he could remember, he says "I can't even remember where *I* sleep." A flash of genius.

July 14 — Sunday, and middle daughter Rachel has been. For lunch. Chicken and salad have been eaten, and I have just left Prof R in his chair because he is totally jerking me around. He has barely eaten all day and it shows.

And after dinner, he rejected his strawberries and cream and so it goes on. Bell ringing. It's a yes-no night. Would you like savoury or sweet? Savoury. Savoury arrives and he won't even taste it.

"Turn that rubbish off", when I try to listen to the Wimbledon men's final, which has gone miles into a fifth set. I'm not trying to watch it. Just listen. I want to be with him. But he won't even let me listen to it. So I leave the room for a few minutes to cool off. Trying to reason with him will work sometimes and not others. And when I went back after 5 minutes, all calm and smiling, he ate his food.

July 15 — Rachel has asked me if she can have his old toolboxes. The ones he inherited from his father. I had to tell her most of them went when we left Wales. But I have kept two. This will happen a lot over the next few months I'm sure. When they realise what they are about to lose. And I will offer them anything we still have, but not anything that has emotional value to me.

Prof R ate normally today, which makes me think Rachel's visit upended his appetite yesterday. It doesn't matter. He is so withdrawn now. I'm finding it harder to connect with him except through touch. How much of what I say does he understand? I know he still wants to give and receive love. That's the easy part.

More old financial files have been disposed of. That is something he would be glad I am doing, if he knew. There is no need to anyone to trawl through his previous finances. They are his business.

July 16 — Tuesday. Another 'ramrod' morning trying to get Prof R's pills safely into him. We are doing what we can. Let's hope it will be good enough for a few weeks yet.

Today he has eaten well for Tina while I continue to trawl the sheds. Two people came today to collect garden tools and the 'failed experiment' – the adjustable back rest. I advertised it as "beach or bed" and it suits the beach far better than the bed.

I've uncovered more garden tools. This will please the woman who missed out on the first lot. Everything is going free. I can't be bothered trying to shift stuff for money. Everyone likes a bargain, and few want to pay.

While I was in town taking my 8mm film to Kodak in the hope of a DVD copy, Prof R rang his bell for Tina. She said, "What would you like?" and he said, "My people". Clearly royal blood will out.

I have just spent time chatting to him before dinner, telling him about my day, and what I have found. I amused him by saying "I can see why you used your nickname on the programmes for your theatre productions. So much more artistic." And he smiled.

But tonight, I made the mistake of feeding him before I had time to eat my own meal. What a difference it makes to my fatigue levels. If we are struggling with toileting or other tasks I can totally run out of steam.

—

In my shed exploring today I had found the event programme brochure for the *Wings Over Wanaka* vintage air display in New Zealand in 2004. There were pictures. Prof R seemed to recall it, so I lay on the bed beside him this evening and read to him from the programme. We both enjoyed it. Facts and figures about different aircraft and their roles during the war of the Pacific.

I still like reading to him, and used to do it quite a lot when I found something I thought would interest him. I wish there was more material that was worthwhile to share with him this way. Tina only managed to produce Peter Rabbit from our bookshelf. I was horrified, but managed not to show it. Dementia does not change someone's essential intellect. Or at least it hasn't for Prof R. Even if he only surfaces occasionally, he does not surface as a toddler.

July 18 — Yesterday was fairly standard, so there is nothing to see or say about it, except that I went to Pilates and found it, as usual, demanding. When we leave the classes, we all weave along the pavement like drunks leaving a wedding reception.

Tina has a day off. She is attending a graduation for her daughter's boyfriend at Cranwell. The preparations have been exhaustive. She has bought two dresses – one for daywear and the second for the evening ball. The dress code is typical MOD. Mad and Out-Dated.

The shed clear-out yesterday has got down to the depressing stage – dead mice and filth under all the boxes and a gracefully rotting and rusted portable tape machine of Prof R's. It almost fell apart in my hands. A museum would have loved it a few years ago.

But I did get a pleasant surprise. A perfectly good espresso machine that seems to have been replaced because it got mislaid in storage. I have tested it, and offered it to Tina and her husband if they would like it. Tina has asked for coffee making lessons first. She would like to be able to make one for Prof R if he asks when I am not here. As an indication of my energy levels, her request exhausts me. Pass.

—

I am still obsessed (diverted?) by food – or the lack of it. A critical tolerance point has been reached with the final 2 kg. No wonder Slimming World offer lifetime memberships. Whether I am suffering from food or comfort deprivation, how to determine the difference is the trick. Or it can just be fatigue. We eat for energy.

When Prof R wakes and rings his bell, sometimes he doesn't know why. When that happens, grooming is my default setting. Cutting his fingernails, washing his hands, trimming his beard.

We had a busy morning. Breakfast, bowel, foot bath, bed linen change. I was exhausted even if he wasn't. Now he should be ready for lunch, but after some TLC he has gone back to sleep. These are times when he just needs me to sit in the chair. Just to be there. No conversation. His eyes closed. So difficult when I don't feel like 'being in the moment'. And if I try to get up and leave the room, at least one eye will open and give me a beady stare.

—

Right now, I'm bored. I've had my lunch; I can't go into the shed in case I'm needed. I do love *Politics Live* but just now the bell went. The cure for housebound boredom is a project, and I don't need to cast my net very far in this house to find one. Both beds needing clearing out underneath and cleaned. Always, there are surprises, most of them rather unpleasant. But now we are ready for the new bed and the loft is ready for guests.

I wasn't the only one feeling active today. Prof R responded to my invitation to join me in a visit to the loft. While there, he decided to use the toilet. His homage to a happy two years. It is always a thrill for me when he goes 'out'.

July 19 — Friday. I almost lost Prof R on the floor this morning. Too eager to get him to the toilet, I didn't allow quite enough time for his legs to fully wake up. We must have been quite a sight, he and I, me shouting "Don't fall, don't fall, strong straight legs!" as his knees began to buckle. We did manage to stay off the floor. Lesson learnt, as the politicians keep saying. Again.

When Prof R is asleep, I can watch his eyes moving rapidly under the lids. Which means he must be dreaming a great deal. Yet he doesn't remember.

Netty brought more war memorabilia today and I found some books in the children's section of the library that are not infantile and have wonderful photos.

The 88 mm film I took to Kodak to be copied onto DVD turned out to be the wrong one. My uncle George appears briefly, and the rest is indeterminate landscape of indeterminate cities and bays. Disappointing for £30 but such is the nature of searching for history. I will take the second reel in on Monday. If they don't reject it for being wound the wrong way on the reel, I may yet get to see my family in the 1950s.

I have discovered the French film director Agnés Varda and intend to view all her films, which I have found on Prime. She has just released what she claims is her last film, *Varda by Agnés*.

—

But the day was not over. After salmon and chocolate ice cream, I read to Prof R from one of my library finds until his eyes drooped. Then I left him to sleep. It was 8.30 pm. Three minutes later, when I was about to pee in the next door bathroom, he rang his bell, and when I, incredulous, got back to the room he said "food".

For some reason this little straw landed like a grenade. I left the room and brought the empty dishes back up to prove to him that he'd had a meal. Then I said I would go downstairs, recover my good humour and return later. If he was still hungry ...blah blah blah. When I did, he was asleep, but still managed to open one eye. He amuses me enough so I can forgive him.

Interesting fact: Prof R can still tell the time on his watch. It's helpful when he is confused about whether it is morning or night, although a 24 hour watch would be more helpful

July 20 — Saturday. I am beginning to catch a glimpse of a commode on the horizon these last two or three days. Even at midday today, the trip to the toilet was made on bent plaiting legs. It doesn't feel safe and it isn't. That's not to say it would be necessary all the time. He must continue to try to walk whenever possible.

Today we are both tired. He extremely so. Breakfast was half eaten at midday, although a coffee and milkshake went down mid-morning. At breakfast, he needed prompting to swallow. He is hungry but no longer interested in what he is eating. Unless he doesn't like the taste.

He has gone straight back to bed after the toilet. Too tired for me to wash his hair, which I am itching to do because I want to tackle the return of the cradle cap. He's just itching.

Then he began to wake up. Lunch and ice cream at 4 pm and dinner at 6 pm. Bell ringing or alarm activating if the meal was too slow coming. Or he had forgotten my request to remain in bed until I returned. I had words. Mainly that he must talk to me. Because I know he can. And if he doesn't understand me, he can say so. He had enough energy to let me trim his moustache.

Dinner, salmon and sautéed mushrooms, was not a success. Only half eaten, so that by 6.45 pm, just as I sat down to my own meal, he was hungry again. I have brought a meal up. (As opposed to 'brought up my meal') One of my emergency Ella's Kitchen toddler supplies, which I can jazz up in an instant. And when I brought it up, he had gone back to sleep.

But I'll need to wake him for his evening pills and bedtime routine. I should stop trying to get him to interact with me, but I can't give up on him. Not when I know he is still in there somewhere.

—

I'm not coping as well as I'd like to with the unpleasant surprises. And then I feel guilty because the power in the relationship resides with me. Or so I like to think. But when he doesn't talk, usually when I am trying to get through to him, I find him very powerful indeed.

And when all else is going to hell in a handbasket, thank heavens for *Dateline London* at 3 am with a cup of tea. The little grey cells salute you.

Sunday 21 — An extremely difficult early morning pill round. Prof R could not wake sufficiently and when I raised him for an extra pillow he winced with pain. Eventually, he swallowed his pills at 8.45. At least, I am presuming they are not jammed onto the roof of his mouth.

This is only going to get worse. I fear how we will cope when he cannot respond at all, or walk. I know how to rip the sides of a pull-up to get them off a prone person but still have no idea how to put a clean one on without violating the patient. Who makes pants with Velcro sides? We will need side fasteners. Like toddler disposables. Even then, I still have to be able to lift or roll him enough to place it under him. When asked, Tina doesn't know. She just says 'slip sheets' again and that would mean no fleece. They use large mattress continence pads in the care home she says. Cheaper if you buy them from a pet shop. Heaven forbid we should have to resort to that.

As usual, Google saves me. There are any number of side-fastening 'slip' products available. But I will still need to learn how to use them. I am assuming 'slip' means what it says. And have visions of sliding them effortlessly beneath Prof R. This fantasy will be extinguished I'm sure, but not today.

At 11 am his legs are locked, and neither he or I can move them. His pull-ups have leaked, and he is wet but it's a very warm day and he is on his fleece. It doesn't matter immediately. What does matter is this: does this mean he needs more medication or less? He was late this morning. But on a previous occasion, this made no difference. The serious leg locking is a new thing. It used to be just first thing in the day, a little stiffness.

By midday he is still semi-conscious and unable to move. I do remember him having occasional days like this, even six months ago, but now it is more concerning because his muscle tone is so much weaker. We have tried CrampStop homeopathic spray, which works instantly with cramp. But this is a different animal.

Just to make life even more delightful, Lucas is sounding off next door. One of his noisier and more violent visits.

At 1.30 pm Prof R was still not mobile and was hallucinating. Not unusual, but disturbing for him. I tried to give him some super shake by spoon, but his mouth feels strange to him. Water is all I can manage with a toddler cup. Straws are no good.

It's Sunday, or I would call the Community Nurse. But he is not unsafe.

And in the end, desperate to get him into dry pants, I managed to rip the sides of the wet one without hurting his legs, and remove it. Then I ripped the sides of a new one and managed to put it on like a pad, pushing the back underneath his bottom, the front up between his legs. Penis secured, (dressing to the middle) I left his top on and didn't try to do trousers. He is lying like a big baby in a pad but hopefully relatively dry and comfortable.

By 3 pm he'd taken his next pills and a super shake from a spoon. He cannot suck on the straw. I can clean his mouth of mucus, but he cannot sit up yet to cough it out.

The new resealable slip pants have been ordered and will arrive in three days from Age UK. I didn't foresee a day like today coming so suddenly without more warning.

It was after 4 pm before he brightened the day by saying he could get up. It was ambitious as it turned out. We barely kept him off the floor crossing the finger-width from bed to chair. And he had a bare bottom, so it was a giant leap of stamina for Prof R to stand while I dragged up a fresh pull-up. He has no legs for the toilet. But ate his breakfast and spat out the pieces of pill that had indeed adhered to the roof of his mouth. Before he retired, I managed to get trousers on him. So much nicer than just bulky paper pants.

While I tried to keep him on track through all of this, I knew someone should be filming it. But it wasn't going to be me. Unless I wore a headcam. Now there's an idea.

What do we think of it so far? A truly awful day. And dinner was as fraught as lunch, with Prof R trying to go to the toilet but not finding his feet and fighting me when I physically propelled him back onto the bed to prevent a fall. It's very upsetting to think he might feel I am the enemy.

But he did eat, and he did smile when I assured him that he could pee in his pants and enjoy it. They were made for it. Designed with him in mind. Which amused him.

July 22 — Monday. At 10 pm last night he suddenly decided to get up. And he managed a drunken wobble to the toilet. My heart was in my mouth. He looked surprised that I doubted his ability. Hopefully he has forgotten our awful day. I gave him a levodopa before he lay down again. Money in the bank for today.

His muscles *are* working again today, but very little else. Tina says "It's just one of those days" but it is so much better than yesterday – he can walk to the toilet – that for me, it is a relatively good day. Telling him to swallow after every mouthful might not be total success but it is good to hear him say he is hungry.

The special side fastening 'slip pull-ups' arrived this morning. It's Monday and I only ordered them yesterday. When you are housebound caring for someone most of the time, internet shopping is a saviour (as I reminded myself while foolishly carting milk home from Tesco this afternoon in 29 deg).

Tina thinks we might get by without a hospital bed. Our motorised one should be enough. It all depends on the 'powers that be' of course and whether they will decide to do things that suit them, whether we like it or not. And whether it is good for Prof R or not.

—

My optician says my eyes are healthy but there is the faint beginning of cataracts.

Given I was repeatedly told by a succession of opticians that having lenses that react to light would prevent cataracts, I have decided to go for clear lenses with UV protection instead. For years, ever since 'transitions' were first invented in fact, I have put up with looking as if I am rudely wearing sunglasses when entering a shop or even having a conversation outside. And on an overcast day, I was in the gloom when everyone else basked in soft light. Forty years is a long time to be fooled. I will get retro clip-on sunglasses instead.

—

Although it's hot, the bedroom is on the morning side of the house, so Prof R is not overheating. But he sleeps for Britain and the Continent combined.

The Speech and Language (and Swallowing as it turns out) report came through the mail and she (Megan the Therapist) had misreported our in-bed feeding and fluids methods. When she tested Prof R's swallow reflex, he was lying reclined, because we were not giving him food or liquids at the time. And she did the test without requesting me to raise him upright.

She then said in her report I had been 'made aware' that it is dangerous to do this and Prof R should be upright. Fortunately, I was invited to provide feedback. I could have said that she had done 'worst practice', not us. But I reported it as a 'misunderstanding'.

My fear is that having an untruth such as that in writing reflects poorly on my ability to care for Prof R at home. She also didn't mention that Tina was present and was a trained and very experienced carer. My rating for Megan the therapist would be 'disappointing'. And yet she had been very pleasant and apparently professional.

—

Later: trying to wake Prof R early evening for his pills and a meal. Kissing didn't work, nor did the radio. I took drastic action and used the mini vacuum right outside his door. Still nothing. The irony does not escape me. If I wanted him to sleep, he would be awake.

Finally, at 7.30 pm I just woke him with a lot more enthusiasm, raised him up and gave him his pills. He can hear me, but he doesn't open his eyes. I want him to have more food, but he needs to be more awake. He's eaten very little today.

At 8.30 pm I made a determined effort and managed to wake him again. He ate lamb moussaka (Tesco's finest) and Gooseberry Fool (Tesco's, but not necessarily their finest) He ate it all. No toilet. "Later" he says. I hope I don't have to use the new slip-on tie-on's. Preferably without the need to 'tie one on' myself.

July 23 — Prof R did not get up for the toilet, but I have perfected the art of medicating him while he is half awake. He will respond and can help me a little with placing extra pillows and raising him to a safe height. At least one I deem safe. If not necessarily best practice. And he follows swallowing instructions.

What to say about today? I managed to get Prof R's tie-on slip pants onto him while lying in bed. Because he could help me by rolling onto his side. I will get better with practice, but the test will be what a friend of mine used to call "big pants".

Tina has told me how she does it. I don't ask the obvious. Why didn't she tell me about side-fastening adult pants when I asked earlier? Because she fears getting it wrong? I also watched a tutorial on YouTube. But I'm still a little nervous about whether I will be able to do it without accident or incident or sheer disaster. This is a sudden upskilling. It will become the norm quite quickly. But it's not a happy change of circumstance for Prof R.

———

He could not walk to the toilet today for Tina, although he ate most of his lunch and his ice cream before trying to walk to the door. He was too unsteady on his feet for safety and Tina had to tell him so. This loss of legs is going to affect him deeply emotionally and mentally. I'm hoping it is a short-lived blip and not the major step-change that we know will come.

The next pants change will be done in bed again and I'm sure I will get better at it very quickly, before any bigger test. It's harder now for me to remain cheerful.

But oh, the relief when his alarm went off at 5.30 pm and he was able to walk to the toilet. Still a man of few words, but able to eat some of his dinner, slow motion swallowing style, and all of his ice cream. The legs still have 'legs'.

July 24 — Wednesday. Boris Johnson is sworn in as the next Prime Minister and makes an ass of himself at the podium in Downing Street promising lollies for Christmas and a new deal Brexit. Only one word for it – disappointing.

Theresa was almost gleeful on her departure. Good. She deserves to feel good about something.

Prof R's mobility has returned to 'normal'. Tina and I are so relieved.

The best news of the day was the biggest surprise. The new mechanical bed is ready and will be installed next Wednesday. A whole week before Douglas arrives, so Prof R and I can sleep upstairs in the loft the night beforehand. As long as he doesn't lose his legs again.

Tina and I will dismantle our bed in the morning.

—

I discovered that Tina had recorded in her logbook that she had given Prof R his afternoon pill at 3 pm, when it was due, but I knew it was 3.30 pm. Not important in itself. We had discussed the fact that the delay didn't matter, but it's important for me to know the correct time is recorded, so the following dose is correct. I understand why she wants to appear to be doing things when scheduled, but I need to tell her that's not as important as accuracy.

Otherwise, we are doing well here. I tried to discuss the political drama of the day with her but it's not her 'thing'. She walked into the room when Boris was speaking at his lectern and started chatting. I had to say, "Sorry Tina, Boris is speaking". Although as it turned out, he wasn't saying anything very intelligent. Hard to believe that man's IQ is off the scale. Which end??

I had to wake Prof R for his pills and his evening meal. But he did manage to show an interest in the VE-Day souvenir newspapers Netty had left for him. So seldom does he have the energy to take an interest in books, but photos still draw him in. Especially the photos of the street parties and the children. He seems to be looking for people he knows. Or perhaps he is looking for himself. In one photo, a young boy was standing up in the front of a truck and Prof R thought he knew him. And perhaps he did.

July 25 — A fun day for some, with temperatures up to 38 deg, but a terrible day for Prof R. We had trouble getting him sitting enough to keep him hydrated. And Tina worried me considerably when she came downstairs and said she couldn't get him to drink. She had been dripping water into his mouth with a wet cloth.

I went straight upstairs with the toddler cup and talked to him constantly till he sucked on it and drank. His swallow has only recently been checked and is good still, but his fatigue and weakening tongue makes everything more difficult.

I had to ask Tina what she would have done if I had been out. I have to be able to trust her to find solutions, not throw her hands up. It just requires perseverance, and she lacks that unfortunately. And it could be risky for Prof R. She said, "You're so much more confident than me" and I said, "No I'm not, I'm working blind here too, but what choice do I have? I can't give up". In this heat you could get cross but I'm just going to have to trust her or hire a trained nurse.

Something funny did happen which lightened the day. The folding director's chair broke under her – not so she fell on the floor – but her weight was too much. I told her not to worry. But she needs a stronger chair. She suggested bringing a big garden one from her home.

There's nothing like a bad idea to stimulate a better one. The solution for me turned out to be a commode. I have found an armchair style cane one that she can use, and Prof R can sit in it for his meals. I had been thinking it won't be long before we need one and getting one that can hold people up to 24 stone seems like catching two birds with each stone. It will probably have been delivered by the time she returns on Monday.

Tonight, I woke him at 6ish, and he ate a little supper and some ice cream. The most striking thing today, and perhaps yesterday, is that he is not opening his eyes. I'm not sure why.

Thunderstorms are beginning overhead and it's wonderful. Perhaps when it's cooler he will revive.

July 26 — Friday. He did revive. But not until Netty arrived at 1 pm.

Being comatose until then meant that I was able to practice my bed-based changing skills. But Prof R was not happy. Half asleep, he fought to keep his trouser pants up while I cajoled and convinced him that it was necessary. Because it was. In the end I was pleased to achieve some sort of result that was good enough, if not perfect. And he did help me roll him on one side to place the clean one.

Later, Netty succeeded in getting him to the toilet. He was wobbly but he made it. Any day now that he can still do that is a good day for him and us. But he's not eating much. Breakfast cereal and ice cream and a milkshake earlier in the day but no lunch.

He is wearing his new short-sleeved shirt I bought him. Netty took a photo because he looks so good. If only his arms were not so long and angular it would be easier to put it on, but nothing is easy to put on.

I also bought myself something that is probably ludicrous. A so-called nurse's watch, to wear on my front, because I fear scratching Prof R now that I am lifting him so much. And I don't want to keep taking my watch on and off. I'll have to take it off to go out of course, unless I wear it under my shirt.

The weekend looms. No help, no room for mistakes.

Tonight I had to wake him at 7 pm for pills and managed some food and ice cream. He wouldn't get up though. Everything was done in bed.

No desire to go to the bathroom. At 9 pm there was more ice cream and a coffee, so another pill for good measure.

At least his eyes were open.

July 27 — Saturday. I have successfully put on my third prone-fitted side-tie pants, but not without considerable co-operation from Prof R. On a good day, he can roll with help. If he couldn't I'm not sure I could move him alone. Or wash him, which is essential. I am bathed in sweat, even though it is raining outside. And much cooler.

It may be a coincidence that he is more alert today now that the temperatures have blessedly returned to normal. Alertness is an unpredictable science with Prof R's brand of Parkinson's, with the dementia thrown in to clog the wheels.

His middle daughter once said she didn't know how I stayed sane. At the time, I thought it was my responsibility to stay sane. And took it for granted. But when I find myself repeating requests or instructions over and over, ad infinitum, and the food is on a loop to the fridge and back, I too wonder. When he doesn't answer me, when I know his voice is sound.

Every day I vow it won't begin to get to me as the day wears on, and each day I find myself gradually burning the wrong end of the candle. Today my heart started to flutter in protest. Fortunately, a sit-down and a breath of other intellects (*Dateline London*) restores the balance.

He went to the toilet on his own legs at lunchtime, which automatically made this a good day, but meant first pulling down, and then up, the tie-side pants I'd struggled valiantly to fit in the bed. As I need the practice, it was an opportunity to learn another skill. The tie-sides are so much easier to take down than pull up.

—

The loft has been prepared for our Tuesday overnight stay before the mechanical bed arrives on Wednesday. It would be tempting to go upstairs earlier, when Prof R has a window of mobility. I'm so looking forward to this new bed I feel like dismantling our current one around us and sleeping on the mattress on the base. That wouldn't do much for Prof R's mobility. It would be almost as bad as being floored by a fall.

My weight is down to 59.5Kg. 1.5 kg to go. What a tedious process this has been. Three months to take it off. An excellent diversion, but I'm sure I could add 10 kg a lot more efficiently.

Lunch was at 2.30 pm. I say lunch, but it is so punctuated with sips of water, just at the moment, it's a wonder he eats anything. The ice cream gets a once over. A super shake the same. He's like a picky customer in a delicatessen, sampling all the free wares. Then I clean his mouth and back into bed he goes. But at least his legs worked.

I'm going to watch an episode of *Big Little Lies, Series 2*.

At dinner, I became very disheartened. It's a marathon, and all energy goes into trying to meet the needs of the professor. It was beef cottage pie and beans and delicious. He ate some, and we experimented with putting his pills in the food instead of trying to swallow them with water, which is such a thin liquid. The second pill he picked out of his mouth and tried to refuse to take it. I just say "Sorry, it's not an option" and pop it back in. When he'd had a few more mouthfuls he just blocked me with his hand. And I said, "Oh fuck you then" and that was the best laugh he had all day. Nice smile.

Then he ate some ice cream; then he appeared to want to get up; once seated, he decided to lie down again. As if I had imagined it. And when I said, "You did ask to get up didn't you?" He said, "Yes". I know he can talk, but he doesn't for some reason. Even just a couple of words is enough to make things so much easier. I always tell him he can get away with it because I love him, and he knows it. I'm sure he isn't as offhand with Netty and Tina. They say how nice his manners are.

Tina asked me last week who I am able to 'vent' to. Well, what to say?

I have learned that to vent is dangerous. If I am judged 'not coping' and my humour is too black, too honest, even close family who should be safe confidants may judge me for it. And there is always the fear I can be accused of inadequate care. I have two old friends I can email who I can trust. Who both know how much I love him, even if I am emotionally exhausted.

I wish I could cuddle him properly. I miss being a proper wife.

July 28 — Sunday. I have finally discovered why Prof R's left-over breakfast seems to grow in the fridge overnight. It is because I add nutritional yeast. I have thrown it out and started again this morning without the yeast.

As Prof R would say, our morning was like the Curate's egg – good in parts. The drama of the hard parts can obscure the successes. He got up. He sat in his chair to eat. He went to the toilet and passed something significant, efficiently, without fuss.

But on our way back with the zimmer to his chair he almost lowered his undercarriage on the taxiway instead of the runway. That was a shouty moment for me. And then there was the incredible tedium of eating successfully. Some spoonful's of this, a sip of that, a taste of the other. A good cough and a spit in between. Until we were both exhausted.

Usually, I knock myself out trying to find interesting things to tell Prof R. But when he is eating, he can't reply. And when he isn't, he is equally likely not to reply. Netty said on Friday that she has decided not to talk to him while he eats because he seems able to concentrate better on the job in hand if she is quiet. I tried that this afternoon, at lunch. And he ate it all. Eventually. I have to be careful I don't drop off to sleep in the endless seconds elapsing between swallows. But it is less stressful for me and seems to work. He even had the energy to clean his teeth.

July 29 — Evening yesterday was sleepy again – just a few bites of food

– but a trip to the toilet, so he began the night dry and clean. I am continuing to give him a last levodopa when I go to bed, and so far, he is definitely more mobile.

Today I watched Tina move as fast as she could when his bed alarm went off while we were both downstairs. He was slow enough for her to meet him sitting on the edge of the bed. At times like that, when I am here with her, I feel like saying, "Don't worry I'll go" or even "Out of my way!" and running up the stairs in front of her. Because I am a lot faster. And even I am often not fast enough.

—

Netty has alerted me to yet more kit, a sort of sitting travelator. It would enable us to take him on his tours of the first floor or even downstairs for a 'walk' without the stress of hoping his legs won't buckle.

I've found one at the local mobility shop and it will be delivered tonight for a trial run. Just in time for the move to the loft tomorrow in preparation for the arrival of the new bed. Tina worries he won't use his feet and should have foot plates for safety. But that would defeat the purpose. This is not intended to be a wheelchair. So, if he can't use his feet, it will go back.

July 31 — Wednesday. This was supposed to be bed moving day. But after a day of bed demolition, Prof R's removal to the loft, and a big clean-up of the bedroom, a phone call at 11am from the bed people to say they had "misremembered" the delivery day and thought it was tomorrow. Which now of course it will have to be.

I could not be good natured about this, although I remained polite. There is no excuse, as Richard-the-incompetent was told exactly how fragile Prof R is, and knew we had to transfer him to another bed in order to have the new one installed. It seems to me they are unused to supplying beds to truly disabled people, and visualise Prof R and I reading in bed, on a nice gentle incline, before heading off on our overseas cruise.

So, another day in the loft for me and Prof R. We used the new wheelie chair twice to keep him off the floor and it worked. This morning it got him from the loft toilet to the bed when his legs had given way.

But, under-promising and over-performing as always, Prof R got up at midnight last night and succeeded in waddling to the toilet with just my help. He is disturbed, but not perturbed, by being in the loft. We are both happy to be back 'home'. It is a much more spacious and restful room.

—

Without Tina's help there are many things now I could not do. She helped me dismantle the old bed and move it into Prof R's office. And without her (and the new wheelie chair) Prof R would have landed bottom first on the floor of the bathroom this morning. Some things are no longer possible solo.

When I am out all day, as I will be when Douglas is here, she will cope as I do, and she may need sometimes to change him in bed. But at least the new bed will help and not hinder her. It's going to be such a relief.

—

Today I picked up my new glasses and immediately regretted all those years with transition lenses. Now the light is as it should be. I am seeing properly. And on overcast days, when my transitions plunged me into gloom, I will see how bright it really is.

I picked up a cine film that I had paid £30 to have copied and discovered that yet again, it does not contain the footage that I am looking for. Instead, it was endless captive animals and monkeys having tea parties at Auckland Zoo. Uncle George, you wasted an awful lot of film.

—

I'm trying to develop safer ways for Tina and I to move Prof R. She said if he can put his arms around us, we can turn in unison – like trick cyclists – to put him in the right position to sit down. Either together or when I am on my own. I tried it tonight, but Prof R panicked when we turned because he couldn't see the bed behind him. So we were locked in combat until I won, with a massive joint lurch backwards onto the bed. Not very successful. But a safe landing. Trust is the thing that prevents him allowing me to guide him.

While I was out this afternoon, Tina had a rather diverting time with Prof R in a confused state, wandering and saying, "I want to go to Oxford Circus". She understands more and more how difficult his illness is.

But for an hour or so before he ate his dinner, I sat with him and read from the archive material Netty has loaned to us. A children's newspaper from 1941; an English school composition written by a child in 1938 at the time of the appeasement and recipes for desserts which featured mashed or grated potato as the main ingredient. I'm probably enjoying it more than Prof R. It seems to fill in so many gaps of my own understanding of how it must have been on the home front.

August 1 — Thursday. Finally, it is 'bed day'. The bed, which looks smaller than the one it replaces, even though it is supposed to be 4 inches longer, is in, made up, but with no Prof R yet.

We couldn't move him, because he has lost his legs today. In fact, Tina encouraged me to help her take him to the bathroom when it was totally unsafe, and we only managed to get him cleaned and back to bed by our sheer joint brute strength. I never want that to happen again. It had been hair-raising enough just getting him up to the loft, without taking unnecessary risks while there. My goal is keeping him safe. Mobility is a bonus.

As it was, this morning, before she arrived, I had already changed him in the bed, because he was uncomfortable. This is the first time that a poo in his pants has been noticed by him. It was good practice for me, although I could have done without it today. I did manage to clean him and re-clad him haphazardly. But he was clean and dry and happy to go back to sleep.

When the new bed was being installed, I discovered that because it was unique, and custom-made, none of the bed rails we already have will fit it. The tutorial I had watched on YouTube applied to beds with three folding sections, and ours has five.

So halfway through the installation, I ordered a freestanding cot rail that the helpful installer said will not attach to the bed, as is ultimately desirable, but which I will make sure is attached well enough with whatever devices are to hand. Bungy cords 'spring' to mind.

In the meantime, I have used a child rail and a bookcase to secure the bed side. And of course, it isn't needed tonight after all, because we'll still be in the loft, but hopefully, with Netty's help, it will be in use tomorrow.

It was 29 deg here a few moments ago and it is almost 7 pm. The loft is cooking, but we are used to it. Two fans keep us from melting. I need to wake the 'baby' for his evening pills.

When I tell him I love him he says with a smile "snap".

I look terrible at the moment, in spite of my new glasses. It's hard to disguise the tired eyes. But fortunately, I feel better than I look.

August 2 — Friday. Prof R is stiff and sore this morning. Even two hours after his morning pills. He let me massage his limbs and try the CrampStop. Then I suggested a roll towards the middle of the bed and that did the trick. He has immediately dropped off to sleep.

So now is the time to begin turning him in the night. He is not moving himself at all, which wasn't a problem in the past, because he was walking more. But now it is a problem.

I'm hoping that by the time Netty gets here I will have successfully changed his pants. Or better still, he has been able to walk to the toilet. I still feel angry with myself about yesterday when Tina and I nearly lost him to the floor. I should not have allowed it to happen simply because I didn't want to undermine Tina.

She is so sensitive if I suggest anything, such as more detail in her log (my euphemism for 'not leaving things out'). I can only assume it is about liability; as if she fears she will be examined on the contents, (subsequent court of enquiry?) and wants to leave out anything that has been difficult. I appreciate she is a high achiever. But her goals relate to her, rather than Prof R. He is my priority. But she has definitely made the daily record more human. It's great to read. And I always tell her so.

In the care home, she tells me, they have no time to record anything other than basic tasks. Now she has almost too much time.

—

Mr Electric Bed Installer had asked me if I had a nurse to help me. I'm beginning to think that is what I do need now. And after cleaning Prof R in the bed once more, I am more competent but no less stressed. This time he was more co-operative, rolling. But it feels like an inadequate clean when you are mopping up masses of the brown stuff and trying to keep it contained. I certainly manage better with the replacement side-tie nappies. And get his trousers back up as well. But what a physical effort it is.

Netty proved I was right to wait for her before this move downstairs. She is determined and capable and confident. Prof R was totally weak and barely able to stand. But together, working as a team, with the zimmer, the chair walker, and the stairlift, and lots of positive voice commands, we got him back to base. The trust issue made Prof R fearful, but we talked to him constantly and he held on.

We are all three exhausted. Netty said that if the move had not been possible, we would have needed to call the paramedics to do what she called "an assisted move". But cheers to us, mission accomplished. Still some electric bed skills to master. And awaiting a new cot rail. But home safe. Huge relief.

Seeing him sitting safely on the bed with Netty, sipping a drink with a straw, so frail, tears spring to my eyes.

August 3 — This is the reality for Prof R when he has had a very tiring day. He ate no meal last night and all I can get into him is water and pills. Water being as important as the pills.

The new bed, while appearing precarious without a proper rail, is at least fulfilling its promise of raising him up into a sitting position without backbreaking efforts from both of us.

He is comatose today and his legs are locked, so I can't even change his pants. They, the pants, are some sort of miracle, because he is not 'leaking'. And he apparently hasn't passed a motion, or he would be showing discomfort.

In the end I decided to text Tina for advice. She offered to pop round and we changed him together. Prof R grimaced and squirmed, but as it turned out, I was wrong, and he *had* soiled his pants. It had taken some effort to swallow my pride and get help. But I needed it. We rigged up a sling with a sheet and tried to move him towards the centre of the bed.

Now he is at least clean and comfortable. And I managed to spoon a milkshake into him. But he dozes on, and frankly, I'm exhausted too. It's taken a while to hit me after such a stressful week, and the failure to cope alone today.

Cheering myself up meant clearing the loft and all the sickroom paraphernalia so Douglas doesn't arrive to a mini hospital room. The riser on the toilet has gone, and the toilet frame. The rail off the bed finally removed as well. There will be no going back.

In between all the stressful stuff I have watched a large slice of a boxed set on TV. Now I know why people watch them. Total escapism. My medicine.

August 4 — "Houston we have a problem." Prof R has started chewing his pills, depositing them on a tooth, or the roof of his mouth, and then complaining later (by pointing) that there is a foreign object in his mouth. This morning, after a portion of levodopa came back for a second time, I opened the Rivastigmine capsule and put the powder on a spoon and mixed it with milkshake. It sort of worked, in that it was still hard to get the residue totally off the spoon and into his mouth.

I have to do a lot of clear commands at the moment. "Darling, open your mouth. Pill coming in. Don't chew it. Here is the water. Suck on the spout. Suck on the spout (when his mouth remains wide open).

But he did eat most of a meal last night. There is still no sign that he will be able to get out of bed. His legs remain, knees bent, turned sideways, looking for an escape from the side of the bed. No matter how hard I try to move him closer to the middle, he seems to gravitate to the edge. He is wedged in with bookcase, child gate and the new commode chair (because it is heavy it stops him kicking over the bookcase).

We've been almost to this desperate state before and retreated, so I am hoping for the same today. Otherwise, it will be another agonising solo change of his pants via locked legs.

And then I had a small triumph, depending on your point of view. I managed to change his pants, soiled, by talking him through what I was doing, apologising, and then doing it, rolling him, regardless of wincing. It was still a little amateurish, but I did it, and felt much more confident. I have said, and thought, so many times, why don't home carers get offered training from the Community Nurse? It would be so much better for everyone concerned.

Email from his eldest daughter, says "I'm so sorry it's getting so hard. I really want to be there for you and Dad, but it feels like there are so many other demands at the moment. Everyone is very fragile."

I said "Thanks Hannah. Don't worry. Enjoy your holiday."

—

I am reminded of why Prof R was so keen to go to New Zealand in 2003. The girls rarely visited him, before or after I first arrived. Crossing London from North to South of the river is indeed a trial. Although they would come for family meals.

But when we announced we were going to New Zealand, they were angry and demanded an explanation. What they got was a partial truth. That Michael wanted to finish his schooling there. He happily took the heat for a lot our decisions that his sisters didn't like.

—

More and more I dread the aftermath when he has gone. Each of us, he (when he could choose) and I, would be happy with a simple cremation. But there is no way of knowing what his daughters will want when the moment arrives. And I will invite them to decide. I suspect they will find it daunting, if I am lucky, and be relieved if I manage it for them.

At his current rate of decline, dearest Prof R won't even be well enough to use the new commode. So much money literally down the toilet. And I wonder if people actually use slipper pans anymore? Probably only those without dementia.

He has just managed an afternoon pill and some coffee and milkshake. He is too dopey to risk muesli, even though it is very liquid. He is lying to the side, regardless of how I try to rearrange the pillows.

A flaw in the bed design. The pillows too easily slip off the top of the mattress when it is raised; while Prof R drifts down towards the foot. I always think of Mae West and her best line, "I was Snow White, but I drifted".

August 5 — Monday. 5.00 am Such a struggle yesterday to get him to take food. I managed to get most of two meals into him – the muesli ending up being a dessert at 7.30 pm. And at least three milkshakes. So he is getting nutrition still.

If I cannot get his legs moving this morning, I will phone the Community Nurse. We have to unlock him somehow and also register the changes in his condition with someone medical. Trying to get the GP out is pointless unless there is an emergency. Although it feels quite like an emergency to me at the moment, as I try to contain the bent twigs in the bed.

At 6.30 am I tackled his pants and felt far more confident about it, if no stronger. Pulling it out from underneath his bottom resulted in it tearing. But I rolled him with encouraging words and ignoring the face pulling. Telling him it was the only way to make him comfortable. He was fairly soiled, as seems usual now, but I sprayed and wiped, and I hope it made his skin safe and comfortable for the rest of the day.

Putting on the new 'nappy' is the same as doing it with an overweight unresponsive baby. Very difficult. He cannot lift his bottom at all. But we got there eventually. This morning I have ordered a slip pad which I hope will help with all this moving and under-bum slipping in and out.

In spite of the difficulties, I do feel much more able to do this job alone. The bottom and the top of Prof R are the challenging areas. His cleanliness at the bottom end and food, liquids and pills at the top. I'm still using capsules when I think it will work. Because it occurs to me that neither Tina nor Netty will be interested in emptying capsules into a teaspoon of milkshake without medical approval.

I have not yet decided whether to call the Community Nurse. He can be moved, locked or not. At first, I tried the magnesium spray. It didn't work. I will call the CN.

———

The Community Nurse phone line was not answered due to the volume of calls. So I left it until after Tina arrived. And when she did, we rigged up a slip sheet to draw him up to the top of the bed. Then we rolled him onto his back and worked on his legs together, with the magnesium spray as more of a hope than a belief.

Eventually, Prof R managed to straighten his legs at least two thirds of the way. Not before time. He is beginning to show the signs of pressure spots. Now he has a pillow between his legs and lies on his back. It's not a cure. As the day wore on his legs stiffened again. We will have to work on them every day. Both of us fear that he may get a premature trip to hospital if we send up a distress flare when it can be dealt with at home.

The sheer physical effort required to move Prof R this way is unbelievable, given his weight. Even though his circulation is good, and all his limbs can move, he no longer seems able to help us with anything we need to do, including changing his pants.

With Tina's help, I was able to give him a much better wash and skin care of his 'underlings'. Too many days crammed in close confines of a pull-up are not good for these sensitive little parts of the anatomy. From now on Tina and I will do a change and thorough clean together before she leaves in the afternoon, and I will change him solo in the morning.

—

Within days, Prof R's care has escalated to orange alert. It's frightening how quickly it has happened and I blame, in part, the delay in moving back down from the loft. He has lost the use of his legs in the process. It seems doubtful today whether he will ever regain it. The Community Nurse is only a phone call away.

I have 'knives' in my throat on one side, but one paracetamol is enough every 4 hours to keep it at bay. It's "going around" apparently, but nothing to worry about. I've felt better, but I've also felt a lot worse. And if I pass it on to Prof R I will know how to treat it.

He's eaten all his dinner and more ice cream. Which is just as well as he didn't have breakfast or lunch. Just ice cream. His legs are gravitating to the side again. Bending and trying to go their own way. Tina's pillow between the knees will hopefully stop them going too far or fusing together.

While I love him more than I could ever have believed possible, I find

I can also be totally frustrated at this time of the evening, when (not his fault) I have been up since 5 am. I don't take failure well. And he is not opening his mouth or his eyes. I'm using Tina's trick of placing the spoon on his bottom lip. It does seem to stimulate him to swallow the previous mouthful and open his mouth. Not always, but often enough. It would be easy to think he is being wilful, because he can still talk, and very clearly, when he wants to.

—

Earlier today I knocked on the door of the woman neighbour who has beautiful coloured glass stones scattered on her doorstep. I wanted to thank her for putting one through my letter box. She was friendly but puzzled. No, it wasn't her. So, her stones are being nicked by someone and put through letter boxes as a prank. I don't care because it gave me huge pleasure when I found it.

August 6 — Tuesday. A day of considerable improvement in our situation on all fronts.

The first change went well at 7.30 am. Sometimes it seems easier alone than when I do it with Tina. One person is less complicated.

The cot rail arrived and is perfect. I think it may have been a 'second' because it was much cheaper than other suppliers, but when I told them a couple of rubber locks needed replacing, they say it will be in the mail today.

The slip sheet arrived and is also perfect. It has handles and is well made and it was also cheap.

Prof R began to eat more and has had his eyes open. He manages a smile after Tina and I have buffeted him around in ways that hurt his muscles, but he understands we need to do it.

We're both still becoming accustomed to the strengths and weaknesses of the bed. More strengths we feel. But with Prof R suddenly bedridden (we hope temporarily) changing his upper clothing becomes much more difficult. We are leaving that problem to mull overnight before tackling it. And perhaps Prof R will regain some of his strength and be able to sit unaided tomorrow.

Tina's training does not cover locations without hoists and other equipment that we have no space for, don't want, and I'm sure we can manage without. I'm sure I could change his top alone with the rolling method. We shall see.

Currently, while I am here all the time, we do his afternoon change and wash together, but I want her able to do it alone in future. Because I am already doing the morning one at about 7 am, and managing by myself. Though I really enjoy having her working with me to problem-solve a lot of the issues that are now emerging. Two heads really are better than one. And it's less lonely when there is a challenge to overcome.

Tonight, he chewed his pills again. And again, his face made me think he was just fed up and doing it because I'd asked him not to. I leave the room for a few minutes sometimes when we are at an impasse. And when I go back, I say, "Shall we start again?" because any impasse makes me more upset than it does him.

He did eat half a meal and the ice cream, and later a whole milkshake. So this is officially the best day of eating in the last five or so. And I am less exhausted, although still ignoring that sore throat. I am very careful to only kiss Prof R on other areas of his face. No lips.

—

And when I am kissing him, again I wonder if it is normal for a wife to become a little jealous of her husband's interactions with other women who care for them. Tina makes a point of saying, "Oh, lots of nice hand holding today." And of course, I say "That's lovely" but I feel a wrench. Because the danger is the 'good cop, bad cop' roles. The 'parent' who has custody versus the one who visits bringing treats. And because he has dementia, I worry he will eventually forget I'm his wife and think one or both of them are, and love them accordingly.

—

The teeth were cleaned. Prof R quite happy for me to inexpertly wield his toothbrush. Every little achievement is a minor triumph.

August 7 — Prof R's condition declines not by inches but by huge trench-edge falls. A week ago he could still walk. For the last few days, he could barely move, and every movement hurt him. Today, with a huge effort, Tina and I managed to get him to sit on the edge of the bed and lower his legs to the floor. This is a real advance from legs locked in foetal mode. And it meant we could change his top and wash his torso.

Where there is still no improvement, is toileting. And he now soils much more frequently, so I will need to change him once more this evening and again in the morning before Tina arrives.

We've become more worried about pressure points. Rather than ring the Community Nurse, to request a ripple mattress complete with motor (Tina's first thought) I have bought a pressure pad which promises results. And would at least help us keep him from losing ground. He's surprisingly calm and content in spite of all this handling. Not when it is happening, but afterwards. He realises it's a necessary evil.

So far, the condition of his skin has been a source of pride. We clean him thoroughly with each change and put barrier creams on him, but sitting up in a chair is the ideal. And the new commode, rejected and dejected, has been moved to another room. It isn't even comfortable enough for Tina to sit in. She needs more cushioning and it wins no prizes for that. A replacement folding garden chair has been brought into service.

I risked a bath and a hair wash after Tina had left. Sleeping beauty looked settled. My first bath in ages. It's been too hot for baths.

August 8 (Douglas Day) — He arrived before Tina and was such a wonderful sight at my front door. Jet-lagged and tired, but here.

It had been a tough morning. A big clean-up of Prof R, washed fleece and sheet. The works. And he is so hurt by my moving him. Painkiller – liquid ibuprofen – is my first line of defence. Our mothers would have told us "It's hurting me more than it hurts you", but looking at Prof R's silent open mouth, I doubt that very much.

My son thinks the commode is very cool. It does look nice. Should I try to send it back? I've no idea.

Sunday 11 — Without Douglas, I could not have done what I needed to do for Prof R this morning. I had to change his top, which was wet, and put cream on a scrape I have discovered on his mid right shoulder. An unwelcome first.

The District Nurse was phoned and came at lunchtime. She has relieved my mind. The wound is not something worse – namely, a bed sore. But I hate to see any broken skin on him. It is a portent of potential disaster. She has also said the GP should now come out, so armed with that referral I will approach the practice again in the hope of a visit.

His youngest daughter Julie visited yesterday, and was hosted by Tina, while Douglas and I were in London, catching up with the kids. Prof R roused himself for his daughter and has not roused himself since. I can barely get his medications into him and no food yet by early afternoon.

Caring for him alone becomes more and more fraught with risk for both of us. Douglas is only here for two weeks, but at least I know he will help with lifting.

What thereafter? How does anyone cope with a prone man with no muscle power? I can roll and I can change and wash his lower body, but I can't change his shirts. Without Douglas, Tina would have had to be summoned – again. And while she is willing, she will not always be available, and it is not how I wish to treat people on their day off. She is not paid to be on call.

It will all be managed somehow. It always is.

An afternoon spent experimenting. When he was more awake, I discovered his fresh shirt had acted as a wick, just like the first, but this time I was determined to do this solo. And I managed. Just as well no one is doing a survey of how the patient felt, but we got through (more easily because there was no poo).

Then it was food and phlegm. Some breakfast, pills dissolved in a spoon of milkshake, coughing and coughing and him now alert enough and able to help me try to clean his mouth. But the rattle is still there. Not in the chest – yet. Water is the best way to shift it.

He's also not comfortable. I am going to ask Douglas to help with this. Hoisting him further up the bed and putting a flat pillow behind his shoulders to see if that will help.

I experimented with pain relief. Poking holes in ibuprofen capsules and finding a syringe and liquid pain killer kept for a visiting child. He likes the taste. He might end up getting that treat regularly before I try to move him in future.

Douglas has spent the afternoon in the garden making a huge impact. How wonderful to have a son who would rather be doing something than blobbing on the couch. And I have two of them.

Only a spoonful or two of dinner at night, after an hour of trying, and no ice cream. But comfortable and phlegm-free enough to settle and sleep soundly. Prof R may not know me all the time, but he does at least some of the time.

August 13 — The GP finally came today. Dr T, who we knew and had seen before. A very practical man, who understood exactly how we (the Royal 'we') want this thing to go. He also understood, and had nothing negative to say, about blending the capsule contents into milk shakes.

He has prepared a lot of paperwork for me to see the process through, including a certificate for DNR (Do not resuscitate). I told him I had no health LPA and understood the implications of that, but he did it for me. I said what he needed me to say. "It would be cruel to resuscitate him" and he agreed.

I pick up three things tomorrow morning. Morphine so he can be changed without pain in the mornings, emergency medications for use (by a crisis team) if he is very distressed, and the forms, including the care plan, that need to be kept in appropriate places.

I feel trusted by the medical practice to do this and it is such a relief. Dr T saw no reason why Prof R should need to be moved. Unless something untoward should happen, there need be no hospital bed. Or a hospital transfer.

The professional advice I have had to date has often been things that make life easier for the carers, not the life of the patient. I have worried about a hospital bed for months, probably needlessly, after being told agency nurses would not tend him in our bed.

If he continues as he is, he should be able to die in peace in his own bed. Or at least, the new one that is now his own. It is all I have ever wanted for him. The stress of its installation might have hastened the process, but so would a move to a hospital bed. And we couldn't manage without it.

—

Douglas works busily on all my messy shed detritus, some of which has turned out to be his, and has wired up the hive thermostat, which operated on batteries and always ran out.

I'm glad he will get a break when he goes up to London on Friday to stay with Hope. I feel terrible that he has had to be in such a sad house, although I try not to make it so. We talk a lot, but we are careful not to talk a lot about Prof R, unless there is something I need to do.

August 14 — First dose of morphine: 10.40 am – 2.5 ml. Second dose: 11.30 am – 2.5 ml (first dose not sufficient for pain relief). But before I could do that, when Tina arrived, a race to the chemist, and relief the medication was finally there. (A day later than promised, so that Prof R had suffered for longer unnecessarily, and so had I.) Plus paperwork from the GP Practice, including the DNR.

I was running on high octane fuel, too high, mainly because his girls and Doris and Brian were agitating on the phone while I was trying to focus on the job in hand. Serves me right for contacting them.

Morphine is a terrifying medication for the uninitiated. Tina told me how to fill the syringe dropper. But she is not permitted to do it. So I took the plunge. It took two 5ml doses to reach a level where I felt I could leave him with her. If he had been more alert, I would have stayed.

But instead, I took Douglas to Canterbury. It was intoxicating, an escape, and while it rained and blew, we had a lovely few hours. Lunch at Byron's paid for by him. Briefly, I felt like a kid on holiday.

—

Home again, we found Doris and Brian on the sofa. I had phoned to suggest they might want to visit. They hadn't been for a few weeks, so I wanted to warn them that Prof R was not doing well. I had suggested Sunday. But this morning they rang, suddenly panicked, saying they wanted to see him now because Sunday may be too late. It seemed premature.[1] And I heard myself say to Brian, "You know you could have visited at any time". Brian said, "I know".

Later, Tina told me that when they first arrived, they had lamented loudly about Prof R's prognosis, in front of the sleeping patient, so that she had to swiftly usher them out of the bedroom. On the way Doris was mouthing to Tina, "How long?" as if Tina had divine control over it.

---

1.   I was wrong.

They have always been welcome, and at times the best friends we could have, but I must control what is said in front of Prof R. They've always found a good drama far too stimulating.

August 15 — The first smooth day with morphine meds. Morning administered 8.20 am. Afternoon – 1.20 pm. Evening 2.5 ml – 7.15 pm.

The District Nurse visited – a different one, unannounced – and unfortunately, I was at the supermarket. Tina could have phoned me, but she still panics a bit when in charge. And when we returned, she told me this District Nurse said the GP should visit. I know, and Tina knows, that it's not what is required now – that Dr T and I have had that discussion.

But because I wasn't here, doubt floods in. I cannot be sure, and I call the practice. Dr T is short with me. Didn't I understand what had been agreed? Yes of course I did, but the District Nurse . . . ?? In truth, she upended me, although I didn't actually admit it.

And Tina still assures me she is confident, and I can leave the house on Saturday to see Hope and the others in London. I have told her she mustn't feel a failure if she doesn't want me to go. I need permission not to. I am only going because it is my last chance to see Hope before she gives birth.

—

It would be so easy for my overwhelming commitment to Prof R in these last days to overtake everything, and I have to be careful. This is the scary time. A very scary time. I am sick to my stomach with it and totally understand why some people are afraid to continue with care at home for the last days and weeks.

Now that Prof R is only drinking water and honey suddenly there are no meals to prepare. He can no longer swallow them. And water will help keep the dreaded mucus at bay. We are only using the milkshakes for mixing his pills. The morphine is liquid and easy to administer.

The relief that he can be pain-free, so cleaning and changing him is also far less stressful. I can enjoy washing him and talking as I do it. I can take extra care now it doesn't have to be done quickly, to save him pain.

His mouth inside seemed filthy this evening and I thought it might be the chocolate ice cream. The cloth was coming out black. Awful. And that is in spite of the fact that Tina had cleaned his teeth at my request. Perhaps she is not checking his mouth. But she is not here so I cannot ask her. (She later suggested to me that it might have been the oral morphine).

I have asked her to stay on for a week or two afterwards, to help me get the paperwork etc organised. But really, it is so her pay doesn't fall off a cliff.

—

I now find myself waking in the night making sure there are suitable clothes to give the undertaker. And I worry about which undertaker. And will the girls want to ship him to London before cremation? I expect they might. It could be fitting, for him to return to where he was born.

I toyed with whether I would wish to speak at the service and decided no. Not only through nerves, and the threat of tears, but because I was the 'last station'. So much of his life came before. The 20 years we were together now seem compressed to 20 seconds. His first wife will be there. And that will be enough wives.

—

August 18 — He escaped silently in the small hours on Friday. And I almost missed it.

I had been checking him all through the evening and all night, each time I woke, giving him small amounts of water, trying to keep his airway clean. There was no need for pills. Suddenly, it was an easy decision not to give them to him.

And when I woke again at 3.30 am, something had definitely changed.

It was silent. I turned to look at him, and reached out to softly touch his cheek. He was so warm, I couldn't be sure. Just the still chest. No shallow breathing. Or was it my imagination? Perhaps he was still breathing. I said, "You've gone haven't you?"[2]

---

2.   (*Much later, and now it seems bizarrely, I thought of the cat I had found by the side of the road when I was small. I ran home, telling dad I was sure it was still alive. I had seen its chest move. This despite the fact there had been a frost and the cat was frozen solid.*)

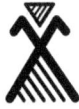

Afterwards

A FEELING OF something momentous. Beyond understanding. And a feeling of privilege, to be there with him. As I had wanted to, more than anything else. We had done it, he and I, this journey together to the end. A triumph.

Immediately I sent gentle texts to all his children. And Netty who was due to come today. But I waited a while before I rang the overnight community nurse number. I knew I didn't have to ring until the morning, but then I found I simply couldn't do nothing. And I'm glad I did ring, because the night nurse was so kind, and rang back at 5.30 am to ask if she could come in half an hour or so, and I was so glad to see her. Confirmation. Even though her recorded time of his death was not the actual time of death. That's the way it works apparently. And I turned away when she checked his eyes.

—

At 4 am I had made a cup of tea and got back into bed and sat with him. Just being with him. Quietly. This is definitely the best time to die, when your loved ones can be alone with you in the peace of the night. No people, no drama until there needs to be. And just for me, for history, so I would know it had really happened, I took a photo of him.

—

My son didn't wake and come down until 7.30 am, as I had hoped. And he was, as I knew he would be, the calm stoic person who didn't make a fuss and just gave me a hug. He didn't want to go up to London as planned but I said he must. It would all be rather grim during the day for anyone not up to their armpits in the process. And grim enough for those who were.

A day for the family history books. As all deaths are.

———

But I still needed to protect myself from his sister. When I texted them to say he had gone, she texted back "Is there anything we can do?" And stupidly I said, "Well you might want to visit". But I added, "His girls are coming at 10.30 am so they will need time to be alone with their dad."

Doris and Brian arrived at 10 am saying they would leave when the girls arrived. As I greeted them at the door, I asked if they would like to see Prof R. Brian said, "No thanks. I've seen plenty of dead bodies". "Haven't we all?", I retorted. Too shocked to say anything else. And grief is so odd. Because I am sure it was grief that made Doris spend the next half hour telling me all the sins that Prof R had committed in his lifetime. And I let her do it.

When the first two daughters arrived, Doris and Brian naturally stayed. The girls were sucked down memory lane anecdotes and raucous laughter. It was a relief for all of them. But it meant I had to go into the kitchen and shut the door when the undertaker rang, so that I could hear when they told me what time the private ambulance could come.

Then I needed to escape. So, I went upstairs to sit with Prof R. But there is no escape in this poorly built house. Sitting with my beloved dead man listening to gales of merriment coming up from below, until I could listen no more. And went downstairs and said, "Do you girls want to come and sit with your dad?" And one said, "I don't know." But she was able to, in the end.

Doris and Brian took the chance to slip away, calling goodbye to me as they went, and the girls came upstairs, and things were as they should be. Peaceful and sad and gentle laughter and tears.

—

I watched the undertaker's men prepare Prof R for take-off, not because I'm a glutton for punishment, but because a need to monitor the men and the process made me vigilant. We don't stop looking after someone just because they have died. And I asked them for his wedding ring before they added it to the inventory as "one yellow metal ring".

I don't think I ever need to watch that again for anybody. Or even any body.

When he was being taken away, the men saw the little boy next door, standing in his window watching, and asked me to warn his mother to take him away, so he would not see the stretcher, or its occupant, being put into the black ambulance.

—

After lunch, when the girls had gone, I went straight upstairs to get the morphine and the emergency crisis kit, hidden high up on top of the bathroom cabinet. The spectre of any inquest – verbal or otherwise – remained a major fear. I almost ran down to the chemist and handed them across the counter. The relief was immediate.

And then I went home to make the bedroom somewhere I could possibly bear to sleep. The bed changed, the ensuite door closed on all the medical paraphernalia. Then I had a long bath and washed my hair. So I could feel almost human.

And that night I slept no better or worse than usual. Radio 4 keeps me company. Nothing seemed real, but I expected that.

When Prof R and I were first properly together, in his London house, he was accustomed, since his wife's death, of going to sleep with classical music. So I embraced it too. Until one night, when a crescendo of percussion had shocked me awake yet again, and I had to say "Darling, I'm sorry, I can't sleep with this anymore."

I hate funerals. Presumably everybody does. There will be no rest until that is over. The youngest daughter is still on holiday with her family, so there will be a delay. Possibly three weeks. Hope's baby may be born beforehand.

I've told the girls I have £6000 for the funeral, so if they'd like to push dad's boat further out, they can paddle it themselves. No, of course I didn't say that.

All I wanted to do the next day, Saturday, was to go up to London to Hope and Simon's to have lunch with them all, including Douglas. And it was a day of solace and love and laughter, as I knew it would be. My eldest granddaughter painted a rainbow on my hand with face paints and I wore it all the way home on the train.

Last night I made the leap of faith, moving to Prof R's side of the bed. It felt friendly. Although I still woke frequently, and at 4 am began planning and plotting. And writing emails and checking the investment hub to see how I can draw down the funds for the funeral. The answer: without any haste from them by the looks of it.

And I'm pottering. More medications leaving the bedroom. Normalising the house without taking Prof R's presence from the room. I'm glad I took his photograph while I waited for the nurse[1]. It will help me believe it has happened. Or even that he really was there for all those weeks and months, in various states of unwellness.

---

1.   *When the time was right, early in 2021, I felt able to delete it.*

My first feelings, on life without him, are of profound loss. Twenty years? Had it been a dream? I feel cheated. Time has concertinaed in a very disconcerting way. The earth has fallen away. And no, there is no relief, although everyone says you do feel some relief. Just the acceptance of a continuum. A sense of completion of one part of our lives and onwards to the next task – looking after his legacy.

Tuesday 20 — I need to keep up. But I am at least accomplishing a great deal. It's necessary.

The crematorium is booked, the venue for the wake is booked, and food organised for multitudes of children – gluten-free, dairy-free and probably pedestrian.

Prof R's death registration time and date is booked. Forms still to pick up today for that. Then, after registration, the green form for cremation to go to the undertaker. Douglas comes back from London today. Lovely.

Prof R's eldest daughter wrote this morning, "Let's all have a conference call at 8.30 am to discuss the order of service and what needs to be done." The order of service needs to be my gift to them. It's important they feel ownership of their dad's farewell. I get to choose the 'how'. So, I said, "Why don't I leave you girls to talk and you can let me know what you decide and what you would like me to do".

—

I will get the order of service laid out and printed once it is written by them. I will organise the flowers. I am happy to do everything else. And they will feel that they have honoured their father in their own way.

Those of us doing the donkey work single-handed at these times know that the legal and administrative hoops you jump through are more than enough. And could drive you to breaking point on top of all the grief. It's a toxic combination. So now I have to draft something for the celebrant for my small segment of Prof R's life.

—

A Dr G rang at lunchtime. I was expecting his call. He is the 'third party' doctor who is called in when a death occurs at home. His job is to oversee what Dr T and I got up to. He seemed satisfied with my replies to his questions. I feel a bit weird this afternoon, a bit upended.

On Wednesday, Douglas went with me to the library to register the death. More and more I appreciate living in a compact town which can cater for almost all of our urgent needs. When we arrived at the library front desk, I told the woman there that we had an appointment with the Registrar. She said, "Of course, let me show you where to wait". Which she did. And then she disappeared.

Five minutes later, she reappeared, with a name tag that said "Registrar". She greeted us, shook our hands, and said "Hello, I'm the Registrar." It was all I could do not to laugh. But she made everything so easy. And because a registered death certificate is set in concrete, and can never be altered, I asked Douglas to double-check that it was correct.

It was tough, but it is done.

Thursday 22 — Today I had to clarify some issues with the manager at Netty's agency.

She, as it turns out, was totally unprepared for any potential legal pitfalls surrounding a death at home. Who knew? A person who's business is based on the principle that no one should lose their loved ones to the care system against their wishes.

It turns out Prof R is the first person to actually die, happily or unhappily, at home under her oversight – even if only partially. Presumably, when the going gets tough, she hides behind the legal skirts of the visiting medical profession – hospice or district nurses.

What divine thought, other than financial, led me to hire Tina? Because goodness knows what I would have done if Netty had not been allowed to help me in his final days. And we were forced to operate alone, or worse, have Prof R whisked away by the strong arm of the NHS.

To underline her panic, the manager then grilled me on the phone about his death, in case she had to report it to the Care Commission. I reassured her that Netty was never in the house when the palliative care drugs were administered. She had not been here since the previous Friday.

Later, she phoned back and apologised for being insensitive, and then sinned further by calling his death 'unexpected'. So that I had to ask her to remove that description from any report, as it was not only untrue but could raise questions about Prof R's death.

It has been a salutary experience, and all my instincts regarding the agency management unfortunately held true. And she will charge me for the day of Prof R's death because he gave her less than 24 hours' notice.

—

But today, after all that, I took Douglas to Whitstable, and we ate fish and chips and walked. And while he is tired, and gearing up for the return flight to Sydney tomorrow, he is good form and hopefully will recover from being my death-bed wingman. Nobody could have done it better.

Friday 23 — Dear Douglas has gone. Relieved of the unrelenting pace of this process.

Whenever I tried to take a couple of hours or days out with him, someone would ring. The Parkinson's nurse finally, not knowing Prof R has died, and the celebrant. I will meet the celebrant here next Tuesday at 3 pm.

The first Mrs Prof R rang me, brave and kind. But talking to her, speech becomes almost impossible. All I could manage, "He has gone on ahead of us". To which she agreed.

—

No new baby yet, but I slept better. I am hoping that she will be born when I can get my head out of death and its duties. A sudden strange foreign thought that occurred to me – "I am a widow".

——

Yesterday afternoon I did my homework on my funeral tribute. It was a very good thing to do. And having read what the girls wish to say, I kept it brief. There were people I wanted to thank, and now I have.

This is what I am going to ask Steve, the celebrant, to read for me:

My dearest friend and loving companion has gone.

In the last days and hours, when his eyes could no longer open, I would press my cheek to his and repeat quietly in his ear "You're my darling, you're my darling, you're my darling" so that if he knew nothing else, he might still know he was loved.

We could not have achieved this peaceful ending we both wanted without help. In the last months, our carers Tina and Netty helped me manage his care in ways I could not have done alone. I will always be grateful to them.

And to the community and district nurses, who came on a Sunday, and later, in the early hours of the morning he died.

In particular I am grateful to our GP Dr T, who in the end, enabled and trusted us to continue our care at home. Without unnecessary intervention.

I appreciate and celebrate that this is a rare and wonderful thing.

I'm happy with that.

I am also happy, because my baby has had her baby.

——

Another dream about Prof R. Somewhere between night-owl time at

4.00 am and in the twilight sleep till 7 am, I lost him in a railway station. So I went to the information desk and asked if a message could go out for him. They asked me if I would like to do it, and I said "sure". And I did, making sure to call him his full name, which he liked on formal occasions.

I woke up before I found him.

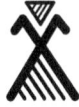

Epilogue

AUGUST 2020 — Now, when I try to remember how it was for us, Prof R and me, for those last months, it still seems dreamlike.

The mixture of the mundane and the divine.

The horror, if I am careless enough to think too deeply.

The love that grew beyond understanding.

The sheer unreality of it all.

It is like trying to catch a cloud.